Cognitive-Beha[illegible]ural Th[illegible] Delu[illegible] and Hallucinations

A Practice Manual

2nd Edition

Hazel E. Nelson

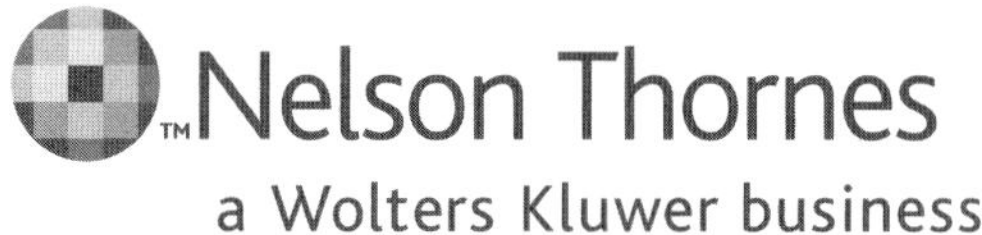

First published in 1997 by:
Stanley Thornes (Publishers) Ltd

This edition published in 2005 by:
Nelson Thornes Ltd
Delta Place
27 Bath Road
CHELTENHAM
GL53 7TH
United Kingdom

06 07 08 09 / 10 9 8 7 6 5 4 3 2

A catalogue record for this book is available from the British Library

ISBN 0 7487 9256 2

Page make-up by Acorn Bookwork

Printed and bound in Spain by GraphyCems

Contents

Foreword

During the past two decades there have been enormous strides in the pharmacotherapy of schizophrenia and schizoaffective disorder so that these patients no longer need to face a lifetime of torment from delusions, hallucinations and disability due to their negative symptoms. While this crucial progress is indeed gratifying for clinicians, it is not generally known, particularly in the United States, that additional approaches to schizophrenia can greatly enhance the impact of pharmacotherapy. In more recent years it has been established that cognitive-behavioural therapy as an adjunct to pharmacotherapy can increase patients' response by an order of magnitude beyond that achieved by drugs. As a clinician as well as researcher, I find it gratifying to learn that tried and true therapeutic strategies based on traditional notions of the therapist-patient relationship and the understanding of the personal struggle of the patients can make a substantial difference in their lives. Moreover, at least one recent study has shown that the administration of cognitive therapy without drugs can, at least, postpone the transition into psychosis of adolescents who are already at high risk for schizophrenia. In recognition of the established value of cognitive therapy, the National Institute of Clinical Excellence in Britain has recommended that cognitive-behavioural therapy be made available at treatment centres for schizophrenia.

This extraordinary volume by Hazel Nelson, representing the latest contribution to the cognitive approach to schizophrenia, fills the need for a hands-on set of strategies and techniques to guide the treatment of delusions and hallucinations. A number of British investigators have previously demonstrated that the role of patients' core beliefs about themselves (their powerlessness and vulnerability), as well as their negative beliefs of others as dangerous and omnipotent, underlie the delusions of persecution or influence. In addition, they have shown that certain thinking problems such as jumping to conclusions, negative biases, and problems in reasoning also contribute to the development of hallucinations and delusions. Moreover, the Canadian psychologist Neil Rector has shown that dysfunctional beliefs regarding social affiliation are associated with the positive symptoms of schizophrenia, and that the negative beliefs regarding the individual's self-efficacy underlie the negative symptoms. In our own work we have attempted to show that the patients' attenuated psychological resources undermine their capacity to test and correct their delusional interpretations.

The New Look in understanding psychopathology has demonstrated the continuity between the thinking disorder in psychosis with that of neurosis and personality disorders. In contrast to traditional theories of schizophrenia, this concept not only makes delusions more comprehensible to the therapist but also provides the tools for the patients to normalize their anomalous experiences. Indeed, the whole normalizing approach destigmatizes schizophrenia and brings the patient back within the human community, figuratively and literally.

Therapists who are familiar with cognitive therapy will find a relatively easy transition from the cognitive approaches with non-psychotic disorders to the treatment of schizophrenia and schizoaffective disorder. Dr Nelson describes the familiar elicitation of automatic thoughts, identification of thought change, beliefs, misinterpretation, biases and so on that constitute the raw material in dealing with conditions such as depression and anxiety. As she points out, the same data are used in the treatment of psychosis. She is particularly informative in describing the formation and maintenance of beliefs through the self-confirming beliefs circles. Other cognitive processes such as selective attention and belief maintenance lead the way to procedures for belief modification. Many of the techniques that have been shown to be effective in the treatment of depression and anxiety, such as the daily thought record, conducting behavioural experiments, listing advantages and disadvantages of the beliefs, can now be applied successfully to the patients with schizophrenia.

Two rather distinct schools of thought regarding cognitive-behavioural therapy of schizophrenia have evolved over the years. The earlier approach based primarily on behavioural principles constitutes the 'peripheralist' approach. This approach conceives of schizophrenia as simply a biological disease and the favoured approach is to try to contain and possibly shrink this disorder through behavioural coping, problem solving and cognitive remediation. These approaches consider hallucinations, delusions and thinking disorders as intrinsic to the biological disease and, therefore, best approached through biological interventions. The 'centralist' approach, which evolved later, emanated from the cognitive therapy of depression and other conditions. This approach views hallucinations and delusions as having a large psychological component that may mitigate symptoms through both direct and indirect interventions. Thus, not only the beliefs about the hallucinations but also their actual content is evaluated and modified through specific techniques such as demonstrating the continuity of the content of hallucinations with the content of automatic thoughts. Similarly, delusions may be tested through behavioural experiments but also evaluated in terms of alternative explanations. Furthermore, various psychological mechanisms such as jumping to conclusions, personalizing and overgeneralizing become the fodder for interventions. Dr Nelson takes a centralist position and outlines, in an impressive way, the cognitive therapy approach.

The present volume provides an important service to researchers and theoreticians as well as clinicians. It not only clarifies the essential nature of delusions and hallucinations but also provides a blueprint for therapists who deal with these difficult symptoms.

Aaron T. Beck

Preface

This book developed from a request to write a second edition of *Cognitive-Behavioural Therapy with Schizophrenia: A Practice Manual*, which was published in 1997. This resulted in substantial changes to the original text to take account of the advances in this area of work, the feedback I had received from clinicians using the original practice manual, and the experience gained from a further eight years of clinical practice and supervision. The title of the book has been changed in order to reflect more accurately the main focus of the therapy described.

This practice manual has been written primarily for clinical psychologists, psychiatrists, psychiatric nurses, social workers, occupational therapists and other professionals working in the mental health field. It aims to provide clear and detailed guidance on how to plan and deliver safe and effective programmes of cognitive-behavioural therapy (CBT) for delusions and hallucinations, and how to avoid or overcome some of the problems that may be encountered. It also offers detailed guidance and suggestions about how the CBT approach can be used in a less formal way in other clinical settings and in ordinary day-to-day interactions with people with delusions and hallucinations.

The first section describes the basic principles underpinning the cognitive-behavioural model and how they relate to the development, maintenance and modification of delusions and hallucinations. The second section considers what it might be like to experience psychotic symptoms, and recommends ways of improving the therapeutic alliance and overcoming problems of engagement that may occur during therapy. The next two sections, which comprise the body of the work, describe how to use CBT strategies to modify delusional beliefs and auditory hallucinations. This is followed by a section on long-term strategies to maintain the therapeutic gains and a section on putting the strategies into practice safely. There are numerous examples from clinical practice to illustrate the points made, including the complete course of therapy for four illustrative cases.

The book is intended to be a practical guide rather than an academic textbook. In order to keep it easier to read and use for clinical practice, literature references have not been included in the main body of the text. Instead, there is a final section that reviews the literature on evidence-based practice and related theoretical issues, the aim being to provide key references for those who wish to pursue these aspects further.

Using the practice manual

The book has been written for use as a practice reference manual as well as an instruction manual. A detailed summary is given as an appendix in order to provide a structure within which the different sections of the text can be placed, and within which the therapy can be planned and delivered. It is recommended that, for the first time of reading, the text is read through in the order given so that the points made are taken in their correct context within the overall structure of the therapy.

Although it would undoubtedly be helpful, formal training in CBT is not an essential prerequisite for using the therapy described in this manual providing the reader heeds the cautions given and respects the need to seek clinical supervision when this is indicated.

My own clinical practice has been mostly with people who have been hospitalized on acute wards or in a specialist unit for enduring, medication-resistant schizophrenia, with some outpatient follow-up work. Although this group includes people who are amongst the most severely affected by their illness, we have found that there are very few people for whom we can do absolutely nothing. The strategies described are equally if not more effective with less severely ill people living in the community and progress is usually faster.

Note on confidentiality

The clinical examples and case studies described in this book are based on people with whom I or my colleagues have worked over the past 18 years. In order to protect the identities of the individuals concerned, in some cases non-significant details of the delusion or hallucination have been changed, as have details about the people involved.

Note on terminology

The work described in this book has been developed with people who meet the diagnostic criteria for schizophrenia, but because of the stigma attached to the terms 'schizophrenia' and 'schizophrenic' most people prefer the terms 'psychosis' and 'psychotic', the broader category of mental illness that includes schizophrenia. For this reason it is now common clinical practice to talk to people about their illness and experiences in terms of 'psychosis' and 'psychotic' and for their diagnosis to be given in these terms. The terminology used in this book reflects this popular change in word usage. The term 'schizophrenia' is only used when it is specifically schizophrenia that is being referred to, for example in case examples where the person concerned had been told this was their diagnosis.

ACKNOWLEDGEMENTS

I have engaged in therapy with many people with psychosis over the past 18 years and it has been a very real privilege and pleasure to do so. The best in this book is what they have given to me.

I have learnt a great deal from the many psychologists and nurse therapists with whom I have engaged in clinical supervision: they are too numerous to mention by name, but my thanks go to all of them.

A very special 'thank you' goes to Dr Hamish McLeod, not only for his very helpful comments on the penultimate draft of this book but also for all his support over the years.

My acknowledgements would be incomplete without mentioning Peter, Hilary and John, to whom I send my love and gratitude.

1 THE COGNITIVE-BEHAVIOURAL MODEL OF THERAPY

Most people who seek psychological therapy do so because of the unpleasant way they *feel*. Although the principal aim of cognitive-behavioural therapy (CBT) is to alleviate the distress by alleviating the unpleasant feelings, CBT does not tackle these feelings directly; rather, it seeks to achieve the required changes by modifying the thoughts (hence the term 'cognitive') and beliefs that underlie them. It may also seek to change actions and situations (hence the term 'behavioural') that are adversely affecting the thoughts and feelings.

THE RELATIONSHIP BETWEEN THOUGHTS, FEELINGS AND BELIEFS

Of central importance for the cognitive-behavioural model of therapy is the relationship that exists between thoughts and feelings: the way we feel about a situation or experience depends on what we think about it and how we interpret it. For example, two people are given surprise birthday presents of a balloon ride. One thinks, 'That will be exciting, how kind of my partner to go to such trouble and expense', leading to feelings of pleasurable anticipation and affection, whereas the other thinks, 'I will feel frightened the whole trip, what a waste of money, how thoughtless my partner is', leading to feelings of fear and annoyance.

Another core concept for cognitive therapy is that the thoughts we have about a situation and the way we interpret it are inextricably linked to our beliefs about ourselves and the world. In the example just given, the first person believed that ballooning is exciting rather than dangerous and that his partner cared enough for him to try to give him a present he would really like. In contrast, the second person believed that ballooning is dangerous and that his partner was insensitive and had made little effort to find a present that would please him.

Although it is the influence that beliefs have on thoughts (the left hand 'influence' arrow in Figure 1.1) that is usually the focus of CBT, the beliefs that the person brings to a situation can also influence the basic *situation→thought→emotion* process by influencing the emotional response to those thoughts (the right hand 'influence' arrow in Figure 1.1). For example, a child and an elderly person, seeing a thick layer of snow on the ground, may both think, 'It's slippery out there, I will fall over if I go out', but the emotional responses to this thought will be quite different. The child, believing that sliding is fun and that falling over will cause her only minor discomfort, will be unconcerned or even excited by the thought of sliding on the snow, whereas the elderly person, believing that he could be seriously hurt, will be fearful at the same thought.

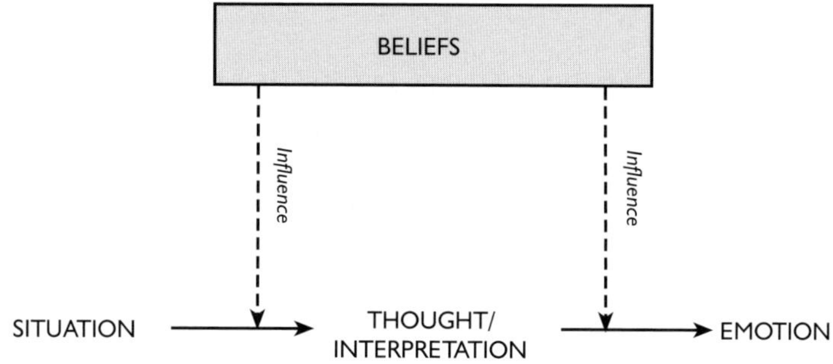

Figure 1.1 The relationship between thoughts, feelings and beliefs.

The symptom maintenance cycles

Our brains are constructed in such a way that our emotions colour our thinking and how we interpret things. For example, when we are depressed our thoughts and interpretations will tend to be pessimistic and negative; when anxious they will be worried and fearful; when happy they will be positive and optimistic, etc. So when our thoughts affect our feelings, our feelings can then affect our thoughts, and so on. This powerful two-way effect is made even stronger by what is called 'mood-dependent memory', whereby our mood state affects which memories come spontaneously to mind and how readily mood-related memories can be recalled. For example, when we are depressed not only will our spontaneous memories tend to be of negative events but we will also find it harder to recall happy memories when we try to do so: when we are feeling happy the reverse is true. If someone is very seriously depressed, they may be unable to recall any happy memories at all – life has always been awful – so it is not surprising if they view their future with pessimism and hopelessness.

Another key relationship for the CBT model is the two-way relationship that exists between thoughts and behaviour; our thoughts affect our behaviour and this in turn affects the thoughts that we have. An important relationship also

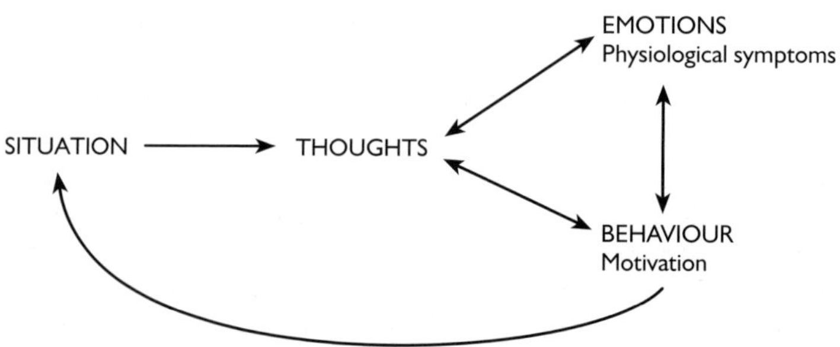

Figure 1.2 The symptom maintenance cycles.

operates between our behaviour and our situation because when we act we change our situation and this in turn influences our subsequent experiences and thoughts/feelings. In the example given previously of the balloon ride, the recipient who interpreted the gift as a sign of his partner's caring thoughtfulness is likely to respond in a warm, affectionate way, thereby creating more opportunities for positive experiences and thoughts/feelings. In contrast, the recipient who interpreted the gift in a negative way is likely to respond in a cold, hurt or angry manner, thereby eliciting a hostile response from his partner, which he will interpret with more negative thoughts.

The tight relationship that exists between thoughts, emotions and behaviour acts so as to maintain or exacerbate the existing emotional state. The triad also tends to maintain the situation(s) that are compatible with it. These maintenance cycles are at the heart of the CBT model, and breaking them is a central part of therapy.

Although the symptom maintenance cycles are generally talked about in CBT writings with regard to the maintenance of negative thoughts, emotions and behaviour, the same process also works to maintain positive thoughts, emotions and behaviour. This means that if, during therapy, you are able to modify the symptom maintenance cycles so that they become positive rather than negative, then the thoughts/emotions/behaviour relationship will work in the person's favour to maintain this positive state of affairs.

Our thoughts can also produce physiological changes which, in turn, can affect our behaviour and thinking in a self-perpetuating way. For example, an agoraphobic man interpreted his racing heart as a sign of an impending heart attack and so became even more panicky; another man who was frightened that he was being invaded by aliens interpreted the unpleasant sensations in his body as confirmation that they were getting into him, which made him even more frightened and thereby increased the sensations.

Thought chains

Thoughts flow through our minds in a steady stream, so it is not surprising to find that thoughts can also produce other thoughts that lead to other thoughts and so on. For example, an A level student waking up in the early hours on the morning of their exam might think, 'It's only 3 a.m. → I've only had four hours sleep → if I can't get back to sleep, I will be tired in the morning → if I'm tired, I won't do well in the exam → if I don't do well in the exam, I won't get my university place → if I don't get my university place, I will be unemployed and have to stay at home → I'll be a failure and my life will be ruined'.

The importance of these thought chains is that each and any one of the thoughts in the chain can produce its own set of 'symptoms'. In the example just given, it is not the thought that it is 3 a.m. that is producing the strong emotions of panic and dread, or even the thought that the exam is only seven hours away, but rather the thoughts further down the chain about the student's life being in ruins if they are unable to take up their university place. Thus, the wider implications of a thought are often as, or more, important than the immediate thought itself.

Automatic thoughts

The term *automatic thought* occurs frequently in writings about CBT, often as part of the term *negative automatic thought* (NAT). Automatic thoughts can be positive, neutral or negative in their effects on a person, but since psychotherapy is primarily concerned with those thoughts that have the negative unwanted effects, negative automatic thoughts are the ones most commonly talked about in connection with CBT. (*Note*: When used in CBT, the terms *negative* and *positive* refer only to the effect the thought has on the person concerned; they do not imply any moral or other value.)

Our brains are generating thoughts all the time that we are awake. These thoughts can be about any aspect of the situation that we are in, including what it means, how it might develop and how we might respond to those developments; or they can be about other things quite unrelated to the present situation. This constant stream of thoughts is necessary for our survival and often acts as the trigger for our more purposeful thinking. Automatic thoughts are constantly monitored by the part of our brain responsible for the overall executive control of our thoughts and actions. This central executive part of the brain selects the most relevant automatic thoughts for further attention, at which stage we become aware of them as conscious thoughts. Unlike purposeful thinking, when you follow a deliberate train of thought within conscious awareness (e.g. when working out the solution to a problem), automatic thoughts are not under our conscious control but occur spontaneously and effortlessly, much as dreams occur spontaneously and without conscious control during sleep.

In Figure 1.4 (p. 15), the direct line from *beliefs→thoughts* represents how automatic thoughts operate and come into conscious awareness.

Characteristics of automatic thoughts

1 Automatic thoughts occur spontaneously and without effort from the person concerned. They cannot be switched off or consciously controlled.
2 Though often verbal (i.e. occurring as words), automatic thoughts can also occur as images or in a vague, preverbal form. They often occur as fragments or partial thoughts, flashing rapidly through the brain.
3 Automatic thoughts may be sensible but they can also be unreasonable, impossible or even bizarre.
4 If automatic thoughts do not come to conscious awareness, their content cannot be recognized or subjected to rational evaluation, but nevertheless they may still evoke a strong, emotional reaction.
5 Automatic thoughts may reflect the thinker's underlying belief system about himself and the world, *but not necessarily so*. One can have an automatic thought about anything within one's memory or knowledge system, i.e. about anything one has ever seen, heard, read or imagined. Having a thought about something does not mean that the person 'secretly' wants to do that.
6 Automatic thoughts that produce a strong emotional response are more likely

to recur. This is why thoughts that are contrary to the underlying belief system can recur if they cause the person anxiety, embarrassment or shame, etc.

The role that automatic thoughts may play in producing an emotional response or mood state is a key feature of the CBT model, especially as the latter was originally developed for work with depression. It was recognized that a depressed feeling or mood could be triggered by a thought flashing through the person's mind, even though they were not consciously aware of the thought. In cases like this a key part of therapy is identifying the negative automatic thoughts so that they can be worked with and changed. CBT with people with psychosis tends to concentrate more on the thoughts and beliefs that are in the person's conscious awareness. Nevertheless, you should be aware of the possibility that automatic thoughts, of which the person is not consciously aware, or which are difficult to convey in words because of their non-verbal nature, could be relevant. You should be particularly sensitive to this possibility where the emotional response does not appear to be consistent with the thoughts and beliefs being reported by the person.

Although automatic thoughts are not usually targeted directly in CBT with psychosis, an understanding of what they are and how they operate may be very important for some aspects of the therapy, for example in taking away the shame of hearing obscene voices (see Chapter 6).

BELIEFS AND BELIEF SYSTEMS

The function of beliefs

We all have a unique set of beliefs that represent our particular way of making generalizations about the world and our part in it. Beliefs are our 'best bet' estimates of how things operate in the world. Without beliefs we would be unable to cope with the complexity and variability of our lives. Because we are social animals it is essential that we are able to manoeuvre our way through the ever-changing social situations around us and so it is not surprising that many of our most important beliefs concern ourselves, others and interactions between ourselves and others.

The principal function of beliefs is to enable us to understand accurately what is going on and to respond appropriately, without having to treat each and every situation as if it were new. For example, I have developed the belief that someone smiling and approaching me with an outstretched hand is a sign of friendly non-aggression and so I am able to respond appropriately to this situation whenever it occurs; but if I had no belief about this behaviour, I would have to consider all the possible reasons for the outstretched hand, smile and movement towards me and weigh these up before being able to work out a suitable response. It is easy to see that we would be overwhelmed if we did not have beliefs to short-cut the lengthy process of rationally analysing every situation we encountered. Because we have developed beliefs to cover most situations we only have to resort to analysing a situation more thoughtfully on the very rare occasions when the situation is so novel that no existing belief appears to apply or when it is not clear which of two or more beliefs is the appropriate one. Even in these latter situations, the existence of partially relevant beliefs greatly reduces the range of possibilities that have to be weighed up and thought through rationally. Beliefs about the consistency of things also enable us to plan ahead. For example, I believe that I will not be dismissed from my job unless I am guilty of professional misconduct so I can take out a mortgage or book a future holiday because I know what money I will have available. I also believe that my partner will stay with me, so I can include him in the holiday plans, etc.

Another important function of beliefs is to enable us to interpret and respond quickly to situations as they arise. Beliefs that are held with certainty are more efficient in this respect than beliefs that are only 'probably true'. For example, if I am thirsty and am offered a glass of mineral water from a freshly opened bottle, which I believe is safe to drink, then I will be able to quench my thirst immediately, but if I am offered a glass of well water, which I believe is only 'probably' safe to drink, then I am likely to hesitate and ask some more questions about the well before weighing up the risks and deciding whether to drink it or not.

From a logical perspective, very few of our beliefs can be held with absolute certainty, but in practice, when the possibility of being wrong is small, we hold and use our beliefs unquestioningly, as if they were 100% true. It is functional for us to do this because it enables us to make quick decisions that are appropriate in almost all situations. Put another way, when the possibility of being wrong is small, then the benefits of allowing for the possibility of error are outweighed by the costs associated with the uncertainty and doubt. In the example given above, I cannot be absolutely certain that the mineral water in the bottle has not become contaminated, but if I doubted the safety of all sources of water in this way, then at the very least my daily life would become a very stressful affair, and at worst I might even die of dehydration if I would not take the risk of drinking 'possibly contaminated' water.

We do not make a conscious choice to treat some beliefs as 'certain' in this way; this is done automatically by our brains. People differ in their tendency to hold absolute beliefs, and within an individual a particular belief can change in this respect. For example, most people who get into a car assume, without question, that they will arrive safely at their destination; if they are involved in an accident, then this sense of safety can be shaken for a while, but if the accident was only a minor one, then the assumption of safety develops again over time.

Knowledge

The distinction between *beliefs* and *knowledge* is an unclear one, and may be largely semantic when applied in the context of therapy. The term *knowledge* is generally used to refer to factual matters about which one is certain whilst the term *belief* tends to be used to refer to matters about which one cannot be certain; but there is considerable overlap in the way that the terms are used. For example, one person may say that they know that God exists whilst someone else may say that this cannot be proved and therefore is a belief rather than knowledge. As far as CBT is concerned, knowledge can be treated in essentially the same way as beliefs, the major proviso being that knowledge that can be proved to be correct can be developed and extended but it cannot be modified as such; for example, you could not modify my belief/knowledge that I am a psychologist, or my belief/knowledge that if I drop a cup, it will fall to the ground.

Functional and dysfunctional beliefs

Beliefs may be described as functional or dysfunctional. Functional beliefs are those that are useful to the person and that serve a positive function. For example, the belief 'If I put my hand in a fire, it will hurt' protects my hand from physical damage, whilst the belief 'Everyone makes mistakes sometimes, even really successful people' protects me from feeling a failure when I make errors. Dysfunctional beliefs are those that are unhelpful to the person holding them and have an overall negative effect. For example, the belief 'I am an even better driver when I'm drunk' increases the risk of self-injury and a drink-driving charge, whilst the belief 'It's a sign of weakness to cry' means that on some occasions I may feel not only very sad but also ashamed for showing those feelings.

As with the terms *positive* and *negative*, the terms *functional* and *dysfunctional* do not imply any moral assessment about the belief but are a purely practical description of how helpful or unhelpful the belief is for that person.

Most beliefs are not purely functional or purely dysfunctional: they have both positive and negative aspects, to varying degrees, depending on the circumstances.

1 *A belief may be functional in some contexts but dysfunctional in others.* For example, the belief 'It's OK to retaliate with physical force if attacked' may be functional if you are trapped in an alleyway by someone threatening a violent assault but it would be dysfunctional for someone working in a mental health setting.
2 *Similarly, a belief that is functional at some time in a person's life may become dysfunctional, or vice versa.* For example, the belief 'I should put myself first' might be functional for a young person striving to achieve independence and career success but would be highly dysfunctional for a parent.
3 *Within a single context, the belief may be both functional and dysfunctional at the same time, that is, it may be functional in some ways and dysfunctional in others.* For example, the belief 'It's dangerous to go out after dark' is functional in that it avoids the risk of getting attacked but is dysfunctional in that it limits social activity.

Beliefs that would be appropriate and functional for most occasions may be dysfunctional if they are held in an extreme or rigid way that does not allow for human frailty or the exceptional circumstances that can occur in life. For example, there may be times when following the belief 'It's wrong to behave aggressively' would not be in the best interests of me or other people. Beliefs of this kind are often expressed in absolute terms of 'always', 'never', 'every', 'none', etc., and often include the word 'should'. In contrast, functional beliefs tend to be expressed in less extreme forms and to allow exceptions to the general rule, for example 'It's wrong to kill (except as a soldier in wartime)'.

By their very nature, functional beliefs tend to benefit the person holding them, and it is a sign of a normal, healthy psychological state that we tend to believe things that go in our favour and to ignore or reject things that go against us. Thus, we tend to have a rosier view of ourselves and of other people's opinions of us than is actually true, the so-called *self-serving bias*. We are also biased in that we tend to adopt beliefs that have the potential to show us in a good light. For example, you may have noticed amongst your friends and acquaintances that people who are good at sport tend to value sporting prowess as an important achievement and worthy of status whereas people who play musical instruments consider musical ability to be a more important and praiseworthy characteristic, etc.

The organization of beliefs

Although we have no direct evidence of where or how beliefs are organized and stored in the brain, their apparent resistance to the effects of focal and generalized brain damage strongly suggests that they must be stored in some diffuse way, involving complex interconnections between many subsystems and areas of the brain.

The key function of a belief system is to bring cohesion and order to the world, to enable us to make predictions and to act accordingly, so it is important that our beliefs do not result in conflicting interpretations or predictions. Therefore, although some inconsistencies can be tolerated within a belief system, for the most part directly opposing or conflicting beliefs are not tolerated.

Contradictory beliefs can coexist if undetected, but once a situation occurs that brings this conflict into awareness, then it is usual for either or both the beliefs to be modified to return harmony to the system. Modification may require one belief to be discarded but is more often achieved by adding provisos to one or more of the beliefs. For example, if you were to hold the beliefs 'It's wrong to tell lies' and 'It's wrong to hurt people's feelings', then these would be called into direct conflict if a friend asked you how you liked her new (unattractive) hairstyle, since you would have to act against one of your beliefs. In practice you are likely to resolve the conflict either by modifying your belief about telling lies ('It's generally wrong to tell lies – but it's permissible in order to save someone's feelings'), which would allow you to answer, 'Yes, it looks good', or by modifying your belief about hurting people ('Sometimes it's necessary to hurt people's feelings – in order to be truthful'), which would allow you to answer, 'Your old style looked better'. Note that if you did not modify one of the beliefs, then you would have the unpleasant feeling of guilt, either for telling lies or for hurting someone's feelings, depending on which 'rule' you broke.

Situations in everyday life are complex so that more than one belief or belief system may be activated. Despite developing belief systems that are, on the whole, internally consistent, these activated beliefs may lead to contradictory interpretations of events or to opposing actions. For example, a mother taking a child for inoculation may bring to the situation a belief that she should protect her child against illnesses and also a belief that she should not cause her child pain. In such cases the potential conflict is resolved by one belief taking precedence over the other. Which belief takes precedence will depend not only on the relative strength of the beliefs but also on the circumstances and the possible outcomes. Thus, in the above case, the mother might decide to proceed with even a very painful inoculation if the illness were severe, whereas she might decide against it if the illness were a mild one. Alternatively, if the injection caused only mild pain, then she might decide to go ahead with the inoculation even for a mild illness.

Some of our beliefs, especially those about social matters, can be remarkably fluid. For example, on some occasions I may feel full of self-confidence but on other occasions I may have a much poorer opinion of myself. Similarly, most of us do not have stable beliefs about our attractiveness, work competence, popularity, etc. Fluctuations in our beliefs can be affected by external factors, for example where we are and whom we are with, and also by internal factors. A very important internal factor affecting beliefs about ourselves and others is our mood; for example, if I feel happy, I am more likely to believe that I am attractive to other people, competent at work, etc. than if I feel depressed.

Belief formation

Our beliefs develop from our experience of the world, using the term 'experience' in its widest sense. As soon as we are born we start to develop beliefs and expectations about ourselves and the world around us. Although we continue to develop and modify our beliefs throughout our life, our childhood experiences are pivotal in determining the development of our core beliefs (sometimes called *schema*). The beliefs we develop are heavily influenced by the cultural (including religious, social and political) beliefs of those around us. The beliefs of personally significant others, such as our family, friends and peer groups, etc., are particularly important in this respect.

Humans are unique in the animal kingdom in that language enables us to learn from other people's experiences as well as our own, through education, books, TV, etc. The beliefs we develop are also affected to some extent by our biological predisposition, which can be likened to the hard wiring of a computer and include both the predispositions that we all share as human beings, for example to protect members of our own family, and those that vary from one person to another, for example the tendency to be anxious. At a more temporary biological level, mood state may also influence the development of beliefs; for example, a person will more readily develop negative beliefs about himself and the world when he is depressed.

New beliefs are heavily influenced by the existing belief system because the existing beliefs bias the perception and interpretation of new information. In this way, new beliefs tend to develop that are compatible with the existing belief system and will fit in without causing inconsistencies. However, should the new belief contradict and be held more strongly than an existing belief, then it is the existing belief that has to be changed or adapted in order to incorporate the new belief (see 'Belief modification', pp. 12–13).

Belief maintenance: the self-confirming belief circles

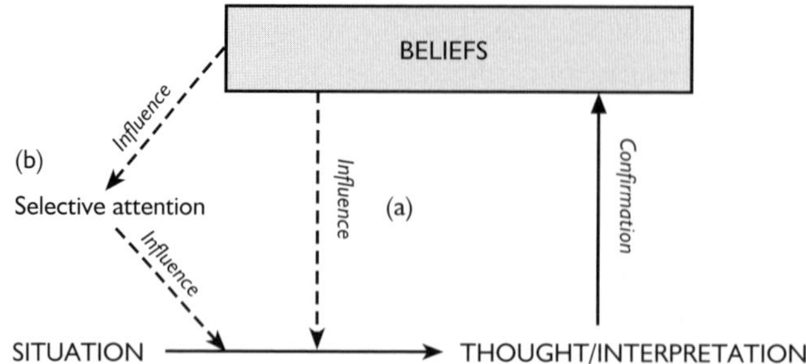

Figure 1.3 Beliefs confirm themselves by influencing the perception and interpretation of evidence.

Biased interpretations (see Figure 1.3(a))

Situations are interpreted according to the beliefs we bring to them. These interpretations then serve to reinforce our existing beliefs because they are consistent with those beliefs. In this way beliefs are self-perpetuating. A clear illustration of this effect from everyday life is that of belief in the accuracy of horoscopes. Suppose the New Year's 'Star Predictions' claim that a world leader will be assassinated in the early part of the year. In May, the ruler of a minor country is killed in a military coup and there are no other assassinations of political leaders that year. The reader who believes that horoscopes can predict the future will point to this assassination as the event foretold by the horoscope, an interpretation that the reader will triumphantly assume to provide further evidence to support their already existing belief in the accuracy of horoscopes. Another reader believes that it is impossible to predict the future from the stars and equally triumphantly points out that once again the horoscopes were inaccurate since the only political assassination that year was of the leader of a small country, not a world leader, and that May is not the early part of the year. By this interpretation the second reader's belief in the inaccuracies of horoscopes has also been confirmed. Thus, the same event has been interpreted in completely different ways but in both cases in such a way as to reinforce the existing belief.

If a belief is very strongly held, the distortion can be so extreme that even blatantly contradictory evidence is interpreted as supporting the belief. For example, if someone firmly believes that they are unattractive, then even a compliment may be interpreted in a negative way: 'She's trying to be kind because she feels sorry for me. I must look even worse than usual'. Such distortions are entirely understandable and reasonable given the strength of the belief. In the example just given, our subject *knew for certain* that they were unattractive so the compliment *could not* be true, and so there *had* to be another reason why it was given.

Selective attention (see Figure 1.3(b))
A second important factor in the maintenance of beliefs is that of selective attention, whereby people tend to notice evidence that confirms their existing beliefs and to ignore or trivialize evidence that is contradictory. For example, people who believe in the ability of spirit mediums to pass on messages from the dead will pay attention to and subsequently recall the instances when a medium seemed to be uncannily accurate with a name or piece of personal knowledge ('She couldn't possibly have known his name was Harry!'), whereas the unbeliever would notice all the mistakes and messages that did not make sense ('No one knew of anyone who had died recently in a car accident' and 'The message about washing the dishes didn't make sense to anyone').

The belief maintenance cycles
The self-confirming effects of selective attention and distorted interpretation are powerful indeed for belief maintenance since the joint operation of these processes ensures that contradictory evidence is either ignored, dismissed or, in extreme cases, interpreted in such a distorted way as to be no longer contradictory. At the same time, attention is given to confirmatory evidence, or neutral evidence that has been interpreted in a confirmatory way, so that the belief is strengthened.

The stronger the belief, the more likely it is that evidence contrary to it will be ignored or distorted. The fact that we distort evidence in this way is not, as one might at first think, a weakness in our psychological system. One of the key functions of a belief is to bring stability to our world and enable us to respond consistently to it. In this variable world in which we live it is advantageous to us to have beliefs that, once formed, can resist the influence of isolated contradictory evidence. If this were not the case, our beliefs would be in a constant state of change and their stabilizing function would be lost. For example, if I think I am a good psychotherapist every time a piece of therapy goes well but a bad psychotherapist who ought to resign every time it does not, then I will be in an unpleasant state of emotional uncertainty and flux, and also risk inappropriately resigning when a piece of therapy has not gone well.

Furthermore, since our beliefs are normally based on a lot of experience and evidence accumulated over time, it is generally appropriate not to change them on the basis of the occasional contradiction. By their very nature, beliefs are generalizations about how things are in the world and so exceptions would be expected. Normally, it is only when contradictory evidence becomes overwhelming that we change our beliefs to accommodate it; the more firmly held the belief, the greater the contradictory evidence required to bring about this change.

The self-confirmation of delusional beliefs

Thus, we see that it is not just people with delusions who do not treat evidence concerning their beliefs in an objective way; none of us do. Indeed, with respect to their distorting effects on evidence interpretation and selective attention, delusional beliefs appear to behave in very much the same way as any other strongly held belief. It is only because the delusional beliefs of a person with psychosis are alien to our own beliefs that we can so readily see the distortions that are going on in the deluded person's thinking. One only has to think of friends or acquaintances that hold different views from one's own to see how 'blind' people can be to contradictory evidence and how they can distort the facts – and how frustrating it can be that they are apparently quite unaware of their prejudiced thinking! On the other hand, when we are with people who share our beliefs, it will be virtually impossible for us to detect the biases in our thinking, because they will not be exposed as such: instead, our beliefs will be gently and reassuringly confirmed.

Of course, it is important to realize that although we may feel confident that we see things clearly, objectively and without bias, this is not the case. We cannot avoid bringing our beliefs to every situation that we encounter or distorting our interpretations of situations according to our own beliefs. This includes our therapy sessions, which is why it is so important for us to try to be aware of our own beliefs and prejudices and the influence they may have on our work as therapists.

Belief modification

We have already noted that some beliefs, especially those about personal and interpersonal matters, are not fixed; they can vary and fluctuate according to our mood and circumstances. For example, our self-confidence can vary according to the situation we are in and according to biological factors such as alcohol intake, hormone levels or mood state. We can even hold apparently opposite beliefs that can be elicited in different circumstances. For instance, as I sit at my desk writing this paragraph, I am convinced that ghosts do not exist; but I have a suspicion that if I were left alone at night, in the dark, in an allegedly haunted house, then this level of conviction would evaporate!

The fact that incompatible beliefs can be triggered in different circumstances (e.g. I am good at my work/I am poor at my work; ghosts do not exist/ghosts might well exist) has an interesting implication for the theory of what we are actually doing in cognitive therapy when we say that we 'modify' a belief. If opposing beliefs can be elicited from the same person in different circumstances, then this suggests that both beliefs must be held somewhere within the overall belief system and that the belief that is triggered to operate in any one situation, i.e. the belief that predominates in that situation, will depend on a complex of internal (mental) and external (environmental) factors. It seems likely therefore that what happens during therapy when we modify a belief is not that the old belief is irrevocably changed into the new belief but rather that the new belief is established and strengthened so that in most circumstances it is this new belief that will be activated rather than the old one.

The notion that new beliefs are superimposed on old ones rather than erasing and replacing them would account for the apparent fluidity of beliefs that can be seen in our everyday lives, as well as the fluctuations that can occur with delusional beliefs. For example, the overlaying of beliefs would account for my irrational fear if I were to be left alone in the haunted house. I was brought up in a culture where ghost stories were read and incidents of hauntings were seriously discussed, so as a child I believed that there was a strong possibility that ghosts existed. As I grew older I realized that the ghost stories were fiction and that my parents could be mistaken, and my scientific training and research into the paranormal convinced me that ghosts could not exist as physical, visible entities. Although it is this later belief that is activated now in almost all situations, the earlier belief about ghosts is still stored somewhere in my nervous system, ready to be reactivated given the right circumstances. Since I have always understood that ghosts tend to haunt specific places, being in a reputedly haunted house at night would be just the sort of external situation most likely to trigger my old belief about ghosts. Even so, this might not be enough on its own to activate the belief, but if I were in a state of anxiety, provoked by being on my own in a dark and unknown place, then the external and internal conditions taken together would almost certainly be enough to trigger the old belief. Once the old belief had been triggered, then neutral events would be interpreted and distorted in line with that old belief. For example, once I believed ghosts to be possible, then the cool draught of air and creaking sound from the stairs would take on a new and a sinister significance.

Biases in thinking (thinking errors)

Our thinking and interpretations of events are influenced not only by the beliefs that we bring to the situation but also by the ways in which we think about things. We all exhibit biases[1] in thinking from time to time, for example jumping to conclusions on the basis of inadequate evidence, and we have already considered the important role that selective attention has on distorting our perception and maintaining the status quo of our belief system. Our thinking is probably at least mildly distorted for most of the time, though we are not aware of most of these distortions since they tend to lead to conclusions that are consistent with our existing beliefs and hence are accepted by us without question. As we have already seen, it is generally only those thoughts that contradict our beliefs and expectations that alert us to the need to consider them more critically.

Biases in thinking are a particularly important factor in depression because when people are in a depressed mood they are particularly likely to be biased in their thinking; for example, so-called black-and-white thinking may lead the person to conclude she is either a total success or a total failure, with no position possible in between. These biases can be severe, leading to significant distortions in rational thinking, for example categorizing oneself as a total failure because of one error made at work.

[1]What were called 'thinking errors' in the early CBT literature.

People with psychosis do show biases in thinking, especially related to their delusional beliefs, but this is a feature common to all strongly held beliefs. The biases associated with delusional thinking are more apparent because the conclusions produced by the distortions are more obviously 'wrong', but most of us are capable of equally prejudiced and distorted thinking when it comes to our strongly held beliefs, for example with our political and religious beliefs. People with psychosis do concentrate on evidence confirming their delusions and pass over evidence that contradicts them but, as we have already seen, this is a feature of normal cognitive processing. In experimental conditions, people with schizophrenia have been found to jump to conclusions on the basis of less information than people without schizophrenia, but the difference is not a dramatic one and the implications for therapy are still not clear.

Another error of thinking that occurs more significantly in psychotic than in non-psychotic people is that of 'personalization' or 'self-reference'. Although we all tend to attribute more significance to ourselves in the grand scheme of things than is objectively justified, people with psychosis can be extreme when making this distortion. In its most extreme form, this bias is what the psychiatric literature calls *a delusion of self-reference*. However, as far as treatment is concerned, it is not possible to approach delusions of self-reference as one would approach biases of thinking in depression or anxiety-based disorders because, without insight, the person is unable to use the concept in a therapeutic way; they *know* their conclusions are correct and therefore they *know* that their thinking is sound. It would only be possible to work with biases of self-reference in the standard CBT way after the person had gained insight about the nature of his or her thinking, by which time treatment would already be well advanced.

In my experience of working with people with moderate to severe schizophrenia it has not been productive to try to work with biases of thinking in the standard CBT way, with thought diaries and homework assignments. One reason for this is that people with schizophrenia tend not to engage in detailed homework tasks of this sort, but another important reason is that they find it difficult to work at the abstract level of thinking about thinking. For these reasons, this particular part of the standard CBT model is not described further in this book; readers interested in this aspect of treatment should consult books on the CBT treatment of depression.

A GENERAL MODEL FOR CBT

Figure 1.4 draws together the different aspects of the cognitive-behavioural model described in the earlier parts of this chapter. People referred for CBT usually come for treatment because of some unpleasant mood state (e.g. depression) or emotional response to situations (e.g. anxiety), or because of the behavioural consequences of the emotional response (e.g. phobic avoidance). Treatment does not target the emotional state directly but attempts to modify it indirectly, by modifying the factors that cause or influence it.

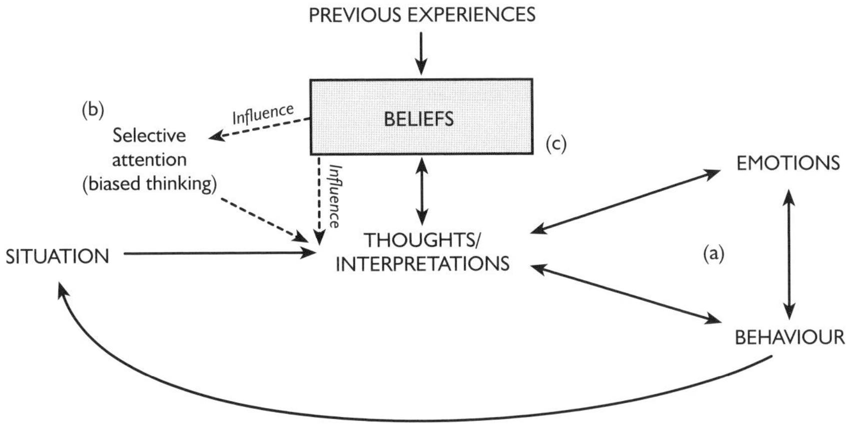

Figure 1.4 A general model for CBT.

Using the model for CBT depicted in Figure 1.4 there are three main lines of treatment:

(a) Breaking the symptom maintenance cycles

As we have seen earlier, thoughts, emotions and behaviour interact closely to maintain the status quo, so changing this self-reinforcing triad from a negative to a positive one is a major aspect of CBT treatment for a wide range of disorders. The interventions are directed at the thoughts and/or behaviour because these are more directly accessible to CBT than the emotions. For example, a depressed woman lacks energy and withdraws from social contacts, thinking that she is boring and that no one wants to bother with her: this lowers her mood even further. Treatment in this case would seek to change her negative thinking about herself (in order to make it easier for her to meet people again), and also to reintroduce her to social situations (so that she could discover that people did want to be with her).

Interventions at the physiological level (e.g. relaxation training and controlled breathing) may help with anxiety-based disorders if the unpleasant symptoms of anxiety are part of the maintaining cycle. For example, if the fear of having a panic attack is preventing an agoraphobic woman from leaving home, then she would receive relaxation training and desensitization to help control and reduce her physical symptoms of anxiety, and also cognitive strategies to modify her panicky thoughts.

The symptom maintenance cycles are also important in psychosis. For example, a paranoid woman gets the thought that people are following her when she walks along the street. Her typical response is to angrily accuse them of being part of the conspiracy. This behaviour usually provokes a negative response from the person accused, which confirms her belief and also provokes her to more paranoid thinking and aggressive behaviour. In this case, treatment would be aimed at changing the woman's paranoid thinking, at least to the extent of introducing a degree of doubt about whether she could be *sure* she was being followed by that person, and also at changing her aggressive way of responding, which is exacerbating the situation.

These symptom maintenance cycles also have an effect by altering the external situation. CBT may attempt to change the external situation directly to make it more favourable (e.g. introducing a night light for someone who panics in the dark) but usually the situational change is brought about via a behavioural change on the part of the person (as with the paranoid man, above, where changing his aggressive response changed the responses of other people).

(b) Detecting and modifying biases in thinking

This aspect of CBT treatment is particularly important for depressive disorders because depressed people are particularly prone to making significant distortions in their interpretations of situations and in their thinking. In these cases treatment is aimed at helping the person to recognize when they are making an error of thinking, to identify what distortion this has led to, and to challenge the thoughts. In this way they learn to generate more rational and positive interpretations of situations, which in turn leads to an improvement in mood state.

Although CBT with psychosis does not directly target biases in thinking in this way, reducing the effects of biased thinking and belief confirmation are a very important aspect of the work. When evaluating the evidence for and against a delusion the therapist seeks to ensure that the person is aware of the evidence that they would otherwise ignore through selective attention and that they are aware of, and can re-evaluate, the distortions that they make in the interpretation of situations.

(c) Modifying the underlying beliefs

With depression and anxiety-based disorders it is normal practice with CBT to concentrate on the more surface treatment levels of the above two approaches and bring about change in the negative beliefs via the *thoughts→beliefs* feedback. However, if belief modification does not occur as a result of treatment at levels (a) or (b), then some more direct belief modification work will be necessary in order to progress the treatment and to avoid relapse after treatment ceases. This approach tends to be the last of the three used because beliefs, particularly those that are deeply held or have been held for a long time, may be difficult to identify and modify, and so treatment at this level tends to take much longer. Personality disorders are rooted in dysfunctional beliefs at the core schema level (i.e. fundamental beliefs about the self and the world) and treatment at the belief level in these cases typically takes years to show significant positive effects. Although CBT is often described as a 'here-and-now' therapy because it focuses on what is happening at the present time, when it is appropriate and necessary the therapy will explore and work on the early experiences that produced the dysfunctional beliefs.

Working directly on the dysfunctional beliefs is the essence of CBT with delusions, but although delusional beliefs may be held very strongly, the fact that they developed later in life means that they are potentially less embedded and enmeshed with other beliefs than dysfunctional schemata are and so, in this respect, they are potentially easier to shift. However, in some cases, in order to bring about significant and lasting benefit, the CBT will need to address core beliefs as well as the delusional beliefs. Typically, this would be where the core beliefs are underpinning the delusions and/or causing the patient distress.

CBT with accurate and inaccurate interpretations of reality

When planning a course of therapy, it is essential to know whether the person's interpretation of events is accurate or not because the line of therapy is different for accurate and inaccurate interpretations. Much of CBT is concerned with factually inaccurate interpretations of reality, for example the depressed young man who thinks his partner is about to leave him because the partner came home late from work, or the social phobic who fears that everyone will look critically at her when she enters a party. In these circumstances, helping the person to make more realistic and accurate interpretations of situations will result in more positive thoughts and hence more positive emotions. As a general rule, if an interpretation of an event or situation is factually inaccurate, then it is appropriate to work on modifying the inaccuracies of interpretation.

However, if the interpretation is factually accurate, then it would be inappropriate to attempt to modify the interpretation itself; instead, therapy would attempt to relieve the unpleasant emotions by changing the beliefs surrounding the interpretation. For example, if the young man just mentioned is correct in his interpretation of his partner's behaviour, then it would be fruitless to try to show that his partner was not intending to leave him, and in these circumstances his despair about ever being happy again could only be relieved by modifying his belief that he could never be happy with anyone else.

THE ABC MODEL

The ABC model was developed within behaviour therapy to help identify the significant factors that are maintaining an unwanted behaviour. The Antecedents are the factors or situations that lead up to and trigger the Behaviour, and the Consequences are the factors or events that follow the behaviour and reinforce it. The ABC acronym has been adapted for use in cognitive therapy; in this case, the B represents Beliefs (which may be detected in the person's thoughts). It is used in two rather different ways in the CBT literature.

1 *To describe the ongoing, here-and-now situation.* (This is similar to the way it is used in behavioural therapy.) In this case, the Antecedents are the situations or events that trigger an underlying Belief, which is apparent in the thoughts or interpretations that it produces, and the Consequences are the behavioural, emotional and physiological consequences of the thoughts. When used in this way, the ABC model corresponds to the horizontal line in Figure 1.4:
situations (A)→thoughts (B)→emotions + behaviour (C).

2 *To describe the long-term development and effects of beliefs.* In this case, the Antecedents are the early history and experiences that led to the Belief, and the Consequences are the ways that the belief affects thoughts or interpretations and the emotional, behavioural and physiological consequences of this. When used in this way, the ABC model corresponds to the vertical line in Figure. 1.4: *experiences (A) →beliefs (B) →thoughts (C).*

The ABC model is a simple but effective way of conceptualizing what is going on, so it can be a helpful aid to case formulation in the clinical setting, but care must be taken not to confuse which version of the ABC is being used.

THE THERAPIST IN CBT

The therapy

CBT is a joint venture between the patient/client and the therapist. Both participants in this venture are of equal status; generally speaking, the patient/client is the 'expert' about their experiences, thoughts, feelings, beliefs, etc., whilst the therapist is the 'expert' in possible ways of changing these.

CBT seeks to achieve the *patient/client's* goals: the only exception to this would be if these goals would adversely and unfairly affect others. If the initial goals are not realistic or practicable, they are discussed with the person so that achievable and useful goals can be set.[2]

The therapeutic process

One of the basic principles of the CBT method of working is that the therapist does not tell the other person how things are, or give information directly, but rather guides their thinking along the right tracks, to helpful conclusions, by asking appropriate questions. This is known as the method of *Socratic dialogue* or *questioning*, so called after its use in texts written over 2,000 years ago by Plato. In these texts Plato would develop his philosophical argument by reporting a dialogue between Socrates and a philosophy student. In these dialogues Socrates would expose the illogical thinking of the student and show him the correct way of thinking by asking pertinent questions. Typically, a Socratic dialogue starts with the student making some reasonable-sounding statement about some matter of philosophical interest and ends with the student making another statement along the lines of 'I see now, Socrates, that I was wrong when I said that . . .', and then summarizing the arguments brought out in the dialogue. The dialogues of Plato make impressive reading for the aspiring CBT therapist but it must be remembered that in some ways Plato's task was easier than ours, not least because he supplied both the questions and the answers, whereas we therapists have control of the questions only – and our patients/clients do not always answer as obligingly as Plato's philosophy students did!

A regular and frequent feature of CBT is the therapist's *rephrasing*, *recapping*

[2]But see Chapter 3 for some of the problems in discussing goals for delusional beliefs.

and *summarizing* of what the person has said. This practice not only enables the therapist to clarify that they have understood what is going on but is also an essential part of the therapeutic process as it helps the person to focus on the key issues. When rephrasing or summarizing what the person has said, it is essential that he or she feels able to correct the therapist if that rephrasing is not accurate, so the therapist constantly questions along the lines 'Have I understood that properly?', 'Have I got that right?' or 'I think we agreed that ... or could I put it more accurately?', etc. If the therapist has not understood or has expressed something inaccurately, then she should take the responsibility for this herself; she should in no way imply that the other person was inarticulate or otherwise at fault.

The therapist should be logical and structured in her thinking, planning and delivery of the treatment, and systematic in monitoring the effects of the different strategies used so that appropriate refinements can be made.

As with most psychological therapies, *good rapport* and *trust* are essential ingredients of CBT. Therapists should have a positive regard for their patients and adopt a non-judgemental attitude to what they are told during therapy. They should be honest, warm and empathic, and blame neither the other person nor themselves when progress is slow.

2 The cognitive-behavioural model applied to delusions and hallucinations

Introduction

Biological and psychosocial models of psychosis

Theories of mental illness have traditionally stressed either the biological causes (the so-called *medical model*) or the psychological causes (the so-called *psychosocial model*), and in the past there has been a tendency to compare and contrast these models as if they were contradictory and incompatible. This was inappropriate on both theoretical and practical grounds. We cannot separate the psychological experience from the brain activity that produces it because they are different sides of the same coin; they are the subjective and objective descriptions of the same thing. Furthermore, it is now known that not only do the biochemistry and activity of the brain affect the psychological experience but also the psychological experience can affect the biochemistry and activity of the brain.

As far as psychosis is concerned, both biological abnormalities in the brain and stressors in the psychological environment are known to affect the onset and development of the symptoms (see Chapter 6, p. 113 for a description of the stress-vulnerability model), so at a clinical level it is more useful to regard the medical and psychosocial models of psychosis as complementary rather than as alternatives. In practice this means considering both the biological and psychological factors that might be relevant for a particular person and seeking to produce a beneficial change by the use of biological and psychological treatments (e.g. medication and CBT respectively).

In order to apply CBT to the symptoms of psychosis it is necessary to appreciate the effects that a biological dysfunction of the brain can have on someone's subjective experiences and cognitions, but it is not necessary to know exactly what the biological abnormality is or how it has arisen. Therefore, for the purposes of this book, we will not be considering the nature of the biological abnormalities associated with psychosis or the range of biological treatments that are currently available: interested readers are referred to standard psychiatric texts covering this area.

The use of diagrams and models

Since CBT is a psychological therapy we will be considering in some detail the psychological processes that are involved in the development and maintenance of delusions and hallucinations, taking into account not only the role played by abnormal functioning but also the very important role played by the normal functioning of normal psychological processes.

There were two main reasons for developing the cognitive-behavioural models described in this chapter, apart from the intrinsic fascination and challenge of trying to understand how and why delusions and hallucinations can take such different forms in different people, and to describe this in diagrammatic form. The first reason was to provide therapists with a framework within which they can structure their thinking about a particular delusion or hallucination experienced by the individual person and within which they can plan the appropriate line(s) of treatment. The second reason was to provide the person themself with a framework within which they can understand their experiences in a helpful way.

In order to keep the models (relatively) easy to comprehend and use in clinical practice they have been kept as simple as possible, but inevitably this means that some relevant factors have had to be omitted. For this reason, they have been called 'working models', to reflect their practical use, rather than theoretical models. In practice these simplified models do seem to be applicable in most cases but if an omitted factor, for example high arousal or a physiological symptom, is particularly relevant for an individual person, then the model can be adapted accordingly.

Some other explanatory models, relevant to particular aspects of the CBT therapy, are described in Chapter 6 and Appendix 2. Although these models may look rather different, and focus on slightly different aspects of the thinking and believing processes, they are entirely consistent and compatible with the models presented in this chapter. Nevertheless, if you are sharing your case formulation with the person themself, it is suggested that you do not risk confusion by trying to introduce more than one model at a time.

DELUSIONAL BELIEFS

A WORKING MODEL FOR THE DEVELOPMENT AND MAINTENANCE OF DELUSIONAL BELIEFS

Adaptation of the general model for CBT

The general model presented in Figure 1.4 (p. 15) to illustrate the formation and maintenance of new beliefs in non-psychotic people can be adapted to account for delusional beliefs by the simple addition of a 'psychotic experiences' factor, which represents the subjective experiences that result from the biological disturbances that underlie the psychosis (see Figure 2.1). This adaptation implies that whereas in normal belief formation the person's subjective experiences are closely related to their situation or environment, when someone has psychosis the subjective experiences that the psychosis can produce may significantly influence or even overwhelm the subjective experience that is coming to their brain from the external environment. The totality of this subjective experience is interpreted in the normal way, using the person's beliefs and knowledge about the world; but although the interpretations will be entirely reasonable given the total subjective experience, they may appear inappropriate or even inexplicable to others who are only aware of the external situation and not of the inner psychotic experiences. Once acquired, delusional beliefs will affect subsequent interpretations of events and will be maintained by the same psychological processes as are involved in the maintenance of normal beliefs (see Chapter 1).

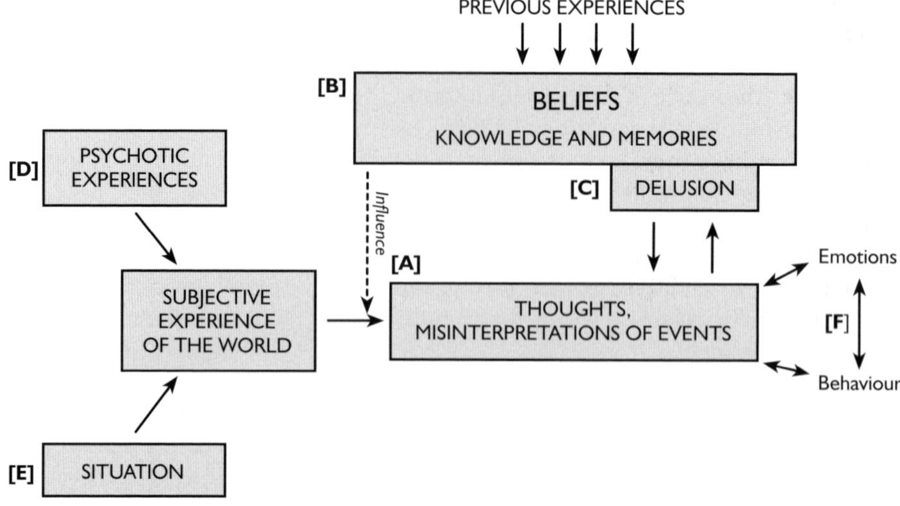

Figure 2.1[1] Working model for the formation and maintenance of a delusional belief, showing areas for CBT intervention.

Psychotic experiences

The *psychotic experiences* of Figure 2.1 fall into three broad categories.

1. Mood disturbances

These include mood states such as paranoia and grandiosity as well as the harder to define feelings such as 'strangeness' and 'significance', often of a mystical or religious kind. Abnormal moods and feelings can occur spontaneously as a direct result of the brain dysfunction that underlies the psychosis. The occurrence of a delusional mood state as a prelude to the onset of specific delusions is well established in the psychiatric literature and some people, particularly in the early stages of relapse, are able to recognize that their feelings are a symptom of their

[1]*Note*: The diagram given in Figure 2.1 is essentially the same model as that described in the first edition of this treatment manual, but it has been rotated through 90 degrees to make it more obviously compatible with the theoretical model described in Chapter 1 (Fig. 1.4, p. 15). This has been done to make it easier to see where additional relevant factors which have been omitted from the 'delusions' diagram might be operating. The 'external events or situations' factor, which had been omitted from the first edition model for the sake of simplicity, has been reinstated. The 'influence of early experiences' factor has also been included in this present diagram, in recognition of the potential importance of this aspect and the need to consider it in case formulation. For the sake of simplicity, the influence of the 'biosocial systems' on psychotic mood state has been omitted from this present version.

illness and do not accurately reflect reality. Some people who relapse after receiving CBT may be able to continue to distinguish between what they *feel* to be the case (e.g. that someone wants to harm them) and what they *know* (e.g. that they are not under any threat), even when the psychosis is severe. Indeed, this is likely to be one of the long-term goals of therapy when the illness is a recurring one.

Of course, once the delusional belief has been established, it will tend to exacerbate the existing mood state by the operation of normal cognitive processes, i.e. by distorting the interpretation of events and by producing delusion-congruent automatic thoughts.

2. Changes in levels of consciousness and awareness

These are some of the most distressing and frightening effects of psychosis. They include experiences of breakdown in the sense of personal identity (e.g. 'I am not the same "me"'; 'My actions are not mine'; 'Everything I experience is caused by someone or something else'; 'My thoughts are inserted/stopped/removed') and breakdown in the boundaries between self and the world (e.g. 'There is no clear boundary between myself and people/objects around me'; 'I am fragmented'; 'Parts of me have been reproduced elsewhere'; 'I am empty, a shell, nothingness').

Changes in levels of consciousness may also affect the person's ability to keep focused so that they slide off the point or move from one loosely related idea to another. Logically discreet concepts may become blurred, 'like a dreamer awake'. At its most severe, thought disorder may make verbal communications with the person effectively impossible.[2]

3. Hallucinations

The most common type of hallucination is auditory, usually in the form of spoken voices though they can be of other sounds, for example whispering, phone ringing, gunshots, etc. Tactile hallucinations are probably more common than we think, but we do not always ask about them. Visual and olfactory hallucinations are often a sign of a frank neurological disorder, but they can also occur in people for whom psychosis is the only identifiable brain disorder.

Hallucinations are very often indistinguishable from real events as far as the subjective experiencing of them is concerned. Our brains are programmed to accept sensory data as accurate (when did you last think it worthwhile checking whether you had 'really' heard your colleague talking to you? or 'really' felt that drop of rain?) so it is not surprising that hallucinations are experienced as, and assumed to be, 'real'. Hallucinatory experiences can be a very significant addition to the external situation that the person experiences themself to be in.

[2]Thought disorder does not necessarily affect all areas of thinking. One woman provided an impressive illustration of this. When she was unwell her thinking and language became chaotic to the extent that it was impossible to communicate with her in any meaningful way; nevertheless, she was able to concentrate for periods of 20 to 30 minutes at the chessboard and played a good, solid game.

External events/situations

The psychotic experiences occur within the context of an external event or situation, so this latter also forms part of the person's total subjective experience. The external environment may be affected indirectly by the psychosis. For example, if someone is responding to voices, then other people may react with alarm and move away, or someone may isolate themself as a result of paranoid beliefs.

Beliefs and memories

All experiences or events are interpreted in terms of the person's beliefs and knowledge about themself and the world. Memories of past events are also used as reference points to help interpret the present situation.

Previous experiences

Our beliefs and knowledge are derived from and determined by our previous experiences, using this term in its widest sense. Our earliest experiences are particularly important in shaping our core beliefs (schemata) about ourselves and the world and about our relationships to others. Adverse early experiences may leave us more vulnerable to psychosis in later life. For example, a child brought up in an abusive environment may develop core beliefs that she is abhorrent and that other people are punitive and uncaring. With these underlying beliefs it will be easier to develop paranoid beliefs than if the core beliefs had been that other people are generally kind and helpful and that she is worthy of love and protection.

As we move through life we acquire knowledge about how things operate in the world and what is and is not possible. This 'knowledge' is an important factor because it will affect how the total subjective experience is interpreted and thus affect whether and how the delusional belief is developed. For example, someone who has heard that lasers can go through solid matter may interpret their burning skin sensations as the effects of lasers from spy satellites, whereas someone who has learnt that lasers cannot penetrate thick buildings would look for another explanation.

Thoughts and misinterpretations of events

Automatic thoughts are being generated by the brain all the time. They are influenced by the underlying belief system (including any delusional beliefs), the external situation and the internal psychotic experiences. Automatic thoughts form part of the total subjective experience. Imagination will also affect thinking and interpretation of the situation.

The misinterpretations that occur are the person's best attempt to understand their total subjective experience of what is going on. They may be influenced by biased thinking, particularly the tendency to select evidence that is consistent with the person's mood state.

More cognitive processing is required to reject something as untrue than to accept it as true, so the cognitive deficits associated with psychosis might mean that people are more likely to accept their first interpretations without question.

The delusion

The interpretation of events made by the brain may, in some circumstances, feel so convincing to the person concerned that it takes on the status of a belief without additional evidence being required and, being experienced as self-evidently true, will not therefore be subject to rational or critical reasoning. Although delusional beliefs can appear quite suddenly in this way, they are often built up more slowly, as a result of an accumulation of evidence provided by the repeated occurrence of misinterpretations driven by delusional mood and/or other psychotic experiences.

Although shown as a separate box in Figure 2.1, the *delusion* belongs within the general *beliefs* box. The brain makes no distinction between delusional and non-delusional beliefs: they are stored in the brain in the same belief system and act in the same way.

'Bizarre' delusions

In some cases, it appears that delusional beliefs may develop directly from automatic thoughts, without involving events in the external world. In such a case it seems that the automatic thought is not subject to the normal filtering and selection of ideas that occurs in the conscious brain but, as part of the psychotic process, is directly invested with 'confirmed-belief' status. This could account for the occurrence of delusional beliefs that are quite bizarre and unrelated to the real world. The process involved may be similar to that seen with LSD, where subjects under the influence of the drug may receive sudden revelations of 'profound truths' (e.g. 'the world is made of cheese') which are then held with complete conviction despite their factual absurdity. The whole question of when and why the brain confers confirmed-belief status on particular ideas is a very interesting one, though at this time we can only speculate about it. However, we saw in Chapter 1 why it is functional for our beliefs to be held with a greater sense of certainty than the evidence would perhaps warrant (a) because this means that we no longer have to keep seeking and weighing up evidence as to their correctness, and (b) because it enables us to use these beliefs without question or hesitation. This suggests that there must be some function within the brain that decides when 'probability' is converted to a feeling of 'certainty'. It is interesting to speculate that this may be the 'normal' process that is inappropriately triggered in psychosis in the formation of apparently bizarre delusional beliefs, turning fragmented automatic thoughts into significant, firmly held beliefs.

Maintenance of the delusional belief

Once established, the delusional belief affects subsequent *interpretations* and a major belief maintenance cycle is formed. The delusional belief will also be maintained by the normal bias of selective attention, i.e. by noticing and remembering things that seem to confirm the delusion and by ignoring or distorting things that contradict it.

There is also a maintenance circle via *memories* (not shown in Figure 2.1); the more often events are interpreted in line with the delusion, the more remembered 'evidence' there is that the belief is true.

Another maintenance cycle (not shown in Figure 2.1) operates between the delusion and subjective experience, mediated by *mood state* and *emotional responses*. For example, if you believe there is a conspiracy to kidnap you, then it is highly likely that you will feel frightened and suspicious as a direct result of this belief. This feeling will be an important part of the total subjective experience that the brain seeks to understand. Making sense of the environment in this fundamental way takes place at a more basic, automatic level of brain functioning than purposeful thinking, though thoughtful speculation may influence the outcome.

Other maintenance cycles may operate through the other parts of the symptom maintenance triad, described in Chapter 1. The person's *behaviour* is likely to be affected by the misinterpretations. In the example given above, if you are suspicious that someone is following you with intent to kidnap you, then it is sensible to go to the police to ask for help and protection, but their unwillingness to take any action against the criminal that you have pointed out to them will be further evidence of the extent of the conspiracy. Similarly in this example, if you think that the world is a dangerous place, then you will not have the *motivation* to seek out friendships: but your isolation will confirm that people do not like you. *Physiological factors* may also serve to reinforce delusional beliefs. For example, if your muscles feel weak when you are pursued by the kidnappers, then this may mean that they are able to invade your body and influence it in some way – so they must be really dangerous.

EXAMPLE OF THE MODEL IN ACTION

A man is sitting in his room at home with his wife and a Community Psychiatric Nurse (CPN) who has visited to give him his depot injection. His brain produces the psychotic experience of being under threat, so his subjective experience is of being under threat in this situation.

Like all human beings, his brain will be predisposed to see other people as more probable sources of threat than inanimate objects such as the furniture in his room, so the 'source' of threat will crystallize around either his wife or the CPN. His early childhood led him to believe that family were trustworthy and his more recent experience with his wife has led to the belief that she is caring and loving, so it is unlikely that the fear will attach itself to her. But he was taught as a child not to trust strangers and he knows the CPN less well than his wife, and perhaps he has some reservations about his injections. In these circumstances it is likely that the CPN will be perceived as the source of the threat. Thus, the first misperception of events, driven by his feeling of threat but influenced by his existing beliefs about his wife, the CPN and the injections, has occurred.

Once a belief about the CPN wanting to harm him has emerged, then it will influence his interpretation of subsequent events so that they conform to and thereby confirm the belief. For example, supposing the CPN visits the next day to offer to take him to the shops. The offer is kindly meant but, believing that the CPN wishes him harm, it is interpreted by the man as a plot to get him away from the safety of his home and the protection of his wife. This interpretation will increase his feelings of paranoia and confirm his delusional belief that the CPN wants to harm him. The self-confirming circle has been brought into effect.

Other confirming circles will also operate, for example through the feelings generated by the delusional belief and through behaviour in response to the belief. In the example we are considering, perhaps the man barricades himself into his flat, which leads to the CPN gaining entry against his wishes, which confirms his belief about the CPN. The delusion may also fuel other psychotic experiences, for example voices warning the man of the CPN's evil intentions, which further reinforce the delusional belief.

Once the belief that the CPN wants to harm him has been firmly established, then these self-confirming belief cycles will act so as to maintain it even after the (psychotic) brain activity responsible for the initial feelings of threat has ceased. The man now has a chronic delusion that can only be overturned by breaking the maintenance cycles that are reinforcing it.

COGNITIVE-BEHAVIOURAL INTERVENTIONS FOR DELUSIONS

(See later chapters for details of the interventions.)

According to the model depicted in Figure 2.1, there are six potential areas of intervention, [A] to [F] using CBT.

[A] Break the cognitive cycles maintaining the delusion by modifying the misinterpretations of events that serve to reinforce the delusional belief. Treatment strategies may include:

- logical reasoning, to prevent interpretations being distorted
- providing alternative explanations
- not allowing contradictory evidence and/or explanations to be minimized or ignored
- providing new evidence that contradicts the delusion.

[B] Modify the non-psychotic beliefs and knowledge that underlie and enable the development of the delusion. Treatment strategies may include:

- CBT for belief modification
- re-evaluation of the memories of past events and situations that were perceived (through misinterpretation) to support the delusion
- increasing or changing knowledge and understanding through discussion and learning.

[C] **Modify the delusional belief.** Treatment strategies may include:

- developing a shared understanding about how and why the delusion developed
- evidence evaluation
- logical reasoning
- reality testing.

[D] **Work on the psychotic experiences.** Treatment strategies may include:

- providing an alternative way of understanding how and why the feelings or experiences have occurred, so that they are no longer mis-attributed to the external situation
- coping strategies to reduce the psychotic experiences.

[E] **Change the environment and events (situation).** Treatment strategies may include:

- practical/behavioural and cognitive coping strategies.

[F] **Break any maintenance cycles that may be operating via the behavioural, motivational, physiological and emotional consequences of the misinterpretations associated with the delusion.** Treatment strategies may include:

- understanding how the maintenance cycle is operating
- cognitive therapy strategies (evidence evaluation, logical reasoning, reality testing)
- behaviour therapy strategies (e.g. graded exposure, desensitization)
- practical and cognitive coping strategies.

Biological interventions

Antipsychotic *medication* can prevent the occurrence and reinforcement of delusional beliefs by preventing the biological disturbance that drives the delusional mood state and other psychotic experiences ([D] in Figure 2.1). Medication may be used also to help to control the emotional consequences of the misinterpretations, for example for anxiety or anger control ([F] in figure 2.1).

EXAMPLE OF A TREATMENT PROGRAMME

If the treatment model is applied to the example given above, it indicates several different lines of treatment that might be helpful in bringing about a modification of the delusional belief about the CPN. [Letters in square brackets refer to the model depicted in Figure 2.1.]

1 To change the misinterpretations of events from the past **[B]** and of on-going events **[A]** that are reinforcing the delusion about the CPN. For example, one goal would be to change the man's interpretation of the CPN's offer to take him to the shops to the more likely explanation that the CPN intended this to be helpful as part of his rehabilitation programme.
2 To change the underlying delusion about the CPN, the goal being for him to believe that the CPN was trying to help him and had his best interests at heart **[C]**.
3 To alter the belief about medication doing more harm than good **[B]**. If the man believes medication is bad for him, it is not unreasonable for him to conclude that the person who gives him the medication does not have his best interests at heart and may even wish him harm. The aim would be to change his dysfunctional belief about medication to a belief that medication is generally beneficial for him (providing that this was the case), whilst acknowledging and trying to minimize any unwanted side effects there may be.
4 To change his interpretation of his voices, so that he understands them to be his own thoughts, reflecting his fears about the CPN **[C]**.
5 To control his voices using coping strategies **[D]**.
6 To change his understanding about why he felt under threat in the past and why he feels under threat now **[C]**, and to develop coping strategies to help him deal with these feelings **[E]**.
7 Medication would be used to control the biological basis of his paranoid feelings **[D]**. If the medication were not effective, then the best position would probably be for him to be able to use his reasoning to counter the feelings thus: 'I feel as if the CPN wants to harm me but I know he doesn't really because . . .' and 'These feelings are caused by my illness and it might help if I did . . .' **[A, F]**.

Implications of the model for treatment effects

1 For many people, medication is able to eliminate delusional beliefs without the aid of CBT. In these cases, once the psychotic experiences that alter the subjective world, and thereby drive the delusion, have been eliminated, then the conflicting evidence from everyday events and the person's non-psychotic beliefs are enough to change the delusion. In effect, the CBT part of the treatment has occurred naturally, because the subjective experience is no longer being distorted by psychotic experiences.
2 A delusional belief may persist even when the biological cause of the originating psychotic experiences is no longer active, because cognitive-behavioural factors are maintaining it. In this case, it should be possible for CBT to completely eliminate the delusional belief and thereby the unpleasant feelings produced by it.
3 However, when the psychosis is active at a biological level, the CBT strategies may be able to hold the delusion at bay, by working on the maintaining factors, but the unpleasant feelings and experiences (which may include voices) produced by the psychosis will remain and these will increase vulnerability to

delusional interpretations and thoughts. The optimal therapeutic position at such a time is for the person to be able to make the distinction '*I feel as if ... but I know really that ...*'

4 (a) Having the understanding '*I feel as if ..., but I know that ...*' helps to prevent the build up of evidence supporting the delusion and also to prevent the development of secondary delusional beliefs.
   (b) This understanding is also important in enabling the person to act according to what they know to be the case rather than what they feel to be the case, thus avoiding unhelpful behaviours and facilitating helpful coping behaviours.
5 (a) Even if a delusional belief has been effectively eradicated, it may re-emerge if the psychosis becomes active again because the mood state and psychotic experiences that were responsible for its development, and that were associated with it, have occurred again. Because belief modification is achieved by strengthening an alternative, incompatible belief rather than by total elimination of the delusion, the delusional belief that re-emerges is likely to be the same as, or very similar to, the one held before.
   (b) This being so, treatment should not only deal with the present situation but should also provide the person with CBT strategies they can use to counter the delusional belief if and when it recurs in the future.
6 Because of this potential for delusional beliefs to be reactivated in the future, CBT has a role to play even if the person is quite well again by the time you meet with them and they no longer believe their delusions to be true. At this time, very useful work can be done to strengthen the current non-delusional beliefs, focusing on and developing the person's own reasons for believing their delusions to be false. This is also a good time to do relapse prevention work.

AUDITORY HALLUCINATIONS

THE 'INNER-SPEECH LOOP' MODEL

Voices are thoughts that are heard as if they were coming from an external source. The model depicted in Figure 2.2 explains why this happens, why the voice may be recognized as someone that the person knows and why it may not be recognized as their own thoughts. The explanation given with the diagram can be adapted for the individual from that given below.

Listening and talking

When we hear someone talking, the nerves in the ear (via the eardrum) send messages to a part of our brain that recognizes the sounds as individual words **[L]**, but at this early stage no meaning is attached to the words; for example, it would merely recognize 'book' and 'flad' as two separate words. The message is then passed to another, very important part of the brain where the meaning of the word is understood **[M]**. So it is at this stage that we would get the meaning of 'book' but, finding no meaning for 'flad', realize that this is a nonsense word.

When we want to reply, we think about the meaning we want to convey **[M]**; at this stage it is not in the form of words. This is then passed to another part of the brain where the meaning is converted into words **[N]**. Neurological messages then go to the lips and tongue in order to articulate the words **[O]**. Listening to our own words is an important feedback loop since it enables us to monitor what we say and to keep focused.[3]

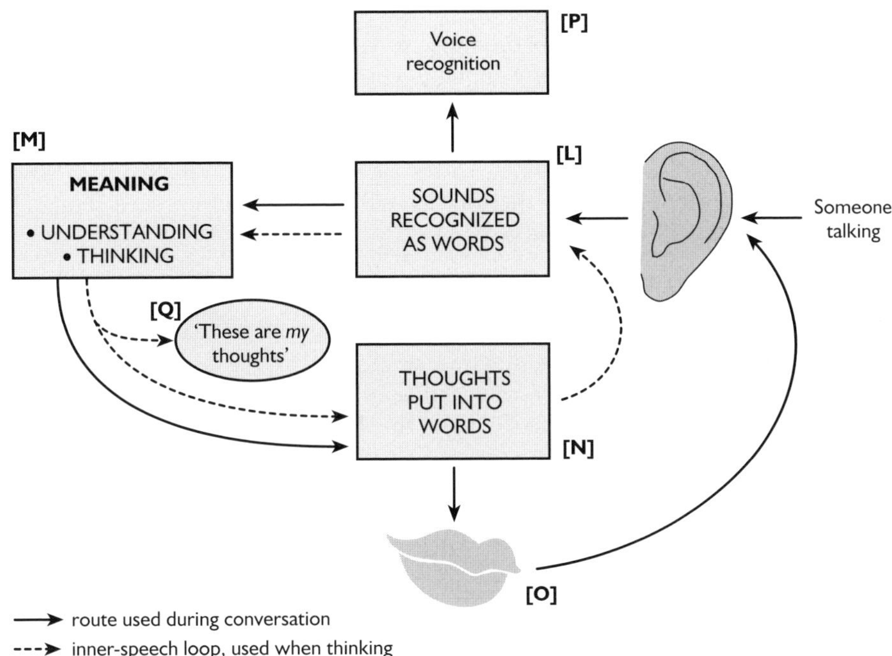

Figure 2.2 The inner-speech loop model for voices.

Thinking

When we are thinking, the meaning of our thoughts comes first **[M]** and then is translated into words **[N]**. This is essentially the same process involved in talking out loud, though when thinking only some of the words, the key ones for meaning, may be formed.[4] This translation of thoughts into words is done

[3]It is surprisingly difficult to keep talking fluently if this feedback is blocked, for example, by white noise coming through headphones.

[4]Interestingly, although we do not speak our thoughts out loud, some neurological messages 'leak' through to our lips and tongue so that minor movements may be detected during thinking.

automatically by the brain because although language has its limitations, nevertheless it is a very important tool that helps us to clarify our thinking and enables us to manipulate and develop our ideas. The word version of the thought is then fed back through the 'word detection' part of the brain **[L]** to the meaning/understanding part **[M]**. This inner-speech feedback loop helps us to clarify and monitor our thinking and this is why, when we think, we can sometimes be aware of using words or of talking to ourselves in our thoughts.[5]

'Voices'

As Figure 2.2 shows, some parts of the brain that we use when we listen to other people are also used during our thinking, so it is relatively easy for the brain to make a mistake about where the input is coming from. This occurs at a basic neurological level, so once the words have been erroneously attributed to an external source, then the subjective experience is to 'hear' them as real sounds coming from outside. This is similar to the phenomenon of referred pain where, for example, a referred pain in the foot is really felt in the foot even though the neurological cause is in the spine.

Why do 'voices' sometimes sound like somebody known to the person?

The area of the brain that has learnt to recognize and distinguish between different people's voices **[P]** is situated very near to the area that recognizes sounds as words **[L]**, so it can become activated by the words coming through the inner-speech loop. If this happens, then the brain will produce the subjective experience of actually hearing that particular person speaking the words.

The voice recognition units for voices that have been heard recently or for voices that are more familiar to the person are more likely to be activated. The recognition units for people who are of particular importance for the person are likely to be more sensitive to activation and hence also more likely to be 'recognized'. This may be why hallucinated voices that can be recognized as someone known often fall into one of these categories.

Of course, in many cases the voice recognition part of the brain is not activated by the words coming through the inner-speech loop and so the hallucinated voice is not recognized as coming from someone known. Furthermore, in some cases it may not be possible to recognize the voice's tone or accent, its direction, whether it is male or female, old or young, etc. This occurs when the parts of the brain responsible for detecting these qualities in heard speech are not activated by the words coming via the inner-speech loop.

If the voice is a memory from the past of someone speaking (see 'The content

[5] It has been suggested that many thousands of years ago, when humans first started to think reflectively, they always heard their thoughts out loud, which helped them to concentrate on the relatively weak neurological messages. It was only later, when this route became stronger, that we lost this ability, but the potential remains in our inherited brain structure, more strongly in some people than in others. I do not know enough about these matters to be able to judge whether this is likely to be true or not, but it is certainly an intriguing notion.

of the voices', below), then 'vivid memory' or 'traumatic memory' is an alternative explanation for why the voice sounds like that person.

Why are 'voices' not recognized as the person's own thoughts?

There is a part of the brain that detects and recognizes what is coming along the inner-speech loop [Q] and this gives us the feeling that these are *our* thoughts, generated by us and belonging to us. So, even if we hear our thoughts out loud (as quite a few of us do, see Chapter 12), we still experience them as our own. When voices are attributed to an external source, there must be an additional mistake being made by the brain, namely that of bypassing this part of the brain [Q] and therefore failing to detect and 'own' the words coming via the inner-speech loop. This mistake is caused at a neurological level and is part of the biological dysfunction causing the psychosis.

FACTORS INVOLVED IN THE DEVELOPMENT OF 'VOICES'

Although all of us will hallucinate if the conditions are right, some people are born with a stronger biological predisposition to do so. (It is still a matter of debate whether environmental factors, e.g. a difficult or traumatic childhood, can increase this innate predisposition at a biological level.) For some people, their predisposition is so strong that they will hear voices even under optimal conditions for not doing so, but for others additional environmental factors will be required.

Voices are more likely to occur if the person is highly aroused. High arousal can occur as a result of the biological dysfunction underlying the psychosis, and it can occur as a result of stress caused by environmental factors, particularly if this stress is sustained over a period of time. (*Note*: Although stress is usually thought of in terms of negative stressful events, apparently enjoyable events, for example Christmas celebrations, can also increase arousal and thereby lead to an increase in voices.) Lack of sleep, food and water are physical stressors that will also increase the likelihood of hearing voices.

Drugs can directly affect brain functioning and produce hallucinations; indeed, in some cases this is the very reason why people use them. LSD is notorious in this respect.[6] Other recreational drugs, for example marijuana, can also cause some vulnerable brains to hallucinate.

A WORKING MODEL FOR THE DEVELOPMENT AND MAINTENANCE OF AUDITORY HALLUCINATIONS

The model depicted in Figure 2.1 to describe the development and maintenance of delusional beliefs can be adapted for auditory hallucinations by the single

[6]LSD is a particularly nasty drug because for some unlucky people one 'trip' is enough to push their brain into a severe and irreversible psychotic state.

addition of the 'brain dysfunction', described in detail in Figure 2.2, that causes some thoughts to be heard as if they were coming from a separate, external source. Hearing one's automatic thoughts in this way is likely to give them greater importance and significance than they would otherwise have, and trying to make sense of the experience leads to the development of delusional beliefs about the origin and power of the voice. Other parts of the model are the same.

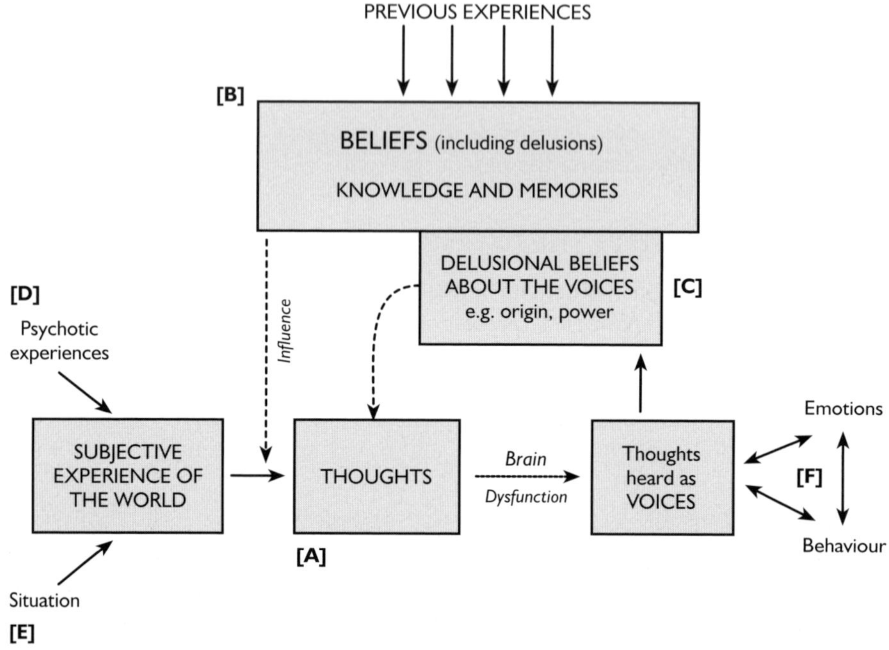

Figure 2.3 Working model for the development and maintenence of auditory hallucinations, showing areas for CBT intervention.

The content of the voices

Voices arise for the same reason that automatic thoughts do (see Chapter 1), and involve the same psychological factors, including the internal and external factors that make up the person's subjective experience of the world, their beliefs and knowledge about themself and the world, their memories and past experiences, and their purposeful thinking and imagination. Examples of how these different factors may influence what the voices say are given in Chapter 11.

Maintenance of the voices

Voices are maintained by (a) the biological dysfunctions that enable thoughts to be heard and to be identified as coming from an external source, and (b) the environmental factors that increase the brain's sensitivity to these effects. There is a maintenance cycle for distressing voices because when the content is distressing this will increase arousal and this in turn will increase the occurrence of the voices.

Once a voice has been heard and experienced as a real event, then it will be stored in memory as a real event, and it may recur on this basis. In some cases the voice may be experienced as a traumatic event, especially if it is heard in the context of other psychotic experiences, during a period of acute psychosis, and in these circumstances it may recur as a post-trauma type phenomenon. When the voice repeats the same things over and over again, then this 'habit' effect will make the brain more likely to produce the same thoughts/voice again.

COGNITIVE-BEHAVIOURAL INTERVENTIONS FOR AUDITORY HALLUCINATIONS

(See later chapters for details of the interventions.)

According to the model depicted in Figure 2.3, there are six potential areras of intervention, **[A]** to **[F]**, using CBT.

[A] & **[B]** Work with the content of the voice, i.e. what the voice says. This is likely to include work on the beliefs and/or memories that underlie the particular thoughts or concerns that are heard as voices.

[C] Work with the beliefs about the nature/origin of the voice, and about its power and/or authority.

[D] & **[E]** Work on the factors that contribute to the person's subjective experience of the world; this is the same as that described for delusions.

Medication is the principal treatment for the biological dysfunctions that enable voices to be heard. From the CBT repertoire, some practical coping strategies, for example the use of a personal stereo or an earplug, may also be effective in stopping or reducing the voices. Other CBT strategies that reduce the distress associated with the voices may have the secondary benefit of reducing their occurrence.

[F] Work on the thoughts/emotions/behaviour maintenance cycles. In addition to the strategies described for delusions, this includes work on command hallucinations and changing the behavioural responses to the voice. Reducing arousal, for example by relaxation, may help to stop the thoughts being converted into voices.

3 Talking to people about their delusions and hallucinations

In order to engage with people in therapy and build up trust and rapport it is essential to know how to talk to them about their psychotic experiences in a way that they find helpful and supportive. Even if you are not involved in formal therapy, your casual, informal interactions and conversations can have a significant impact on someone's overall well-being, so this skill is a very important one to develop.

Listening

An essential prerequisite for talking in a helpful way is listening to what is being said to you. Listening to someone and trying to understand them (sometimes called 'deep listening') is important for the following reasons:

- It provides human contact for the speaker and the opportunity to 'share their load'. It also may be comforting for them to know that someone else is aware of what is happening.
- By showing non-judgemental acceptance, the listener can validate the person's experiences and suffering.
- Taking time to listen to someone affirms the importance of what is happening to them and their worth and value.
- Seeking to understand the other person's point of view affirms their reasonableness.
- In a mental health setting, deep listening may indicate that the people and environment around them are safe and caring, and it may provide the opportunity for the listener to give reassurance, if appropriate (see p. 276–277).
- By listening, misunderstandings that have arisen may be detected and clarified.

Of course, listening may also provide you with important information about the person and their illness, but that should not be seen as the most important reason for listening deeply.

Listening empathically is one of the most powerful therapeutic activities that you can engage in. Listening can be beneficial even when the person is so thought-disordered that you cannot understand what they are trying to communicate and therefore you do not know what their problems are or what might be a helpful response. This was brought home to me on a couple of occasions when I met with people whose thought disorder was so severe that I was unable to get a sense of even the gist of what they were trying to communicate to me; nor could I gauge whether they could understand me, or whether my lack of understanding was frustrating for them. In these circumstances I was unable to do more than listen and respond with non-verbal signs of interest, concern and empathy for any emotions expressed. At the time I thought that the sessions had probably had no more benefit for the person than providing them with a welcome cup of coffee and time away from the ward milieu, but later, when they were better, they spontaneously reported how much the sessions had helped them, though they were not able to expand or explain beyond 'They helped me to get better'. Since then I have had a couple of similar experiences with people with pressure of speech. One woman talked continuously through three consecutive sessions so that I was unable to interject anything at all[1] but in the fourth session she said how much the earlier ones had helped, by enabling her to sort out her feelings about things that had happened in her life.

These were particularly valuable experiences for me as I had previously assumed (erroneously) that if I could not communicate verbally with someone in a way that seemed meaningful to me, then there was no chance that they might gain anything by my taking time to listen and talk with them. When I observed other people making the same assumption, I realized how isolated thought-disordered people can become from human contact. Now I take the pragmatic position that if someone who is very thought-disordered wants to spend time talking to me, then they must be getting *something* out of the interaction, even if I do not know what that something is and cannot describe it in terms of CBT.

DISCUSSING DELUSIONS AND HALLUCINATIONS

Basic skills

The core skills used when talking to people about their delusional beliefs and psychotic experiences are the same ones that form the basis of the non-directive therapies, namely empathy, warmth and unconditional regard. These are expressed verbally, through what you say and how you say it, and non-verbally, by nods and smiles and other appropriate gestures.

Empathy means being able to appreciate the other person's situation and feelings from their perspective. However, when listening to people talking about their psychotic experiences, it is important to be aware that it will not always be possible for other people to understand these experiences or what it is like for the person concerned. Have you ever tried to imagine what an extra 'sense' might be like, other than in terms of seeing, hearing, touch, etc.? For most of us it is quite impossible to imagine what this would be like because we can think only in terms of the senses that we have experienced. Similarly, since some of the feelings and experiences produced by the psychotic brain are likely to be outside the realm of our non-psychotic experiences, including our dream experiences, they will also be beyond our powers of imagination and understanding.

At the best of times our human vocabulary is relatively imprecise when it comes to describing internal subjective experiences, so the problem of under-

[1] It is no mean feat to stop a trained CBT therapist from saying anything during a CBT session!

standing may be compounded because words to adequately express the experiences just do not exist. It may also be impossible to understand what the person is feeling if their explanation is in such idiosyncratic or thought-disordered language that it makes no obvious sense (e.g. 'It's the transmigration of the intergalactic figures, sitting still'). Despite these problems in communicating feelings and experiences, even if you cannot understand or imagine what the person is describing, you can ask questions to ascertain whether the experience is pleasant or unpleasant, frightening or comforting, important or insignificant, etc. so that you can have an empathic appreciation at least at this very basic level.

Perhaps the most important thing to remember for empathy is that it makes no difference to how the person feels whether or not their beliefs or fears are actually true in the 'real' world; this is so for all of us, of course, not just for people with psychosis. For example, if a policewoman were to knock at your door now to inform you that your partner, child or parent had been killed in a car crash, you would probably be very upset. The fact that you will be told in an hour's time that there had been a terrible mistake, that your loved one is actually quite safe and well, would not in any way affect how you feel *now*, since you have no way of knowing now that this is not true. Similarly, for the person with schizophrenia, the fact that their voice will not succeed in carrying out its threat to kill them next year, or the fact that their internal organs will not rot away, will do nothing to relieve their feelings and fears *now*. What tends to happen when we are talking about a delusional belief is that we take into account our own evaluations of the person's situation and this affects the empathy that we feel ('It must be awful for her, of course, but she's not *really* in danger of dying, etc.) But as far as empathizing with the person's feelings is concerned, the same empathy is appropriate whether the belief is true in fact or not, since the person's experiencing of the situation and the intensity of their feelings will be the same whether it is true in fact or not.

It may be particularly difficult to sustain empathy with delusions that are obviously incorrect when they recur frequently. This was brought home to me many years ago when I attended my first case conference on a continuing care ward and heard a patient describe his intense fear that his voice would carry out its threat to cut off his head in the next day or so. I was deeply moved by his distress and was surprised therefore when the rest of the team calmly discussed his progress and opted to wait for another week before reviewing his medication. Even though we are aware of this 'fading empathy' effect, this does not make us immune to it. For example, an inpatient in our hospital would wake up every morning believing she was going to die later that day and seek me out, in some panic, to tell me of her fears. After a 20-minute session of CBT she would leave, feeling greatly reassured. But the next morning her fears were back almost to their original level. Despite being aware of the fading empathy effect, it was difficult for me to be as patient with her interruptions or as sympathetic to her need for impromptu CBT sessions at the end of a fortnight of daily interruptions as it had been at the beginning. It is almost as if we expect the person to realize 'somehow' that because these things keep happening they cannot *really* be true, and therefore that they should not be *so* upsetting; but of course the very essence of these delusional beliefs is that they do retain their immediacy and conviction even over long periods. The lesson I have learnt over the years with recurring delusional beliefs is that it is particularly important to remind myself to imagine the situation afresh from time to time, to feel again what it would be like if these things were true and about to happen, and to remember how sympathetic I felt when the person first described what seemed to be happening to them.

It may also be difficult to feel spontaneous empathy for a belief that appears impossible or even ridiculous. One way of trying to engender appropriate empathy in these circumstances is to imagine that the impossible has actually happened or, if this is not possible, try imagining a similar but possible situation. For example, a woman believed that a shark might get into her hospital ward and attack her. This is clearly beyond the realm of possibility, but if I imagine that I am swimming in the sea with a hungry shark circling around me, then I get a much better sense of the fear that this woman's belief engendered.

There may be a temptation to try to joke the person out of a 'ridiculous' belief, a temptation that should always be resisted; not only would the attempt be unsuccessful but it would also be grossly insensitive and unkind. Humour does have a part to play in therapy and, indeed, it can be an important part, but this must be led by the person themself. Even when someone has developed enough understanding to be able to laugh about one of their previously held delusional ideas, you should always acknowledge and re-express your empathy with the feelings that this generated at the time and for their reasonableness, given the situation at that time, in believing it was true. For example, 'I suppose, looking back on it now, it does seem a funny idea, the shark flapping its tail in its attempts to move across the open field and then trying to climb up the flight of stairs to your ward, because you're absolutely right when you say that no shark could live or move out of water ..., but, nevertheless, it must have been a terrifying thought when it seemed as if it could actually happen'.

Similarly, it can be particularly important to re-express empathy with the person's feelings immediately after they have made the intellectual step of rejecting their delusional belief. Your empathy will signal your recognition that their current understanding in no way diminishes the distress they felt when they believed their delusion to be true, and that they were not foolish for believing or feeling the way they did at that time. You can also use this opportunity to summarize and rephrase what they have discovered. For example, 'From the work we've done it does look as if you were wrong when you thought your sister had tried to poison you. I am sure you are right when you say that she wouldn't visit you and buy you presents if she hated you enough to want to poison you. But it must have been really frightening when you thought that she wanted to do this, because you had no reason to think at the time that the coffee might have tasted funny because it was a different brand'.

A word of caution. Empathizing with feelings whilst disputing the explanation or cause of those feelings may not feel very empathic to the person concerned. It may even provoke in them a feeling of irritation or anger, or a sense of being patronized or wilfully misunderstood. Imagine that you have just been told by your doctor that you have cancer and have only four weeks to live. You tell a close friend. She is not upset by the news but remains calm, smiles reassuringly and says, 'You don't really have cancer you know, you'll be fine. But I believe that *you* believe you have cancer, so I really *do* understand how very upset you must feel'. How empathic does that feel? This sort of situation is one which comes up frequently in both formal and informal discussions about delusions and hallucinations and requires great sensitivity in response. It may be a helpful exercise to consider scenarios such as that given above, where the other person does not believe that the cause of your distress is true, and to think about what responses from the other person and what phraseology *you* would find empathic and supportive in these circumstances.

Feelings of *warmth* towards the person follow naturally from an awareness of how it might feel from their perspective and from an understanding of the factors that have led them to be in the position that they are in, especially the recognition that they are not 'to blame' for this. (Even someone's 'personality' is the result of the interaction between innate biological predispositions and environmental influences, so in this sense they cannot be blamed for their personality or ways of reacting and behaving.)

Unconditional regard means positive regard for the person, as a unique and intrinsically worthwhile human being, regardless of what they may have done, thought, felt, etc. In the context of psychosis, unconditional regard follows easily from the understanding that delusional beliefs and associated behaviour are entirely reasonable, given the person's psychotic and non-psychotic experiences within the context of their previous life history and belief system. This means that even if a belief or behaviour does not seem reasonable to me, I know that they *are* reasonable and therefore that they appear unreasonable to me only because I am missing an essential piece of the jigsaw.

Unconditional regard means being non-judgemental and accepting and respecting the person as they are. This will often involve affirming the person's experiences and suffering, and affirming the reasonableness of their conclusions and/or actions given the totality of their circumstances and understanding at that time.

Whilst accepting the person as they are, in some circumstances it is appropriate and functional not to accept or sanction their behaviour, either for their own or for other people's sakes.

Difficulties in feeling empathy, warmth and unconditional regard

If you do not have these feelings towards the person you are working with, do not feel guilty about it. There will be a good reason and it is likely to be very useful if you can identify it. For example, one man I worked with in therapy often made me feel irritated during our sessions, and so, having overcome the guilt feelings resulting from my dysfunctional belief that perfect therapists should always feel sympathetic towards their patients/clients, I set myself to observe closely what was going on. I discovered that my irritation was triggered by the man's persistent habit of asking me questions and then almost immediately interrupting my attempts to reply. This was a valuable observation for the young man's therapy because it transpired that this was the behaviour that was causing him to irritate friends and family as well, and it was very easy for us to alter it once we were aware of it.[2]

If I find myself being judgemental or unsympathetic, I find it helpful to remind myself that if I were in the same circumstances as the person concerned, with the same genetic make-up and life history, then I would have developed *exactly* the same delusional beliefs and behaved in *exactly* the same way as they have done. Furthermore, I would have developed *exactly* the same personality characteristics, including those that affect their attitude to me and to treatment.

As a general rule, if we do not have feelings of empathy, warmth and unconditional regard towards the person, then it is likely that either (a) we do not have, or are failing to appreciate, some important factor(s) about the person, their life history and/or present circumstances (in other words, our case formulation is incomplete), or (b) the issues raised have particular significance for our own life story and have hit a vulnerable spot. These issues should be brought up and discussed in clinical supervision (see Chapter 17).

Be aware of your own beliefs and prejudices

As we saw in Chapter 1, we cannot avoid bringing our own experiences, beliefs and expectations to every situation we are in, and this also applies to the therapy situation. To give just a couple of examples, one therapist told me that he could not see how it was possible to make the diagnosis of schizophrenia acceptable to his patients (see Chapter 6) when it was such a terrible and socially unacceptable illness to have, whilst another therapist felt unable to work with someone who believed he was inhabited by the devil because she believed she could be putting her own soul at risk by doing so.

As therapists, it is important to be aware of the possible effects of our beliefs and prejudices on our work, but we may be unaware of our beliefs or may not realize that they are 'beliefs', which could be wrong, rather than 'facts'. This latter is particularly likely to occur when we share our beliefs and opinions with the other people around us, for example other members in the care team. Even when we are aware of our beliefs and prejudices they will still have an impact on our work, possibly in ways that we do not recognize. By their very nature, it may be impossible for us to take a detached and objective view of our own beliefs, assumptions and values, so this is another important reason for engaging in clinical supervision.

Believe the person until proved otherwise, or at least suspend your disbelief

If you were to tell me that I am not a trained clinical psychologist, I would probably conclude that you are either ignorant, stupid or deliberately trying to

[2]Of course, it was also useful for me to consider the implications of my own reactions to this situation – but that is another piece of therapy.

wind me up. If a number of people repeated the same thing and threatened to take me into hospital for stating what I know to be the truth, then I might quite reasonably conclude that this was some bizarre experiment or that there was some nasty conspiracy going on. It is not surprising if people with delusions react similarly when their beliefs, which they know to be true with as much certainty as I know I am a clinical psychologist, are refuted. Openly denying the truth of the person's beliefs, describing them as delusions and attributing them to an illness, is probably the most common reason for poor rapport with people with psychosis. At best, frank disbelief may indicate to the person that you have failed to understand how things really are for them and at worst it may imply callous disregard, or even some wilful and malevolent reason for your denial. Therefore, if you are able to do so, it is better to believe that what you are told could be true, until you can prove otherwise. This does not mean that you have to believe that what you are told is definitely correct or even probably correct, only that you reserve the possibility that it *could* be correct, even though that possibility seems, to you, to be very small, i.e. you do not come to a definite decision at this stage but instead suspend your disbelief.

I believe that adopting the approach of suspending disbelief is in the true spirit of CBT because by so doing we are not jumping to conclusions or assuming that we know better than the person concerned what is going on. It is a genuine stance, not a phoney one. It is appropriate for a wide range of beliefs because in practice there are very few things that we can be absolutely certain about. As we saw in Chapter 1 (see p. 6), many of our 'certainties' are actually firmly held beliefs that we *assume* to be definitely true despite the fact that this level of conviction cannot be justified logically. For example, I may jump to the conclusion that someone's belief that they are inhabited by a ghost must be a delusion because ghosts do not exist – but can I really be certain about that? Or that someone is not being tracked by a foreign secret service? Or that God does not send messages via the shape of the clouds? And even if everyone else shares my belief or interpretation, this does not guarantee it is correct: 500 years ago everyone 'knew' for certain that the earth was flat.

Whilst you are keeping open the possibility that the other person's interpretation of events just might be correct, you should of course be speculating about other possible explanations for their experiences and other possible interpretations of situations and events, because these speculations will guide your questioning. For example, are the neighbours next door really shouting abuse at him; or has he misinterpreted a family row or their noisy conversations; or is he hearing voices that have nothing to do with the neighbours? You can then ask the relevant questions to help clarify which, if any, of your speculated alternatives might be correct. In the above example, you might ask, 'What time of day/night did this happen?', 'Where were you when this happened?', 'Could you see them when they are doing this?', etc. In my clinical experience I have found it very rare for people to imagine events that have no basis in fact at all, although their perception and interpretation of the events can be grossly distorted. Therefore, I usually find it helpful to approach even situations that clearly cannot have happened as described with a view to trying to work out what 'really' happened. In the example just mentioned, if the man reported that he could see the neighbours in the garden at the time he heard them shout abuse, then I would be confident that they had been there, but I would reserve my judgement about his report that they looked threatening, or that they were being abusive to him, until there was more evidence one way or the other.

Caution: There is a theoretical risk that genuinely holding open the possibility of the other person's belief being true could cause you to be influenced by that belief to such an extent that you are no longer able to appraise it rationally. This effect is most likely to occur if the delusional belief (a) is largely compatible with your own beliefs, and (b) evokes a strong emotional response in you (e.g. fear) so that your emotional reasoning works against your logical reasoning. For example, if you are dealing with a belief about devil possession and your religious education taught you that the Devil can interact directly with people, then by suspending your disbelief you may start to fear that the Devil really is involved, with all the implications that would have. In practice I have seen this effect working in only a couple of cases, and in neither case was it the result of deliberately suspending disbelief, but nevertheless it is better to know what to do if you should start to lose your objectivity in this way. In order to protect and distance yourself from the dysfunctional belief you should, in your own mind at least, deliberately reverse the open-minded approach of suspending your disbelief, and reframe and label the belief as 'definitely delusional' and 'a symptom of mental illness/psychosis', or even 'obviously mad'. Using these terms will also help to disempower the belief. You will be able to get reinforcement for this unequivocal position by reading the medical notes and by discussing the 'case' and 'diagnosis' with your colleagues in the mental health team.

Do not jump to the conclusion that the person's experience is a symptom of their illness, even if it seems to be compatible with it

Over the past years I have come across a number of incidents that were, perhaps understandably, assumed by family or care staff to be delusional or hallucinatory but that later turned out to be entirely accurate. These cases include the man who reported seeing a tiger in the garden next door (his neighbour had kept cubs illegally and as they got bigger he needed to let them run in the garden at night); the woman who reported that her husband was poisoning her (he was putting weed killer in her tea to help calm her down); and the man who could hear clearly what was going on in the office next door (the heating vents conducted and amplified the sounds).

Another problem that can arise is that once someone has received the diagnosis of schizophrenia or psychosis, then a wide range of their behaviours and beliefs may be put down to their 'illness'. For example, if you lose your temper after being badgered non-stop for cigarettes, then this may be interpreted as a significant worsening of your schizophrenia; or if you believe in ESP and the power of crystals, then this may now be interpreted as evidence of a delusional system.

Do not assume that what is written in the notes is correct

Notes are often written in haste, and psychiatric interviews may be brief, so if the person disagrees with what is written in their notes, or remembers incidents differently, do not assume it is the notes that are correct – check them out. For example, a man who was sectioned on the grounds of being very thought-disordered claimed he had only been drunk. Fortunately, the psychiatrist had recorded exactly what he had said, as evidence of the thought disorder. It certainly appeared thought-disordered to me, too, but when he was shown what he had said, the man recognized it as verses from an obscure modern poet that he must have quoted when being interviewed. On another occasion, a man's notes clearly indicated that he had been found to be carrying a knife on two separate occasions, although the man himself denied this, saying he had done this on one occasion only, because it made him feel safe, but after he realized how other people viewed it he had never done so again. Because of his diagnosis, his version of events was not accepted. This was not easy to check out, but what appeared to have happened was that someone new to the case had collated two letters, reporting the same incident rather differently, and assumed that they referred to two separate occasions. Thereafter, subsequent letters and notes referred to the two different occasions, until there were many references to them in the notes, which had significant consequences for his discharge back into the community.

Allow for the possibility that the person may be speaking figuratively

Our everyday vocabulary may be very inadequate to describe psychotic experiences, so we should not be surprised if people sometimes resort to using words in a poetic or figurative way. It is a feature of psychosis that figurative descriptions can become crystallized, so that they are believed to be true in a concrete way (e.g. 'My stomach feels as if it is on fire' becomes 'My stomach *is* on fire'), but do not assume that people are speaking literally and that the belief is a delusional one. For example, a man was referred for therapy because he repeatedly stated that his head and arms were empty. He confirmed this during the CBT assessment and a belief modification treatment plan was drawn up. In order to establish the basic facts prior to using them in a line of logical reasoning, the man was asked, 'What would someone see if your arm was cut across, would it be just a shell of skin?'. He looked both surprised and irritated before replying, 'No, of course not; there would be bone and blood like anyone else'. He had been emphasizing this extreme description because it most closely matched how his arms and head felt and he wanted people to understand how awful that was, but because he had a diagnosis of schizophrenia it had been assumed that this was another delusional belief.[3]

Situations where suspension of disbelief is problematic

Needless to say, if you decide to adopt the approach of suspending your disbelief, then you should genuinely do so, which means maintaining this position whoever

[3]This 'delusion' was re-evaluated as a symptom of depression, and he subsequently responded well to a course of antidepressant medication.

you are talking with, including your colleagues in the care team. This will prevent you being hypocritical and also, importantly, will enable you to continue to hold your position of suspended disbelief if you are called to a meeting where both the person and other care-team personnel are present. If you feel it is necessary to discuss details of your therapy with other staff in these early stages, then explaining to your incredulous colleagues why you cannot be absolutely sure that the belief is delusional may be a helpful way of reminding them how easy it is to jump to conclusions about people's experiences and beliefs, especially once they have been labelled 'psychotic'. However, whilst I am still at the stage of suspending disbelief, I must admit that I usually try to avoid this issue by reporting, quite truthfully, that I am 'still in the assessment phase' or 'still trying to complete the case formulation' and so have not come to any definite conclusions.

Suspending disbelief is a very useful approach for CBT with psychosis, especially in the early stages when you do not have a lot of 'hard' evidence on which to judge the person's beliefs and explanations, and when not disagreeing is important for building rapport. There are a number of circumstances in which it will not be possible to adopt this approach (see 1–3, below), or not advisable to adopt it (see 4–7, below), but in many cases you will be able to choose whether or not to adopt it, your decision being based on whether it is functional for the other person for you to suspend your disbelief at this time. It is important to note that choosing whether or not to suspend your disbelief is *not* incompatible with genuinely suspending your disbelief if that is what you choose to do. As we saw in Chapter 1, our brains attribute certainty to a belief when the possibility of that belief being untrue is so small that it would be dysfunctional in our everyday lives to keep open the possibility of error. Therefore, in many cases when we make a choice about suspending our disbelief, what we are doing is choosing whether to go along with that 'common-sense' attribution of certainty, or whether to override this with the more logically accurate position that allows for the possibility that the other person's beliefs and/or interpretations *could* be the correct ones.

1. When your professional role (e.g. as prescribing doctor) requires you to make a decision that the person is ill and to act on that decision, then suspension of disbelief is impossible and you should be honest and upfront about this. You should explain why you have come to the conclusions you have, given the information that *you* have (which will not include the subjective experiences of the person themself), and that you have the duty or responsibility to make decisions and act on the basis of the information as you have it. It may be helpful to acknowledge that you cannot be absolutely sure that your decision is the correct one, but that nevertheless you have to act on what seems to you to be the most likely situation, and that your actions, whether or not they turn out to be the optimal ones, have been motivated by concern for their distress and/or the unpleasant situation they were in.

2. You will not be able to suspend your disbelief when you are convinced the belief cannot be true (a) because it conflicts with the laws of nature and science

as you understand them (e.g. I could not believe that someone had walked around on Mars without a space suit, as they reported, because no human could survive in such extreme cold and with no oxygen), or (b) because it conflicts with your own firmly held beliefs (e.g. I could not believe that someone was condemned to eternal damnation because it is my personal belief that hell does not exist). In these circumstances it may still be appropriate to talk about the delusional belief from within the other person's belief system (see below), without challenging the belief, but if asked directly, then you should be honest and explain why you have come to a different conclusion from theirs, noting that it is natural and not uncommon for people to see things differently, and that you are not claiming your view is necessarily the 'correct' one or based on superior knowledge or understanding (see 'Agree to differ', p. 54).

3. If the work you have done together to test a delusion indicates that the delusion is not true, then it is usually appropriate at this stage for you to 'come off the fence' and use the evidence obtained so far to argue against the delusional belief, stating why you are persuaded that the belief is not true. Coming off the fence does not contradict the earlier held position of suspending disbelief because it is appropriate to come to a more definite conclusion once the possibility of the belief being true has been reduced to a very low level by the CBT work you have done together. Nevertheless, in the early stages of coming off the fence it may be appropriate not to be too dogmatic about your conclusions, couching them in terms of 'possibly' and 'probably', and 'That's just how it seems to me', rather than in terms of 'definitely'.

4. Although it is often possible to act on the assumption that the person's belief could be true (e.g. checking the newspaper item that the person thought had mentioned them by name), in some cases this is not appropriate (e.g. the man who wanted me to phone the police to report that he had been tortured in a bath of boiling water). Where it is not appropriate, you should explain why you are not able to act according to what you have been told (e.g. in the case just mentioned, I explained that without any burn marks or other evidence to substantiate the complaint the police would not believe me). Another explanation that may be relevant is that because of the magnitude of what you are being asked to do (e.g. evacuate the hospital in response to the fear that terrorists had planted a bomb) you would have to be absolutely certain before you acted, but since you cannot be absolutely certain at this stage, from the hard evidence that you have, you cannot act as requested.

5. If the person is reassured rather than irritated when other people disagree with their belief, then it is appropriate not to suspend your disbelief but rather to explain why you think their belief is untrue (e.g. the woman who was comforted by reassurance that there were no gunmen in the hospital grounds).(See 'Reassurance', p. 276–277.)

6. When you are into the therapy and have built up a trusting relationship, then you may, as part of the planned treatment, decide not to suspend your disbelief any longer. One reason for this might be to demonstrate to the person that someone else, who knows all about the situation, does not come to the same

conclusions they do, i.e. suggesting that it is at least possible that there could be other interpretations and explanations than the ones they have. Another reason might be to enable you to put forward other arguments and evidence that contradict their belief.

7. It is unlikely to be helpful to suspend your disbelief about a delusion when talking to family members, as they may become very confused if, their family member having been diagnosed with a mental illness, you now say that their delusions could possibly be true. If you can avoid interacting with family members (perhaps this task could be done by a colleague), then you can continue to suspend disbelief, but if you have to come off the fence in order to talk to family members, then you will have to come off the fence with the person as well, as you could no longer be genuine in your suspension of disbelief. You can, of course, continue to talk to the person from within their belief system (see below) but you should explain your doubts if you are asked directly whether you believe the delusion to be true.

8. Therapists who do not have a dual role in the care team are in an easier position with respect to adopting the stance of suspending disbelief. However, there may be concerns that if they suspend disbelief, this could conflict with other team members and the role of 'the team'. If the care team believes that it should always 'speak with one voice', it may be viewed by some members that if you suspend your disbelief when the collective decision is that this is a delusion and part of an illness, then this will undermine other members of the team. Personally, I think it is the sign of a strong, assured team if different members can take different positions. Furthermore, from the patient/client's point of view I think it is more likely to be reassuring than otherwise to discover that, as in the wider world, different people can genuinely hold different opinions, and also that these can be respected and discussed calmly and rationally. However, teams may differ in how they see this issue. Needless to say, if you are suspending your disbelief, this does not mean telling the person that you believe they are correct and your colleagues are wrong: it is just acknowledging that you do not have enough information at this stage to come to a definite conclusion one way or the other, and therefore that you are keeping an open mind.

Whilst suspending your disbelief, you should always support the good intent of your colleagues. Suspending your disbelief will actually put you in a stronger position to do this. By standing apart from their decisions and actions your opinions will be perceived as being less biased when you explain how other team members view the situation and why, from their perspective, it seemed to be in the person's best interest for them to act as they did. It may be helpful to point out that your colleagues often have to act 'on the balance of probability' and cannot wait until they have absolute certainty about the matter, as you can.

Working from within the other person's belief system

If you are unable to suspend you disbelief, it is recommended that you adopt the approach of working from within the other person's belief system, especially in the early stages of therapy. This means viewing and feeling the other person's world and experiences from *their* perspective and talking about these things using *their* concepts and vocabulary, rather than your own. The approach is similar in practice to that of suspending disbelief, but it is possible to work from within the other person's belief system even when you are sure their beliefs are delusional and the voices they hear are hallucinations.

Working from within the other person's belief system is primarily, I believe, a matter of social courtesy and respect. In everyday life we do not feel it necessary or appropriate to impose our interpretations and opinions on friends and colleagues who feel strongly about something, and we certainly do not insist that ours is the 'correct' view. For example, if I meet someone at a party who tells me of some strange course of exercises she is attending in order to help her get pregnant, I do not feel obliged to tell her I think it will not work and that she is wasting her money, and nor do I tell a colleague who reads palms that I think what he is doing is a load of rubbish. So why should we feel it necessary or appropriate to tell our patients that what they believe so profoundly to be true is a load of rubbish? Because, like it or not, that is exactly what we are telling them when we inform them dogmatically, and from a position of assumed authority, that their beliefs and experiences are delusions and hallucinations.

Working from within the other person's view of the world, trying to understand and experience it as they do, will help you feel and express appropriate empathy and improve rapport and engagement in therapy.

Another advantage of this approach is that it will help you ask natural questions based on your concern and interest to learn more, and these questions will not be experienced by the other person as challenging or sceptical. For example, if you are seeing and judging things from a purely medical model perspective, then asking the question 'When did you first notice the ghost inside your head?' would probably feel false and you would almost certainly communicate this falseness, if not by the words you used, then by the way you said them. But to ask 'When did you first think you had a ghost inside your head?' would be tantamount to saying that this never actually happened, which might not be therapeutically desirable at this stage. On the other hand, if you are using the person's own conceptualization, then the question 'When did you first notice the ghost inside your head?' becomes an entirely natural one, which leads naturally on to a series of relevant questions, for example 'What exactly did you feel?', 'How did you know that these sensations were caused by a ghost?', etc. In this way a lot of important information can be gathered from questioning that is experienced as interest and concern rather than as interrogation.

Some staff may not feel comfortable about working from the other person's perspective rather than their own, even to the extent of feeling it to be hypocritical, but if the therapist and patient/client have different models of the world, why should it be the patient/client who has to adapt and work from the therapist's system rather than vice versa? That would seem unreasonable to me, firstly because we are the ones who, through our training, are supposed to have a broader perspective and understanding of what is going on, and secondly because we do not have to cope with the additional distractions and disturbances of psychosis. Working from someone else's perspective only becomes a fundamental problem if we believe that our perspective is 'the truth'. But it is worth remembering that our perspective is as much the result of brain function as that of the person with psychosis. Have you ever wondered what the world would be like if the large majority of the human race had evolved with 'psychotic' brains and only a few had non-psychotic ones? Who would be considered to have the 'true' perspective then?

Ask neutral questions

Asking neutral questions is not as easy as it sounds. It is difficult not to 'leak' what we really believe when we talk with someone. For example, when talking to people about their delusions and hallucinations it is easy to make the mistake of using the word 'think' instead of 'know' when asking them about something that they have told you as fact. For example, 'Why did you *think* they were following you?' implies that perhaps they were not really doing so, whereas 'How did you *know* they were following you?' implies acceptance that this really took place. 'What happened ...' is also a useful format for eliciting information without questioning its veracity.

It is important to recognize that when we speak, we communicate what we think and mean in other ways as well as by the words we actually use. Tone of voice is important in indicating how we feel about what we are saying, whilst the inflection in our voice and the emphasis that we put on different words in the sentence can significantly affect the meaning conveyed. Try expressing the two questions above, about being followed, in different tones, and see how significantly you can change what you imply in the questions. These aspects of our speech occur spontaneously and automatically and so are very difficult to control consciously. Genuinely suspending your disbelief is the best way to automatically control the language and intonation that you use, but practice in talking to people from within their belief systems will increase your sensitivity to the covert messages you are sending, and make it easier for you to temporarily immerse yourself in their view of the world.

Responding in a way that is not jarring is also not as easy at it sounds. It is normal practice in human society to ask questions because you do not know the answer, and therefore it is also normal practice to accept the answer you are given. For example, if a colleague asked me when the canteen was open and I told him it opened at 12 o'clock, I would not expect him to reply that I was wrong and that actually it opened at 12.30 p.m. Therefore, if you question someone about events or experiences, or their interpretations of these, and then imply that you do not believe their answers, it should not be surprising if they take offence. Here again, if you are able to do so, then suspending your disbelief is probably the best way of ensuring that you do not inadvertently signal dismissal of the other person's view of things or appear to be attempting to impose your own.

Sometimes the delusional belief system may be so complex and/or disorganized that you may be completely unable to understand how or why something affects the person as it does. It is important to get this information but asking a direct question to clarify the matter may run the risk of implying not only that you have not been listening but also that you need to ask the question because their response or feeling is so unusual or unreasonable. One way of overcoming this sort of problem is to ask a question about specifics, because implicit in a specific question is your acceptance of the general point; this is true even if you are unsure what that general point is. For example, a man tells you he was very upset by an event in the supermarket, but to you the event appears to have been a perfectly normal, neutral one. To ask 'Why was that upsetting?' indicates that the reason is not obvious to you and thereby implies that being upset in these circumstances is at least unusual, if not downright unreasonable. The questions 'What was the *most* upsetting aspect?' or 'What was the *worst* moment in this situation?' may obtain the information you need without the unwanted implications. Similarly, if you are in the dark about what the distressing feelings were, then you might ask 'What was your *strongest* feeling at that moment?'. I remember one woman who started to refer in therapy to 'that special incident I told you about'. Clearly I had failed to appreciate that one of the incidents we had discussed was not only very special but also very difficult for her to talk about, so I was reluctant to imply this incident had not appeared that way to me by asking her which one it was. Fortunately, I was able to retrieve the situation by asking 'What, for you, was the most significant moment of that incident? This gave me the information I needed to identify the incident and I was able to explore it further.

Answering the question 'Do you believe that what I say is true?'

Although in my experience I have found it unusual for people talking about their delusions to ask me this question directly, nevertheless you should consider in advance how you would answer such a question should it arise. This will enable you to reply in the most helpful way and without implying, by hesitating, that you are hiding something or being untruthful. You should, of course, answer the question honestly, but how much of your own beliefs and opinions you share in your response is a matter of clinical judgement and is likely to change as therapy progresses, so you should keep this question in mind. For example, when first asked this question by the woman who was inhabited by a ghost, I told her that I had no way of knowing for certain; I was only able to go on her explanation of what was going on but that I had no reason to disbelieve what she told me (the approach of *genuine ignorance*). When this question was repeated several sessions later, when rapport was stronger, I was able to share some of my doubts, noting that the doctors believed her symptoms to be due to an illness and so, not having had her experiences myself, I was not sure which explanation was correct. Yet further on in therapy, when we had tested out the belief, it was appropriate for me to explain why I believed the 'ghost' explanation was not the correct one.

Indirectly suggesting alternatives

It is not just in formal therapy that you may wish to suggest that there could be an alternative explanation or interpretation for a situation, or another way of viewing things. This is likely to be an important aim of informal interactions with people with delusions and hallucinations as well. Presenting alternatives for the other person to consider without implying that yours are 'correct' and theirs are 'wrong' is a skill that requires sensitivity and practice.

Floating ideas

Floating ideas is a way of suggesting that other alternatives could exist whilst making it clear that you are not particularly supporting any one of these alternatives or even doubting the other person's conclusions. Some examples of the sort of phrases that we have found useful in clinical practice are given below. Notice how most include a rider that expressly casts doubt about the alternative you are suggesting, in order to make it easier for the other person to reject it and to enable you to remain remote and untainted by it.

- 'I was wondering if . . .? Is that a possibility at all or have I got it quite wrong?'
- 'Do you think there is any chance that . . . or is that not a possibility?'
- 'It seemed from what you were saying that it could be that . . ., but have I got that right?'
- 'Someone else I knew had an experience that sounded a bit like yours and he found in his case that it was due to . . . Do you think something like that could be going on with you or is your experience of . . . quite different?'
- 'I suppose to some people it could look as if . . . Of course, they are not actually in your position, but if you were them, do you think you might look at it in that way too? Or have any doubts about . . .?'
- 'I can imagine that some people in that situation, especially if they did not realize . . . might have thought . . . What do you think?'.

If you are floating ideas, then you should accept the response given, as you would if you were just having a casual conversation and idly wondering about something the other person had said. If your floated idea is rejected with some vehemence, then it is likely to be appropriate for you to admit that you have got it wrong, or that on further thought you agree that it was a bit of a silly suggestion to make in the circumstances.

It is important to remember that the aim of floating ideas is not to persuade the other person that these alternatives are the 'true' ones. In the first instance the aim is to plant the idea as a 'seed', so that even if it is totally rejected at this stage, the idea will be available as an option should they develop any doubts about their belief in the future. If the delusional belief is less strongly held, then the ideas floated may be accepted as 'possibilities'; indeed, this is how the technique is used in CBT when suggesting alternative interpretations of 'evidence' (see Chapter 8).

Floating ideas is a gentle and safe approach because it is easy to back off if the ideas are not acceptable or are resisted.

What does 'X' say about . . .?

In our interactions with one another we do not normally consider it worthwhile to put forward an idea for discussion unless we believe it to be true, or to have at least some merit. For example, if someone asked me for an explanation for a colleague's outburst of temper, I might speculate that perhaps he had been very stressed recently, or had misinterpreted what was going on, but I would not suggest that perhaps he had been eating more red meat recently. Similarly, when talking to people about their delusions and hallucinations, it may be difficult to introduce alternative explanations or viewpoints for discussion without implying, by the very fact of introducing them, that you consider them valid and viable. This will be a particularly important consideration when the person is very sensitive about being doubted, and as such it is likely to be more of a problem early on in your therapeutic relationship. In these circumstances it may be possible to generate alternatives for discussion by asking what their doctor, nurse, friends, family, etc. think is going on and whether they see things differently. This avoids the risk of appearing to support these particular alternatives, and leads naturally to follow-up questions about how they feel when these things are said.

Whilst this strategy is well worth trying, it is not always productive. In some cases, the person's belief is so strongly held that it distorts their perception of what other people say and believe; for example, 'My mother thinks I am in hospital because I need a rest' or 'My doctor wants me in hospital in order to ensure that the hospital stays full so that he gets a fat salary'.

It says in your notes that ...

This is a similar way of avoiding putting forward an alternative explanation yourself, enabling you to discuss it from a position of neutrality. You should, of course, be circumspect about what information you give from the notes and only disclose what the team agrees the person can be told, but in practice this is rarely an issue since the most likely 'disclosures' you will want to make are those around alternative explanations in terms of illness, alternatives that will already have been put to the person by other team members. One potential advantage of using the 'notes' strategy as the basis for generating alternatives, as opposed to 'What does 'X' say?', is that the notes are impersonal and so there is no risk of aggravating an interpersonal disagreement.

Do not assume that 'insight' will be beneficial

There is still a tendency for some professionals to assume that the best, if not only, therapeutic approach is to tell people that they are mentally ill and that their experiences are not real. There are a number of reasons why this approach might not be beneficial (see Appendix 3 for a summary), at least in the short term. Unless there is a good reason why you need to adopt this approach, it is recommended that you stay neutral and do not attempt to impose the medical model unless and until you know that it will be therapeutic to do so. These issues are covered in detail in the sections on goal setting and insight promotion in Chapters 5 and 6.

Do not directly challenge a delusional interpretation of events or a delusional belief

Although we sometimes talk about 'challenging' delusions, this is nearly always done very gently, chipping or nibbling away at the belief rather than attacking it with a head-on assault. Directly challenging the delusion in a confrontational way is rarely correct unless it is done strategically as part of the planned treatment programme. At best it risks damaging rapport and at worst it may actually strengthen conviction in the delusional belief. This paradoxical effect, whereby strong opposition may strengthen rather than weaken a belief, is not peculiar to delusional beliefs but applies to any firmly held belief. We must all have had the experience of having one of our treasured political, social or moral beliefs questioned by someone with opposing views. Did you find yourself suddenly doubting your beliefs or did you just become more dogmatic and heated as you mustered more arguments in order to convince the other person that they were wrong and you were right?

There is also a very real risk of evidence being confabulated if the challenge to the belief is sustained. Again, this is not peculiar to delusional beliefs and it is not done consciously or intentionally; it is a direct result of the way strongly held beliefs affect our thinking. The problem is exacerbated because the fabricated evidence is not recognized as such and so gets stored back in memory as 'a fact'. For example, if you persist in challenging my belief that W. G. Grace was the greatest cricketer who ever lived, then I may support my claim by telling you that he scored more centuries in a season than anyone else. I cannot recall exactly where I learnt that fact but I *know* that it is true. I am unaware that I have deduced this fact from the belief itself (he was the greatest cricketer so he *must* have achieved this record), and that I have never had it confirmed by an independent source (I *know* he achieved this record so I *must* have read about it somewhere). But now, if the topic comes up for discussion again, I have another 'well-established fact' to support my claim.

Paranoia

Trainee therapists are often concerned that if they appear to question someone's paranoid beliefs, then the person will interpret this as a sign that they are part of the persecutory conspiracy, and they will become incorporated into the delusional system. If this does happen, then clearly your ability to function as a CBT therapist is substantially reduced. Indeed, in such cases your immediate goal would probably be no more ambitious than to re-establish trust, to modify the person's paranoid beliefs about yourself and then perhaps to use this modification as a starting point for a CBT programme. However, in practice you can nearly always avoid being drawn into a paranoid system (a) by ensuring that you have established a good trusting relationship with the person before you express any doubts about their version of events or start to attempt belief modification, and (b) by taking care to proceed very slowly and to be on constant alert to back off if there is any indication of distress, irritation or unwillingness to continue talking about a particular issue. It is important to remember in this context that it is not the questions themselves that are likely to make the person feel threatened so much as the way in which you ask them and how you react to the answers.

When interacting with someone who is paranoid, do not rely on subtle social cues to indicate that you are non-threatening. There is evidence to suggest that some people with schizophrenia may fail to detect the more subtle social cues in interpersonal interactions, and if the person is already feeling threatened, then it may require correspondingly more obvious or powerful indications from you that you are not the source of this threat. You should also be thoughtful about the non-verbal signals you are giving; if the person has not asked for and does not really want the interaction with you, then their position is likely to make them particularly sensitive to signals of authority and of dominance or power. Smiling is a universal and powerful way of signalling friendly intent, so it may be appropriate to convey reassurance by smiling frequently. Or it may be appropriate to state explicitly what normally you would only imply, for example by telling the person in so many words that you like and respect them, that you do not want any harm to come to them and that you would like to help them in their present situation if it is possible. It is perhaps surprising how often people with paranoia can be reassured of your good intent by using these basic social strategies.

Therapists engaged in formal therapy are in the fortunate position of not having to force the person to do something they do not want to do (unlike nursing colleagues, for example, who may have to force the person to take medication against their will). Furthermore, they can spend more time with the person in individual sessions, listening and talking with them. It is for these reasons probably more than any others that the therapist is commonly the member of the team most able to build a trusting relationship with a paranoid person. This position may be greatly enhanced if the therapist is able to take the approach of suspending disbelief about what they are told.

Agree to differ

At any stage of therapy you may suggest that you agree to differ. This may be stated explicitly, or be implicit in the way you work together. Although agreeing to differ can be a very helpful stance, indicating mutual respect and avoiding arguments, great care must be taken that it is not done in a patronizing way, and you should in no way imply (or, ideally, even believe) that because you are the therapist your point of view is necessarily the correct one. As rapport and mutual respect develop it will become easier to express a different point of view or to express your doubts about the other person's interpretations without it damaging the therapeutic relationship.

Avoid collusion

Not so many years ago, mental health staff were taught that the correct way of interacting with patients was to tell them kindly but very firmly that their beliefs were delusions and their voices hallucinations, and then to refuse to talk about these 'symptoms' for fear of 'colluding' and giving them credibility. Fortunately, this has changed considerably over the past few years so that now most staff members feel comfortable discussing people's psychotic experiences with them, but the legacy persists.

'Not colluding' is more usefully understood to mean not providing additional evidence to support the delusional belief. When people do collude with a delusion, it is usually for the sake of short-term convenience, but this is rarely correct because in the long term the extra evidence that it provides is likely to strengthen the delusional belief. For example, a woman who believed she had had an immaculate conception had been told some years earlier by her doctor to take her medication 'because it will be good for your baby': it is not surprising that she used this later as authoritative evidence to support her belief that her current doctors were just pretending when they said they did not believe in her pregnancy.

However, not colluding does not mean that you should not talk about the issues that are disturbing people and take them seriously. Imagine that you have just been told that you have a fatal illness that will kill you within weeks; how would you feel if the people you told ignored you or tried to change the subject to tomorrow's lunch menu, or offered you a game of ping-pong? Angry? Rejected? So how must people feel when, for example, they are worried that someone is trying to poison them or are frightened by threats from their voices and they find that the people who claim to care for them will not talk to them about it? Presumably much the same as if these terrible things were really happening and people were indifferent to their suffering. I have always thought it must be particularly galling for people when someone who has not been where they have been, and has not experienced what they have experienced, nevertheless has the temerity to dismiss their version and explanation of events in favour of his or her own!

If I tell you about my career as a clinical psychologist and you ask me questions about it, this does not strengthen my belief that I am a clinical psychologist, just as you saying that you do not believe that I am a psychologist does not weaken my belief. So it is with delusions. Listening to people and respecting their opinions about what is going on will not strengthen their conviction in their delusional beliefs – they already believe them to be true, probably despite many other people having argued, often forcefully, against them and told them they are wrong – but being perceived as an interested and caring person, who has not prejudged the issues, will put you in a better position to engage therapeutically.

Similarly, agreeing to check out the facts where possible (e.g. looking for gunmen to verify the report of gunshots from outside the window) is *not* collusion. Indeed, it may be an important part of therapy because it may provide information about what is being misinterpreted, and lay the groundwork for looking for alternative explanations (see Chapter 8).

Summary

When talking to people about their delusions and hallucinations, try to see and feel the situation from their point of view. If you can do this, everything else will follow naturally – your empathy and your expression of this empathy, your questions and the way you express your questions, and your replies. Whilst part of you is keeping an enquiring scepticism and speculating about alternative explanations of what might be going on, consider that what you are being told might actually be true, at least to some extent, so it should be considered seriously and investigated further before you come to any definite conclusions. Do not worry that you might be colluding with the delusion: concerned interest and talking from within the other person's belief system or suspending your disbelief will not strengthen their conviction in their beliefs, but it will provide a solid platform from which to engage in therapy.

If you do not want to suggest alternative explanations for fear of implying that you doubt what you have been told, you may be able to get the person to generate the alternatives by asking them about other people's opinions and views of what is going on. Floating ideas is a safe and gentle way of introducing new ideas.

4 ENGAGEMENT AND THE COURSE OF THERAPY

ENGAGEMENT

The therapeutic relationship

Unlike other conditions, where people come to the therapist seeking help for an identified and recognized problem, people with delusions and hallucinations may have no insight into their condition, no recognition that they have a problem that could be helped and therefore little reason to engage in a series of therapy sessions. In these circumstances, good rapport with the therapist is essential because the relationship that someone has with you may be the only reason for them to attend your sessions, at least in the earlier stages of therapy.

Good rapport and trust are essential when you start challenging the delusional beliefs. Having the inaccuracies of one's beliefs exposed is generally not a pleasant experience. So when you start the belief modification work, it is important that the person is confident you respect them so that they do not experience your questioning as a personal attack or as being critical of them in any way. Furthermore, if there is mutual trust, then the person is more likely to accept that any difference of views is a genuine one, and be more ready to consider your suggestions of other possible interpretations and explanations.

A strong therapeutic relationship is important because it provides a sense of safety within which someone can explore their frightening experiences and beliefs, knowing that they are supported and respected. Paradoxically, although it may be harder to build up a trusting relationship with someone who is paranoid, the therapeutic relationship may be a particularly important component of the therapy. Furthermore, people with paranoia are particularly likely to interpret challenging questions as a personal threat, so you must have a correspondingly good relationship in order to counter any paranoid ideas about you that may arise when you are doing therapy.

The effects of the illness on the person's life and relationships can be widespread and devastating, with a consequent loss of self-esteem and self-respect. A good therapeutic relationship, and the interest, concern and respect that the therapist demonstrates within that relationship, may be important in helping to reverse these consequences.

Some commonly encountered problems

The person is uncooperative with treatment of any kind

People admitted to hospital against their will, under Mental Health legislation, may have no insight into their illness and therefore see all members of staff as part of the system that is against them, keeping them in hospital and forcing them to take unwanted medication. In these circumstances it may be appropriate for the therapist to distance herself from the other members of the care team in order to build up rapport; for example, 'I didn't have anything to do with your being sectioned', or 'I don't have anything to do with medication', and 'I'm afraid I can't influence your doctor about that one way or the other'. (See Chapter 3 for comments about different members taking on different roles within the team.)

Rapport is built by showing interest and concern. With the most sensitive people you have to be particularly careful not to challenge what they are telling you (see the previous chapter.)

If there are any practical or other issues that you can help with, then you should do so, even if it is not strictly in your job description as a CBT therapist. For example, I have arranged for benefits to be paid to one person and for a church minister to attend the ward to give communion to another. As far as possible, you should do these things yourself rather than delegating them elsewhere, not only because then you can be sure they will be done promptly but also, and perhaps more importantly, because your own efforts will demonstrate your goodwill and genuine wish to help.

The person sees no reason to attend psychological therapy

People's failure to take up the offer of CBT therapy and attend sessions, sometimes described as 'lack of motivation', can be frustrating for the therapist, but it should not surprise us since it follows almost inevitably from the belief that the delusion is true. Would you be prepared to attend psychological therapy because someone said you were mistaken in thinking you were a mental health worker? And if you knew your roof was leaking, would you think it relevant to seek help from a talking therapy, or would you think some practical help from a builder would be more appropriate? Similarly, if someone *knows* their family member is trying to poison them, or that they are going to be damned eternally after they die, then they will *know* that just talking about it will not change anything.

Without the usual motivation for therapy, namely the hope that the sessions will help with what is wrong, you have to provide the person with other motivations. In these circumstances, it is often appropriate to use the distress caused by the person's situation or experiences, rather than the situation or experiences themselves, as the focus for your sessions.

One way of making the sessions more pleasant is to take some time to talk about whatever the other person wants to discuss, including purely social topics. Another very practical way of making the sessions more enjoyable is to offer tea or coffee and biscuits. I know that some people do not agree with giving patients/clients tea and coffee in this way, as a matter of principle. This objection may be appropriate for some other therapeutic models, but I always offer a drink to professional colleagues who visit me for a meeting so I consider it entirely within the CBT spirit of equality and mutual respect to extend that same courtesy to the people I meet with in therapy.

Negative symptoms
If present, the negative symptoms of schizophrenia can significantly impair someone's ability and motivation to engage in CBT, because the effort required to think and talk about the issues is just too much for the person. This is a difficult problem to overcome and requires both patience and persistence on the part of the therapist, and an appreciation of how difficult it is for the person concerned. The aims of therapy are likely to be limited, and keeping the sessions short and as undemanding as possible may help.

Social aversion
Some people with schizophrenia do not find social contact rewarding in the way that most people do, and a few find close or one-to-one contacts positively aversive. In these circumstances you should keep the sessions short and consider seeing the person less frequently.

Eye contact may be perceived as threatening rather than showing interest, so if the person you are with is reluctant to catch your eye you should take the hint and drop yours, only occasionally flicking to see if they want to make eye contact. (See also the comments about arranging the chairs in 'The therapy room', p. 64.)

Forgetfulness
Some people with psychosis are disorganized, or may just forget to attend sessions. For this reason keeping to regular appointment times is advisable. If appropriate, the person may agree to your giving them a reminder, for example by ringing them or a member of staff at their hostel or ward prior to the arranged session. In some cases, it may be simpler and more effective to arrange to go to them rather than vice versa, for example if they rarely leave their hostel or ward (but see 'Therapy in the person's home', p. 65).

Be flexible about appointments

To be successful in engaging people with psychosis in therapy you must be prepared to be flexible about appointments. Be innovative about when and where you see the person, especially when you are at the early stage of building rapport and trust. Do not insist that people come for sessions if they are unwilling; for example, if they say they feel unwell it is better to express concern that they are not so good today, hope that they will soon feel better and then give them another appointment. Try to give priority to fitting the appointments around *their* other commitments rather than your own.

Needless to say, it is not appropriate to adopt the approach taken in some therapies that the therapist's responsibility for meeting with the patient/client ends when they have offered the appointment, and that the patient/client must make a positive commitment to therapy by attending the appointment. When working with people with psychosis, you have to be more active in pursuing appointments because poor motivation and disorganization are an integral part of the disorder, and so your arrangements for therapy sessions must take this into account. One young man never attended any of the outpatient appointments I gave him; this was only partly due to his rather disorganized thinking. However, for over a year he would call in at approximately two-monthly intervals for an urgent appointment whenever he felt he wanted to talk over something. Although this arrangement was far from ideal from the point of view of progressing any planned therapy, since this was the way he was prepared to work, then this was how it was.

THE COURSE OF THERAPY

When to deliver treatment

Medication-resistant psychosis

The most common way in which CBT is used is to treat delusions and hallucinations that remain despite the person being on medication. The optimum time to conduct CBT in these cases is when the psychosis is least active at a biological level. There are three main reasons for this. Firstly, without the psychotic experiences fuelling and refreshing the delusional beliefs and hallucinations, the CBT can be more effective in eliminating the residual symptoms (see Chapter 2, p. 29). Secondly, without the attention deficits associated with acute psychosis, engagement is likely to be better and treatment can proceed at a faster rate. Thirdly, CBT is a time-intensive treatment and trained therapists are a scarce resource, so if medication is given first, then CBT need only be given to those people for whom medication is not a sufficient treatment on its own.

In recurrent psychosis, CBT may be indicated even though the symptoms are well controlled by medication at the time of referral. Providing the person is prepared to discuss their previously held delusions and hallucinations,[1] then it is easy to build up effective lines of CBT for use if the symptoms should recur in the future. This work focuses on the reasons they have *now* for knowing that their beliefs were delusional and that their voices were hallucinations, and on strengthening these reasons. At this stage, the emphasis of the CBT work is on developing relapse prevention strategies.

Although the theoretical ideal may be to wait until an appropriate medication regime has been established before starting CBT, other factors may operate, such as the person being discharged from hospital as soon as the medication begins to take effect, so in practice it is often advisable to take the opportunities to see people for therapy as and when they arise.

If the person has been admitted to hospital, then this can be a good opportunity to engage them in therapy, for a number of reasons. Being in hospital may make the notion of therapy more relevant, and even where illness is not acknowl-

[1]When better, people are often reluctant to talk about when they were ill. This may be because it is unpleasant to remember unpleasant times, but in some cases it is because people are frightened that thinking about the thoughts and experiences they had when they were ill might bring them back. In other cases, people seem to be unable to recall how they thought and felt during that period.

edged people may see the sessions as a way of accelerating their discharge. At a practical level, access to the person for sessions is likely to be easier when they are in hospital, not least because you can go to them rather than vice versa, and your sessions may seem relatively more attractive when compared to hospital routine. Furthermore, in my experience, people are significantly more likely to attend for therapy as an outpatient if they have already met and know me than if my first contact is via an appointment letter.

Seeing people on an outpatient basis can work well, not least because the biological aspect of the psychosis is likely to be under relatively good control if the person is living in the community. However, regular attendance at therapy appointments can be a problem, and when people are living in the community their medication adherence may be more erratic. If you are seeing the person regularly for other reasons, for example as their psychiatrist or community psychiatric nurse, then this puts you in a much better position with respect to regular contacts. However, there is the potential disadvantage of having a dual role, namely that some aspects of the former role may conflict and interfere with the approach and role of CBT therapist.

First episode and early intervention

CBT intervention in the early stages of a psychotic illness can help prevent the consolidation of delusional beliefs, leading to faster and more complete recovery, with fewer secondary impairments, such as decreased social functioning, and a better prognosis. Therefore, it may be beneficial to attempt to start CBT as early as possible with people in their first or second episode, before the medication regime has taken full effect, despite the adverse effects of the uncontrolled biological activity and despite the fact that they may be hard to engage, easily distracted and/or thought-disordered.

One of the main difficulties in this area of work is that people in their first episode of illness may not come to the attention of health workers for months, or even years, after the onset, so the opportunity for early intervention is missed. A key area for the health services at present is the development of programmes to enable earlier detection of people developing psychosis so that both medication and CBT treatments can be started earlier.

CBT as an adjunctive treatment to medication

We saw in Chapter 2 (pp. 22, 27–28) that CBT and medication work on different factors involved in the development and maintenance of delusions and hallucinations, so it is usual for CBT to be given in addition to, and not instead of, neuroleptic medication. When the psychosis is active at a biological level, CBT may be able to help prevent the symptoms escalating by helping to control the cognitive-behavioural factors that exacerbate them. However, CBT cannot prevent the occurrence of the psychotic experiences: only medication can do this. Without medication, the psychotic experiences may be so overwhelming that any attempt to hold them with psychological techniques alone would be fruitless, and even to consider otherwise is to fail to understand their profundity.

Even in milder cases, where CBT is effective in coping with the adverse effects of the active psychosis, it is likely to require considerable effort from the person concerned to apply it. Although it is, of course, for the person themself to decide what treatment to use, unless the medication is not effective, or unless it has unpleasant side effects that outweigh its advantages, we would expect even mildly affected people to choose to control their symptoms with medication as well as with CBT.

Who is suitable for CBT?

Level of conviction

At the present time, we cannot tell with any degree of certainty who will benefit from CBT and who will not. Clinical experience suggests that CBT will be more difficult and/or take longer the greater the person's conviction in their delusions and the greater their involvement in them, and there is evidence that CBT has a better chance of being effective if the person can consider from the outset the possibility that they could be mistaken about their delusional belief(s). However, these general trends are not accurate enough to enable us to predict at the individual level who will and who will not respond favourably to CBT. It is certainly true in my own experience that some actively psychotic people with firmly held delusions and hallucinations have responded well to treatment, whilst other people, with apparently less severe symptoms and more commitment to the therapy, have not.

'Reaction to hypothetical contradiction' is a test in which you ask the person a question along the lines of 'Suppose X were true [X being something that contradicts the delusion], would this make you have second thoughts about your belief?'. For example, 'If someone else ate the food that had been "poisoned" and remained completely well, would that change your mind in any way about the food being poisoned?'. If the person agrees that it would make a difference, then this suggests that they are CBT-minded and therefore more likely to respond well to a CBT programme. It is not clear to what extent this question may be measuring some aspect of conviction and to what extent it is tapping into some aspect of flexibility in thinking, but in any case it cannot accurately predict an individual's response to treatment, and so people should not be refused CBT on the basis of their response to this question alone.

Complexity of the delusional system

Some people have complex delusional belief systems that pervade many aspects of their life. This does not of itself make the person unsuitable for CBT, but from a practical point of view the aims of treatment are likely to be modest and to address part, rather than all, of the delusional system.

Removing a complex and well-established delusional system (even if you could do it) would almost certainly have some significant negative implications for the person, as well as the more obvious positive ones associated with no longer believing the delusion to be true. In some cases it may not be possible to set a goal for belief modification such that the positives would outweigh the negatives (see Chapter 5), and in these circumstances work to modify the delusional belief should not be undertaken.

Auditory hallucinations

Although auditory hallucinations are subjective in that they come from within the person's own brain, they are experienced as real sound, coming from outside the person who hears them. Therefore, even if someone has a firmly held delusional explanation for the origin of their voice, the *phenomenon* of the voice can be readily agreed and discussed. Furthermore, because the voice is perceived to be separate from the person themself, you may be able to form an alliance with them against their voice and challenge it head on. In contrast, delusions are experienced as being an integral part of the person who believes them, so challenges to a delusional belief have to be more subtle and oblique. Because it is usually easier to talk to someone about their voice than about their delusional beliefs, if someone has both delusions and hallucinations, it is often the case that you can start to intervene more quickly with their voice.

Other hallucinations

The CBT techniques described in the later chapters of this manual have been developed for use with auditory hallucinations because these are the most common type of hallucination in our population, and arguably the most distressing. Tactile hallucinations are also relatively common in this group; visual hallucinations are less common but do occur in some people with psychosis, as do olfactory hallucinations. In principle, many of the techniques used with auditory hallucinations could be adapted for use with these other types of hallucination. The basic approach is the same, namely to accept that the experience of the hallucination is real but then to work with the person to modify their interpretation and beliefs about that experience, and to devise ways to limit the adverse effects.

Thought disorder and idiosyncratic language

When people are thought-disordered, you may still be able to follow the general themes of what they are saying and work therapeutically with these. However, communication difficulties undoubtedly make it harder and the aims of therapy are likely to be modest.

Shorter sessions may be helpful because thought disorder seems to get worse when people get tired. CBT cannot be used while the thought disorder is so severe that you are unable to follow what the person is saying (but see p. 36–37). Fortunately, thought disorder of this severity is very rare, but when it does occur it is not safe to assume that because the person's comprehension and expression of speech are grossly disordered then the thinking behind their words must be equally disordered – we just do not know.

Whether or not the person is thought-disordered, do not assume that they are using terms or language in exactly the same way that you would. If you do not recognize a word, or if they seem to be using a word in a way that does not quite make sense to you, then ask questions to clarify what they mean. I remember one session with someone who became increasingly irritated by my attempts to empathically rephrase what he was saying; it turned out that our definitions of the key word he was using to make his point were exact opposites, so my rephrasing was anything but empathic!

Willingness to engage in therapy
Probably the single most important factor in determining suitability for CBT is whether the person is able and willing to engage in this form of treatment. I have a simple rule of thumb: if the person is prepared to sit down with me, then I will have a go to see if there is anything at all that CBT might be able to help with.

The environment

The therapy room
Where possible you should see people for therapy in the same room every session. The familiar room will help to engender a sense of safety and the expectation that you will be talking about particular issues. Environmental cues may also help people recall what you have done in previous sessions.

It is worth paying some attention to the layout and furnishing of the room in order to create a warm and comfortable atmosphere. Not only will a relaxing environment make the sessions more pleasant for people but it may also help them feel safer. Although you may have standard-issue furnishings you can still make a big difference to the atmosphere by adding a rug, potted plants, ornaments, etc.

Wherever possible you should both sit on the same type of chair, or if that is not possible they should be of similar height.[2] Pay attention to how the chairs are positioned within the room. Having a desk between you is not recommended because it puts a barrier between you and is likely to emphasize the 'doctor:patient' hierarchy. Putting the chairs at a 90° angle will effectively distance you from the other person and will naturally avoid eye contact unless this is actively sought. Depending on the size of your room, it may also be feasible to increase the distance between the chairs. On one occasion I had sessions with someone in a large room with our chairs separated by at least 15 feet; this felt really quite uncomfortable to me, but with this arrangement he was able to stay for periods of up to half an hour whereas previously I had been unable to persuade him to sit down with me in a one-to-one situation.

Having a third person present
It is common practice to have trainees present in some therapy sessions. Whether it is the therapist or trainee who is conducting the session, the presence of a third person undoubtedly affects the situation, and many people with psychosis do not

[2]Needless to say, if one chair is more comfortable than the other, then you should take the less comfortable one.

feel comfortable with this arrangement and do not agree to it. You should be sensitive to those occasions when people may be agreeing to the additional person being present in order to oblige you rather than because they genuinely do not mind.

Of course, in some cases you will be working jointly with another professional and then it is entirely appropriate to meet all together because the content of your session will reflect this joint working. Having joint sessions in these circumstances also helps to ensure that you are working consistently in your respective individual sessions. For example, the hospital chaplain and I had joint sessions with a woman who believed she would burn in hell after she died unless she starved herself. Essentially I was providing the CBT strategies and the chaplain was providing the religious arguments and authority, but then we were both able to use the other's expertise in our individual sessions.

It may be necessary to have someone else present in the session if either the patient/client or therapist feels themself to be at risk, but generally speaking this should be avoided if at all possible. Having someone present that the person knows from another context, for example a family member, is likely to be intrusive and to significantly affect the therapeutic relationship, what is brought up for discussion and how it is discussed.

Therapy in the person's home

If you are seeing someone in the community, you may have the choice between seeing them in their home or on health service premises. It is probably better not to see them in their own home unless you are already visiting them there, for example as their community psychiatric nurse, or unless they are unwilling or unable to make the journey to see you anywhere else. 'Home' is good from the point of view of being a familiar and safe environment for the person, but being in the role of visitor to the person's home can conflict with your role as therapist in the therapeutic relationship. Needless to say, if there is any risk of a violent reaction to your visit or to your questioning, then you should not attempt therapy in the home.

The therapy session

The duration and content

There is no correct length for a CBT session. Normally I plan for one hour per session. This allows 50 minutes for the therapeutic contact plus 10 minutes to write up notes and plan the next session or, if needed, to extend the session. However, the planned session can be shorter, for example if the person finds the one-to-one social situation difficult, or if they are easily distracted by thoughts of other things they have to do.

Because the therapeutic relationship is so important, you may need to spend quite a lot of time building up rapport and trust, both before you start active CBT work and to maintain the relationship whilst therapy is progressing. It may require weeks, and occasionally even months, devoted to building up the therapeutic relationship before you can attempt to do any direct belief modification work. Even when well into therapy, it is not uncommon for much of the session to be taken up with general conversation or discussing other concerns that the person may have, with less than half of the session being used to push the cognitive programme along. Some people may not feel confident or secure enough to talk about their psychotic experiences until they have spent some time talking about more neutral things, whereas other people are keen to talk about their concerns early on in the session but then need time to 'wind down' with more relaxing or reassuring conversation. With less ill people, who have more insight, you can start the modification work sooner, and once someone understands what the therapy is seeking to achieve, then the modification work is rewarding in itself and so more time can be spent on it within the session.

For some people with thought disorder, it is noticeable that they can engage in a meaningful dialogue for 20 minutes or so before their thoughts become too muddled, so in these cases you would aim to cover the CBT work in the early part of the session and be prepared just to listen in the later part.

When the psychosis is in relapse, it may not be possible to progress the CBT at all, but nevertheless the session is not wasted if it can be used to support and help the person through this difficult period.

The 'Ask rather than tell' approach

Like other CBT programmes, as far as possible CBT with delusions and hallucinations uses the principle of Socratic dialogue, i.e. that it is better to encourage the person themself to come up with a line of reasoning, re-evaluation of a piece of evidence, etc. by asking the appropriate questions than it is for you to tell them the same thing. People more readily 'own' a conclusion that they have arrived at themselves, and working in this way brings out and focuses on lines of argument or evidence, etc. that the person themself finds most relevant and persuasive. It also helps to pace the changes so that they go at the other person's rate.

Despite the advantages of using the Socratic method, in practice you may find that you are often unable to elicit the alternatives you are hoping for. Undoubtedly this is partly because strongly held beliefs lead to such firm conclusions that they do not allow for other possibilities, for example if I *know* that the woman standing at the bus stop opposite my flat has positioned herself there in order to spy on me, what other reasons could there be? But another reason is that for some people the psychosis may actually adversely affect their ability to generate thoughts and options. When this latter is the case, you may have to present the functional alternatives yourself, by floating them or offering them as your own view if that is appropriate.

Informality of the approach

When working in a CBT way with non-psychotic disorders, it is usual to start each session by recapping what was done the previous session, discussing the results of the homework assignment, and then setting an agreed agenda for the work to be covered in the present session. However, we have already noted that as a general rule we cannot discuss delusions and hallucinations as targets for treatment in the same direct way that we would use for non-psychotic disorders, and so nor can we adopt such a formal approach to the discussion of treatment aims, plans and progress. It is likely that you will start your session by asking the person how they have been during the week and how they are now, and take it from there.

Although the approach to treatment sessions with people with psychosis is typically much more flexible, informal and unstructured than CBT with non-psychotic disorders, this does not mean that you can be unstructured or imprecise in your thinking or in the notes that you keep. Indeed, in many ways the informality of the treatment session itself means that you must be all the more structured and focused about the aims and plan of treatment.

Flexibility in the treatment

The treatment programme for a particular person could involve one or more of the major components described in the later chapters of this manual, and it could use some or all of the possible strategies within those components. Whilst the stages of therapy are presented in this manual in an order that would be appropriate for a course of treatment, this order should not be considered a fixed one. The various CBT strategies are to some extent interdependent and develop alongside one another, so with any one person you could be working with different strands at the same time, moving from one strand to another and back again in order to pursue and strengthen a particular line of approach. For example, a typical programme with hallucinations would be to work with what the voices are saying at the same time as working to change the person's understanding about where the voices come from. With any one person you might also be flexible in moving from one delusion to another or from delusion to hallucination, working on whichever aspect of each delusion and hallucination seems to be the most acceptable and beneficial for the person at that time. Because of this latter consideration, although it is strongly recommended that you plan your sessions ahead of time, you should be ready to abandon the plan for another occasion if unforeseen circumstances arise, which they often seem to do in this area of work. My own way of working is to make the plan for the following session immediately after the session has finished because then all the nuances of the session are fresh in my mind. I would recommend that at key stages of the therapy you also take an hour or so in between sessions to take stock and plan the broader therapeutic aims and strategies.

The person's conviction in their delusion may vary from time to time, so sensitivity is required to know how far to discuss and question a delusion at any one time. Particularly where the psychosis is fluctuating, you should be prepared to make progress in one session only to find that what was agreed during that session is refuted in the next. Because of this potential for people's insight and delusions to fluctuate, you should be careful to check whether the person's understanding about the issue under consideration is the same now as it was during the last session it was worked on. Asking general questions about how the person has been since the last session should give you a good indication of their current mental state, and if you feel this has deteriorated, then your recapping should be particularly tentative, for example 'Can you remember what we were talking about last week ...?' or 'I'm not sure if I have remembered correctly but I think you were saying something last session about ... Am I right?'.

The skill of being able to move flexibly from one aspect of the work to another is an important one for the therapist to acquire, though in practice it is difficult to teach and is best gained through experience. In CBT with delusions and hallucinations, there is no set way of doing things and usually no 'correct' way with any one individual. The only real guide as to the best approach to adopt in the individual case is your sensitivity to the person's reactions as the different strategies are tried, so you need to be constantly on the alert to detect any resistance or adverse reactions. Providing you have set the goals of therapy, have good reasons for pursuing the approach you are using and are prepared to move slowly, backing off if necessary, you are unlikely to go wrong; the worst that will happen is that you will take longer to achieve the modification than is strictly necessary. Remember, providing you do not lose the person's goodwill and cooperation, you can always come back to an unsuccessful strategy at some time in the future, when different circumstances and levels of understanding may make it more acceptable and beneficial.

Monitoring the effects of the therapy

It is good clinical practice to monitor the effects of the various strategies you use so that you know which are the effective ones for the person concerned. Thinking about how and why they are effective may also suggest other related areas of work that might be useful.

The effects may be assessed informally, from discussions with the person concerned and your own observations, or formally, by using structured measures (see Chapter 18, p. 312–315). Formal measures are preferable and may even be necessary if you need to prove that your therapy has made a significant difference. Standardized measures help to minimize the biases that can occur when therapists are trying to assess the effects of their own work, though in routine clinical practice it is usually the therapist who has to do both the 'before' and 'after' measures and so they are not as free from bias as when used in controlled research studies.

There may also be some negative aspects associated with asking someone to complete a formal assessment, and in some cases it may not be possible to use them without adversely affecting the therapeutic relationship and engagement in therapy. This latter is most likely to occur when the notion of 'illness' is rejected. When you ask someone to rate something, you are implying that you believe this something *could* change and be other than it is. Whilst there is usually no problem in agreeing with people that features such as their distress and preoccupation could vary, if they believe that something is a fact, then from their point of view not only is it not possible for their conviction to vary but also your very suggestion that it could is likely to constitute a 'challenge' and indicate that you think their belief is a delusional one. Other potential disadvantages of using formal measures are that they may irritate or upset the person being rated, and completing them may use up valuable therapy time, though these adverse effects can be minimized by keeping the formal assessments as simple, quick and non-intrusive as possible.

As with all aspects of CBT with delusions and hallucinations, formal rating scales should not be used in clinical practice without first weighing up the advantages and disadvantages of using them for the individual concerned.

Frequency and number of sessions

Normally I see people for therapy once a week, not least because this regularity helps everyone to remember the appointment, but there is no correct frequency. It may be appropriate to see some people more often, for example if they will be in hospital for only a short while, or less often if they find the sessions difficult or are only attending because they feel they ought to. Your clinical caseload may also dictate that you see people less frequently than once a week, but for the sake of continuity it is probably better not to space the sessions by more than two weeks on a regular basis. From limited experience with frequent sessions, I would recommend that you do not have more than two active CBT sessions each week because more frequent sessions can make even the most willing participant feel pressured. Furthermore, people seem to need a cognitive breathing space to consolidate what has been covered in the previous session.

It is impossible to say how many sessions are required 'on average'. In some cases a beneficial change can be effected in only a couple of sessions, whereas in other cases it can take many months to engage the person in therapy and/or many months once the person is fully engaged. In some cases the therapy has no apparent beneficial effects at all, even after months of sessions. As a *very* broad estimate you should probably be thinking in terms of six to nine months for a comprehensive CBT programme, followed by monthly and three-monthly follow-ups. The number of sessions required will depend on the aims of treatment, but you may expect therapy to take longer if the person is difficult to engage, if they deny having an illness, if their psychosis is still very active at a biological level, if the delusional systems are complex and well established, and if there are advantages as well as disadvantages to the symptoms.

Homework assignments[3]

Although setting the person work to do in between sessions is normally an essential and integral part of the CBT model, in my experience most people with psychosis are not good at completing formal homework assignments, especially written ones, and for this reason I use regular homework in only a minority of

[3]Some people have negative connotations for the term 'homework'; for example it may remind them of school, or they may find it demeaning in some way. In these circumstances you should try to agree a more acceptable term such as 'therapy work' or 'practice'.

my cases.[4] People are more likely to be able to engage in homework, and to see the reasons for doing so, in the later stages of therapy. Where they are able to extend the work they do in sessions in this way then this can be of great value, not least because it may help to ensure that the work covered in sessions is transferred to other situations and environments.

If you do want to set a homework task, then the following principle's will help to encourage adherence apply. (a) The person should understand exactly what the task is and how to do it, (b) they must be capable of doing it, (c) they must want to do it, and (d) they should get some reward or reinforcement for doing it. It is important to set the homework so that at least some of it gets completed, so that the exercise can be experienced as positive and successful rather than negative and failure. In practice this is likely to mean starting with very unambitious tasks and attempting to build up the task requirements as the homework progresses.

SUMMARY OF DIFFERENCES BETWEEN CBT WITH PSYCHOTIC AND NON-PSYCHOTIC DISORDERS

- Some people with psychosis may consider any form of 'treatment' to be inappropriate and a 'talking therapy' to be irrelevant.
- It is often the therapist, or one of the care team, who approaches the patient/client to suggest and encourage therapy rather than vice versa.
- Engagement in therapy may be problematic, and is often based on factors other than hope that the therapy will make them 'better'.
- The person may give the therapy sessions low priority, and attendance may be erratic and unreliable.
- The presence of disorganization and negative symptoms of schizophrenia can exacerbate the problems of engagement, and can affect the complexity of work that can be undertaken.
- The problem(s) that the person brings to the therapy may not be the same as, or may not be expressed in the same way as, the one(s) identified by the therapist and/or care team.
- A strong, trusting therapeutic relationship is essential.
- Treatment sessions are often less formal in their structure.
- Where there is no insight, the CBT model of working and aims of treatment cannot be discussed and made explicit in the same way that is normally done at the start of a course of CBT therapy.
- Ensuring that all aspects of the 'goal' are acceptable to the person can constitute a major part of the therapy (see Chapter 6), whereas with non-psychotic disorders the person identifies their own goal so this is acceptable to them from the start of therapy.
- Most of the therapy is targeted directly at the delusional beliefs and voices,

[4]People living in the community are more likely to be able to undertake formal homework assignments.

and the beliefs that influence them and that are incorporated into them. The CBT strategies of identifying negative automatic thoughts and biases of thinking, which are central to work with depression and anxiety, are rarely used as such.
- Formal homework assignments may not play a major role in the treatment programmes. In some cases, no homework is possible.

5 Assessment, Case Formulation and Goal Setting for Delusional Beliefs

Assessment

The way in which a psychological assessment is conducted and the questions asked will depend on the reason for conducting it: it is not the same as a psychiatric interview. For CBT for delusional belief modification, the main aim of the assessment is to enable you to construct a case formulation for the delusional belief, i.e. for you to understand what the relevant factors are in its development and maintenance and how they act and interact with each other.

It may take several sessions to gather the information necessary to make a preliminary case formulation. These early contacts are important times for building up the therapeutic relationship so it is important that they are not experienced as 'interrogations'. Phrase your questions from within the other person's belief system in order to avoid the risk of being confrontational and also the risk of inadvertently challenging the delusional belief before you have determined whether or not this would be beneficial. Try to avoid asking 'routine' questions unless they seem to be relevant to this particular case; you can always come back and fill in the gaps later if necessary.

Basic information about the delusion(s)

The initial assessment aims to identify and collect basic information about the main delusional beliefs. For each delusional belief the basic information required includes:

- What is the delusional belief? Is it a vague, general belief or can specific details be given?
- What does this belief *mean* for the person?
- How does it fit in with their other beliefs about self and the world?
- How firmly is it held?
- How distressing is it?
- How does it affect the person's life?
- What evidence does the person have to support the belief?
- How long have they held it? What led up to it?

Additional information will be required as the case formation is built up.

Obtaining details about the delusional belief

In the assessment interviews, some people are very clear and detailed about the delusional beliefs they report, for example 'Nurse Smith wants to put me in a coffin and burn me alive', whilst others are much vaguer, for example 'One of my family wants to harm me' or even just 'Someone wants to hurt me'.

People may be vague when talking about their delusional beliefs for a number of reasons other than the obvious one that the delusional belief itself is vague. For example, they may be avoiding distressing issues, they may fear the consequences of revealing what they know, or they may fear that you will not believe them and dismiss what you are told, or that it will lead to an increase in their medication if the doctors come to hear about it. In some cases, the delusion may be such that not talking about it may be a direct consequence of the belief itself, for example if the person believes they are a member of MI5, or it may just be that it is difficult to put into words because it involves feelings or concepts that are not covered by our everyday vocabulary.

Whatever the reason, if someone you are assessing is reluctant to talk about their delusions, or finds it difficult to put them into words, then you should be gentle in your probing and not push them for more information than they are comfortable for you to have at that time, even if that means you have to go cautiously, feeling your way with generalities rather than being able to focus in on specifics. In their role as 'patient', people may feel under a certain pressure to tell you personal things that they would rather keep quiet about, so you should be careful not to abuse your role as 'therapist' by persistent or intrusive questioning.

Whether the delusional belief is general or specific in nature, it is important to obtain as precise a description of the belief as possible, as it is held by the person, because this will affect the goal that is set and the treatment strategies that are used. For this reason it is important to determine whether any 'vagueness' in the person's reporting of their delusional belief indicates that the belief itself is held in a vague form or whether it is due to a reluctance to talk about the specific details. If the belief is held in a specific form, then you should obtain as much detail about it as the person is comfortable giving, not least because precise delusions tend to be easier to challenge than vague ones. For example, 'Jackie wants to kill me because I had an affair with our next-door neighbour' would be easier to disprove than 'Someone wants to kill me, I don't know why'.

Do not push too hard for details

Asking for details about a delusion that is held in a vague form may constitute a challenge if the person realizes the significance of *not* being able to provide the information. For example, if a woman remembers being abducted by aliens, she may be disconcerted to discover that she cannot recall any details of what the aliens looked like; or if a man believes that a close family member is trying to steal his money, he may be puzzled when you ask about each member by name to find that he dismisses all of them. Therefore, as you ask for details, the person may become aware of inconsistencies in their responses or of gaps in their knowledge, and realize what this implies, bringing about a challenge to their delusional belief before they are ready for it. Therefore, you must question sensitively, backing off if the person reacts adversely to any questions or is unable to answer.

Another risk of pushing too hard is that it may force the person to confabulate the missing details. This is not done intentionally; confabulation is a normal process and is the brain's way of trying to fill in detail that it 'knows' should be there. The problem here is that once the evidence has been confabulated, it will be stored back into memory as having really happened, and this means it will have to be re-evaluated later as part of the CBT programme.

In other situations, pushing too hard may risk forcing the person to resolve their vagueness with some other delusional explanation, which may be harder to modify than the original one. For example, in the case above, persistent questioning about who is trying to steal his money might lead the man to conclude that if it is not one of his family, then it must be 'government powers'.

If the delusional belief is held in a vague or general form, then this may be useful as evidence that it is based on feelings rather than on hard facts, which may be used later in therapy as a basis for challenging the delusion itself. So for this reason, having ascertained that the vagueness reflects the belief itself, you should accept the vagueness as a fact, being careful not to imply that this vagueness is surprising or unreasonable. For example, you might summarize the man's belief about his family along the lines of 'So you know that one of your family wants to take your money but no one has given you any signs or indications of who that might be – is that right?'

Explanation for the experiences: attitude to 'illness'

As we shall see later in this chapter, it is essential for goal setting to know how the person understands their psychotic experiences, and what their attitude would be towards illness or psychosis as an alternative explanation. However, you do not need to obtain this information immediately, so it may be better for rapport to cover it later on in the assessment process.

In the everyday world of our social existence we do not normally ask questions about something unless we think it is, or could be, relevant, so asking someone direct questions about their attitude to illness/psychosis/schizophrenia is very likely to imply that you think this is relevant to their situation, and as such runs a high risk of being experienced as confrontational.

The strategy of using other people's opinions (see p. 52) is helpful here. Having asked what the other person's opinion is, you can follow this up with questions like:

- How does it make you feel when he/she says that?
- Why do you think he/she sees it that way?
- What do you think/feel about that way of looking at things?

(See also 'Discussing the meaning of psychosis', p. 111.)

CASE FORMULATION

Accurate case formulation is an essential prerequisite for accurate goal setting and for ensuring that the factors targeted for CBT are those causing the person distress and difficulty. These in turn are essential prerequisites for planning appropriate and effective treatment strategies, which in turn are essential prerequisites for carrying out those strategies.

It is usually possible to start to develop a preliminary case formulation, for both the development and maintenance of the delusional belief, based on the basic information you obtain in the initial assessment sessions. Your first attempts at case formulation will highlight some other potentially relevant factors that you need to get more information about; having acquired this information, you adapt the case formulation accordingly, which in turn may highlight other possible relevant areas, and so on.

The working model for the development and maintenance of delusional beliefs (p. 22) may be useful in highlighting some of the key factors that you need to consider for your case formulation, and the ABC model (p. 17) may be useful as a different way of thinking about what is maintaining the belief. However, perhaps despite their appearance, these models are *simplified* representations of the complex of factors that could be involved, and so you need to keep asking yourself questions until you are satisfied you have identified the factors that are operating in the particular case. The skill in this area of work is to be able to sense when there is something about the delusional belief, or about its effect on the person or on their life, that cannot be adequately explained by the factors you have included so far. The sort of question to ask yourself is 'Given what I know so far, would I have expected ... to happen as it has? or for the person to feel as they do? or to respond as they have?'

The case formulation is adequate as a basis for planning treatment when the factors identified can adequately explain why the person holds the delusional belief that they do and why it affects them in the way that it does. Making the decision of when to start on the modification part of the programme is a matter of clinical judgement, which will be affected not only by the completeness or otherwise of your case formulation but also by your evaluation of the potential risks of starting to change the belief too soon.

It will probably not be possible to identify all the relevant factors before starting treatment, though you should have identified the major ones, so you should be ready for new ones to be revealed during therapy, and be flexible about changing your treatment plans or even goals accordingly. In some cases you may sense that you are 'missing a piece of the jigsaw' but be unable to determine exactly what it is. In such cases you should keep on the alert for any possible indications as to what it might be so that you can include it if and when you become aware of it.

CASE STUDY JANE[1]

(See also pp. 95, 99, 136, 143, 188, 277.)

CASE HISTORY

Jane's core delusional belief was that she was an evil witch. She thought that she was responsible for some of the terrible things happening in the world, including the war in Iraq. She knew she must be a witch because she had the power to change the weather. She also reported that people in the nearby town could see she was a witch and responded negatively to her; some people stuck their tongues out at her and others turned away when she tried to smile at them.

She had found that she was unable to use her powers to bring about anything good and so she knew she must be a bad witch, which she hated. She had held this belief for approximately three months when she was referred for treatment. She knew that she had had schizophrenia for the past 10 years but believed that this was well

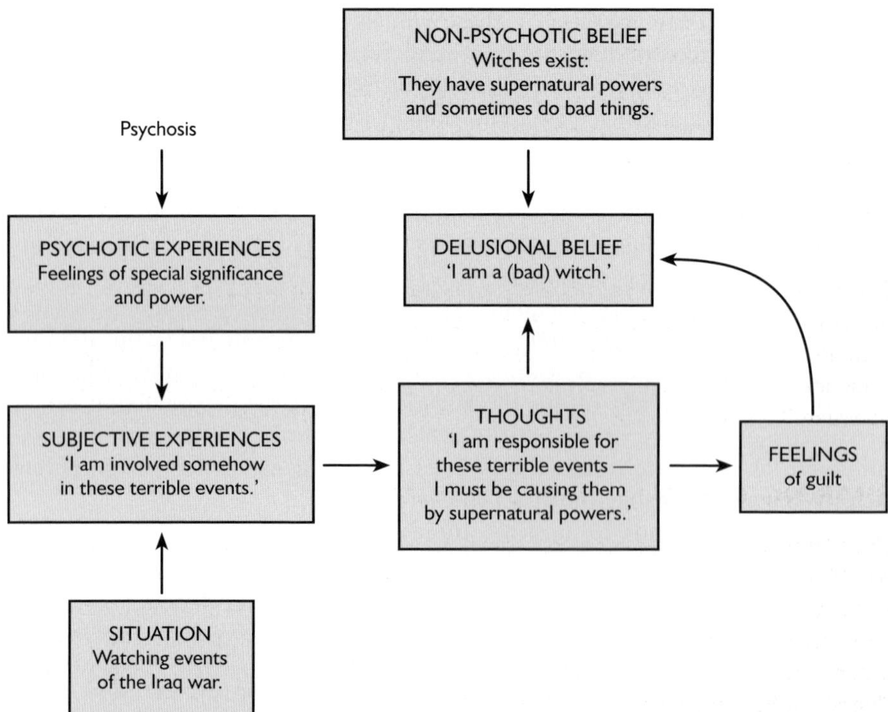

Figure 5.1 Case formulation for the development of Jane's delusional belief.

[1]The course of therapy for Jane is followed through at appropriate points in Chapters 5–8 and 15.

controlled by the medication she took, and so she was convinced that her current beliefs could not be due to the illness.

When asked what 'witch' and 'evil' meant, she described the common understanding of these words.[2] She did not have a special interest in, or knowledge of, witchcraft.

CASE FORMULATION

The development of the belief

Although, as is often the case, it was not possible to determine exactly when or how Jane's delusional belief first occurred, the information from the assessment suggested that the speculation depicted in Figure 5.1was a reasonable one.

The initial delusional belief that she was a witch was limited by Jane's own experimenting: this showed that she could not do good things to command and therefore that she must be a bad or evil witch.

The maintenance of the belief

Once the delusional belief had been established, the self-confirming belief maintenance cycle ensured that she interpreted subsequent events from the war as further evidence to support the belief.

The delusion also caused her to misinterpret other situations and develop secondary delusional beliefs that then reinforced the core delusional belief. These are depicted Figures 5.2(a) and (b) p. 78.

The effect of biased attention explains why Jane failed to notice the occasions when the weather did not follow her expectations (see Figure 5.2(a)).

On initial assessment it seemed likely that the event 'Some people stick their tongues out at me' was a distorted perception, caused by the fact that the secondary belief 'People can see I am a witch' had led Jane to be hypervigilant for 'confirming' evidence. These recurring events then set up a strong belief-confirming cycle between 'I am a witch' and 'People can see I am a witch' (see Figure 5.2(b)).

SHARING THE CASE FORMULATION

Since Jane knew she had a schizophrenic illness that could make her paranoid, it would have been safe to share this case formulation with her at any time. In practice, once Jane started to doubt being responsible for the events in Iraq, she wanted to know how she could have come to believe this if it were not true. She dismissed other parts of the delusional system, once they had been modified, as 'part of my illness', without wanting any further explanations.

[2]When terms like these are used, you should check that the person is not using them in some idiosyncratic way. It is the meaning *they* attach to the words that is important, not how they are used by anyone else.

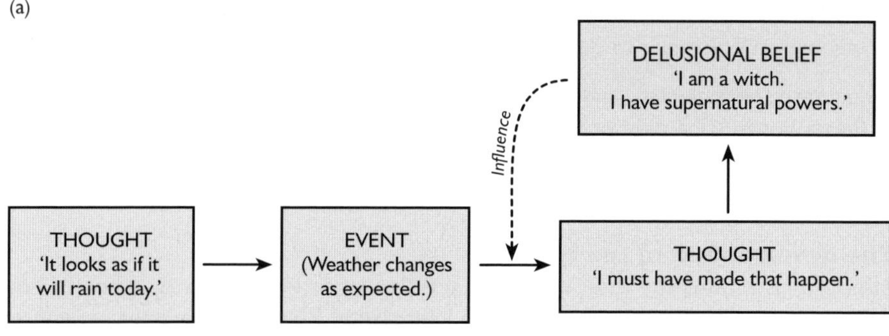
(a)
DELUSIONAL BELIEF
'I am a witch.
I have supernatural powers.'
Influence
THOUGHT
'It looks as if it
will rain today.'
EVENT
(Weather changes
as expected.)
THOUGHT
'I must have made that happen.'

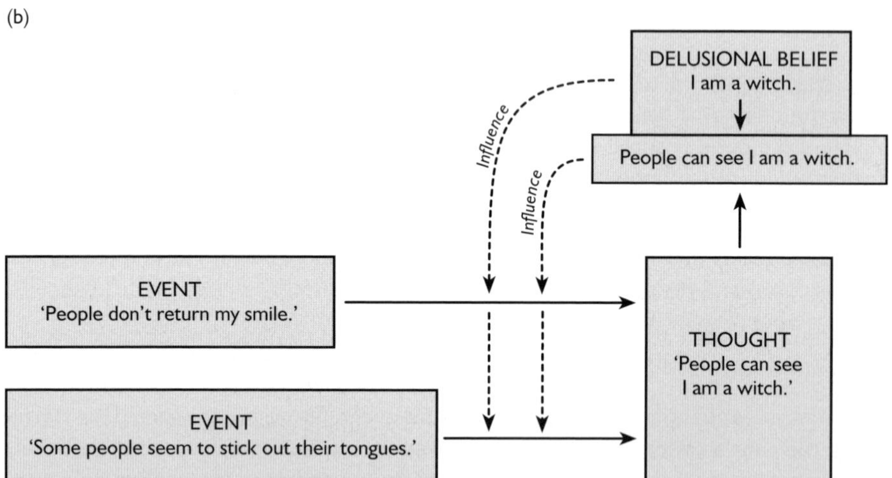
(b)
DELUSIONAL BELIEF
I am a witch.
People can see I am a witch.
Influence
Influence
EVENT
'People don't return my smile.'
EVENT
'Some people seem to stick out their tongues.'
THOUGHT
'People can see
I am a witch.'

Figure 5.2a & b Case formulation for additional evidence maintaining Jane's delusional belief.

CASE STUDY STEPHEN[3]

(See also pp. 97 and 192.)

CASE HISTORY

Stephen believed that he got messages from a benevolent spirit guide who answered questions put to him via sounds in the environment: one sudden sound meant 'yes'

[3]The course of therapy for Stephen is followed through at appropriate points in Chapters 5–8.

and two sudden sounds meant 'no'. He would go away to a quiet place to ask these questions because he had noticed in the past that he could miss a faint sound if he was in a noisy environment and so make a mistake.

Stephen had been ill for many years but strongly denied having a mental illness. He believed that his periods in hospital were to give him a break when housework, etc. got too much for him. He derived great comfort from the presence of his spirit guide and also a sense of being special. The spirit guide was supportive and generally gave good, sensible advice. However, on this particular occasion it was advising him not to continue medication once he was off section and discharged from hospital; previous experience had indicated that he would deteriorate rapidly if he did this.

CASE FORMULATION

Working from within her own belief system and understanding of the world, the therapist considered that the most likely explanation for the yes/no messages was that Stephen was interpreting noises in his environment according to his expectations. The fact that the answers agreed with him on nearly all matters and gave what sounded to him like good, sensible advice would be consistent with this explanatory model. The case formulation was as follows.

The development of the belief

Stephen already believed that he had a spirit guide who had wisdom and powers beyond those of humans. Maybe the first time he felt he had received a message in this particular way occurred when he had been trying to resolve a particular issue and the solution had come to him suddenly. Maybe the feeling of certainty that he had found the right conclusion was so great that he thought it must have been sent to him by his spirit guide. (There is also the possibility that there were some psychotic experiences of 'special significance' at that time.) Perhaps he then wondered *how* he could have received the answer and remembered that there had been a loud noise, and so concluded that perhaps this was how the message had been sent: one bang for 'yes' and two bangs for 'no'. This latter conclusion might well have been influenced by the 'folk' belief common in our culture that this is how some spirit mediums receive their messages from the dead.

The maintenance of the belief

However the idea had first occurred to him, once Stephen had discovered that he could ask for the advice of his spirit guide in this way it, is not surprising he used this as a source of reassurance about actions and events. The sort of questions he asked tended to be seeking confirmation of his own views and intended courses of actions, i.e. a preponderance of questions to which he would expect 'yes' to be the answer. The fact that noises in our everyday life usually occur singly, indicating a 'yes' reply, would help to ensure that the underlying delusional belief was usually confirmed. Furthermore, since there was no clearly specified time span between the first and second noises to constitute a double knock, when he expected a 'no' answer he could usually get it by listening for long enough. This frequent confirmation of the accuracy of the messages would be a powerful factor in maintaining the belief.

SHARING THE CASE FORMULATION

Since the therapeutic goal was to *not* undermine Stephen's belief that his spirit guide sent him messages (see p. 99), the therapist did not share this case formulation with him.

PRIOR TO TREATMENT: REDUCING THE DISTRESS CAUSED BY THE DELUSIONAL BELIEF

As soon as you have completed your preliminary assessment and case formulation you should consider whether there are any simple, practical ways of reducing the distress caused by the delusional belief that might be immediately available for the person to try. (See Chapter 15, pp. 273–278.)

SETTING APPROPRIATE GOALS FOR THE MODIFICATION OF DELUSIONAL BELIEFS

Note on the term 'goal setting'. There are many different sorts of goals that you can set in therapy, corresponding to the many different aspects of your treatment programme; for example, 'Attend the social centre regularly', 'Recognize and identify when "voices" occur', 'Do not follow the voices' commands', 'Use the relapse prevention strategies when required', etc. When the term 'goal setting' is used in this manual, it refers specifically to the goals of a belief modification programme.

Ethical considerations

In general clinical practice it is the patient/client who comes to the therapist to request help in changing a particular aspect of their life, be it behavioural, emotional or cognitive, and it is the patient/client who is ultimately responsible for setting the goals of their therapy. But since a cardinal feature of delusions is to believe that they are true, people with delusions are necessarily not able to be objective or to request help for their 'symptoms' in this way. Nor is it appropriate to discuss possible 'treatments' for what they know to be true. Therefore, you have no choice but to take the lead in making the initial decision to attempt to modify the delusional belief, without first discussing and describing the treatments you would like to offer, and without getting explicit consent for them. In these circumstances you must be particularly careful not to infringe the person's right of choice for treatment.

Goal setting for CBT is governed by the overall principle that no one has the right to interfere with another's belief system unless there is good reason to do so. In particular, *the fact that a belief or experience may be considered by others to be a symptom of an illness is not of itself sufficient reason to attempt modification.* The following guidelines are recommended for consideration before starting treatment:

1. CBT may be started if the person understands and requests it or, having had the treatment explained to them, agrees to it. This is the standard CBT position, of course. It can sometimes apply when working with people with psychosis, for example if the treatment is being offered whilst the person is in between episodes, or if the problem concerns a voice that the person knows is caused by their illness.

2. CBT for a delusion or hallucination may be started when informed consent is not possible if the delusion or hallucination is causing distress to the person, and if there is good reason to believe that modification would reduce that distress.

Caution: A delusion or hallucination may cause the person great distress but this does not necessarily mean that they would want it modified or removed. There may be secondary gains that are not always immediately apparent to the therapist, or that may be intricately bound up with the psychotic experience itself. Religious delusions and delusions about special relationships are particularly likely to fall into this latter class. For example, one man was distressed by the invasion of the spirit world into his mind but he did not want this to stop because it was a significant religious experience for him. In another example, a woman would become quite distressed by the critical messages sent over the airwaves by her parents, but although these messages were always unpleasant she did not want to lose this only remaining contact with her mother and father.

Although you may not be able to discuss the issue of modification directly with the person, *it is incumbent on you to find out by indirect questioning whether the modification you are considering would be welcomed if it were successful.* Needless to say these questions should be framed within the person's own belief system (see Chapter 3) to avoid the risk of 'challenging' the belief before the goal(s) has been set. Some questions that I have found helpful in this situation include:

> 'What are the worst things about . . .? or hearing . . .?' '(It must be awful but) are there any good aspects of . . .? or hearing . . .? or is it all bad?'
>
> 'What was it like before you realized . . .? or heard . . .?' 'Overall, was it better or worse . . ., were you happier or less happy . . ., more or less worried . . ., etc. than you are now?'
>
> 'I know this isn't possible, but suppose you woke up one morning and found it had all been a dream/nightmare, would you be relieved? How would you feel? Is there anything at all you might miss?' 'Would you miss . . . at all?'

3. It is not uncommon for delusional beliefs to have both positive and negative aspects and consequences. In this situation it is often possible to use a modification

that reduces the negatives whilst retaining the positives, but where this is not possible the decision has to be made as to whether the positives gained from a modification would outweigh the negatives. Again, as far as possible it is the person themself who should make this decision, so you should try to phrase the necessary questions from within their own belief system in order to ascertain this.

4. The most difficult ethical situation is if a delusion or hallucination is causing distress to others rather than to the person themself. In these circumstances it may be ethical to start CBT without their expressed consent *providing* the expected secondary gains from the modification outweigh any possible negative effects of the belief change itself. For example, a woman, when she became unwell, would believe that another patient on the ward was her 'true biological father', an idea that she found intriguing rather than distressing but that her father found very upsetting. In this case, modifying her belief caused no loss for her but it had a direct benefit for her father and so in the long run it benefited her as well, because her recognition of him as 'father' helped to reinforce his frequent visits and care.

A harder situation arises if the person themself wants to retain their belief or experiences For example a man liked being a reincarnation of a Roman emperor because it gave him the right to have sex with any females that he fancied, but this had led him to be detained in a secure hospital. As in point 3, above, the positive and negative effects of changing the dysfunctional belief have to be balanced against each other.

5. If, at any time during therapy, it appears that the person does not want to lose their delusional beliefs or hallucinations, or is ambivalent about losing them, then therapy should be suspended immediately whilst you review the situation. It may be necessary to adjust the goals for modification, for example from a total to a partial goal (see below), at least temporarily. Alternatively, it may just be that the therapy is pushing ahead too rapidly so that the person is having difficulty accommodating the belief changes involved, in which case the solution is to go more slowly and gently.

If it becomes apparent that there are some secondary gains you have not detected previously, then it may be possible to replace the source of secondary gain by some other source. For example, a man believed he could invade people's minds and read what they were thinking; he found this very distressing because most of the thoughts that he 'read' were critical and disparaging. During therapy, he appeared to be less pleased about the results of some of the CBT strategies than expected. It transpired that a secondary gain of the delusion was knowing he *could* destroy the other person's mind when he invaded it, if it posed a significant risk to him, even though he would never actually do so. Modifying his belief that other people posed a threat to him gave him a sense of safety that replaced the sense of safety associated with the delusion.

6. Grandiose delusions should be approached with great caution. It is probable that a grandiose delusion will not be distressing to the person themself, in which case this primary reason for attempting a modification, will not be there. Modification should only be attempted if the potential benefits of doing so

clearly outweigh the possible disadvantages. The fact that a belief is delusional is *never* sufficient reason on its own for imposing treatment.

Grandiose delusions often serve a very positive function for the person of maintaining or boosting their self-esteem. Therefore, if there are other clear benefits to be gained from modifying a grandiose delusion, then you must seek to determine what the potential effects of removing the grandiose delusion will be on self-esteem, and to work to build up self-esteem from other sources before attempting the modification. For example, a man who believed he was a senior member of the secret service gained a great sense of self-esteem and purpose from the belief, but the disadvantage for him was that he not infrequently came into conflict with the law when he shoplifted electronics equipment that he needed for his work for the government. Inconvenient as this latter behaviour was, it was decided not to attempt modification of the core belief unless and until the sense of self-esteem it gave could be provided from elsewhere.

In many cases of grandiosity it is appropriate to go for a partial rather than total modification (see below), which allows those parts of the delusion that are important for self-esteem to be retained. Total modification of a grandiose delusion would normally be attempted only where a partial modification is not possible or would not be sufficient to produce the required positive effects. For example, if a man believed he had supernatural powers that would allow him to emerge unscathed if he threw himself off a high building, then the modification must ensure that he did not test this out in practice: the partial modification 'I have supernatural powers but they might not be enough to stop me crashing to the ground' could not be relied upon to prevent this happening.

Setting goals appropriate to the socio-cultural-religious background

A guiding principle for goal setting with both delusional beliefs and the non-psychotic beliefs that may underlie them (see Chapter 7) is that the goals are set within the person's socio-cultural-religious affiliation, i.e. the goals are compatible with the beliefs of that group(s). This is particularly important where changes to these beliefs could impact on the person's socio-cultural-religious identity and group membership. For example, a woman was very distressed because she believed the words of condemnation that she heard came from angels. Normally in these circumstances we would set a goal to change the belief about the origin of the voices, but in this case it was not considered appropriate because belief in direct communication from angels was a central belief held by the religious group to which she belonged, and, furthermore, this religious group was her primary source of social support and friendship.

It is always much harder to work with socio-cultural or religious beliefs that are other than your own. Even if you know the main tenets of these groups, you are unlikely to appreciate the different shades of opinion that exist within them, and, perhaps equally importantly, you are unlikely to understand the sometimes subtly different ways that people from different backgrounds can conceptualize and think about the issues. The person you are working with will be a prime source of information, but it can also be helpful if you are able to get information and advice from another member of that person's religious and/or socio-cultural grouping. It may be helpful to call in a minister or religious leader to talk directly with the person if they are concerned about religious issues, not least because the religious leader will have more authority as well as knowledge about these matters than you do. Indeed, I often work together with an appropriate minister or elder in these cases and this can be very effective. However, ministers or elders do vary greatly in their approach to religion and mental illness so you do need to be careful that their intervention will be helpful and not reinforce the delusions. For example, a woman with schizophrenia who believed she was possessed by the Devil was not helped when the priest she visited recoiled from her in fear and horror and told her that she needed exorcism.

Most social and religious groupings show some diversity with respect to their beliefs and values, so it is often possible to modify the dysfunctional belief in question to conform to a more functional view that is still acceptable within the group. For example, a woman from India who had come to live in the UK some years ago believed that she should obey her husband in all things. (However feminists might view it, this was not considered to be a delusional belief but an important non-psychotic belief underlying a delusional one, and this was why it was being targeted for modification.) Other women that she knew from the same cultural group did not hold the belief in this extreme form and so we were able to modify her belief accordingly. As an example from the area of religious beliefs, some members of the Church of England believe in judgement and punishment after death and some do not, so within this group it would be possible to modify this belief and remove the fear of eternal damnation without affecting group membership: this would not be possible for a member of the Roman Catholic Church.

If it is not possible to modify the dysfunctional belief directly because this would conflict with the group's beliefs, then the beliefs of the group itself may be able to provide an alternative, functional option. For example, in the situation just given, a member of the Roman Catholic Church would retain their belief in punishment after death but could avoid the feared consequences by attending confession and gaining absolution.

Some religious or cultural experiences and beliefs can be very similar indeed to those attributed to psychosis, so this can present a particular difficulty when goal setting and working within these group beliefs. Fortunately, the groups themselves often have their own ways of distinguishing between 'genuine' and 'psychotic' phenomena, so you may be able to use these. For example, a spiritualist retained her belief in messages from the dead but was advised by other spiritualists that the voices she heard did not come from this source because they were critical and threatening instead of being not helpful and constructive. Another spiritualist was given reasons by his church elders as to why his fears that his spirit would not leave his body when he died were not valid ones.

Setting goals within the person's own beliefs and values can present problems if by so doing you are reinforcing some dysfunctional aspect of the delusional belief. In such cases you need to be careful to consider the wider implications of your end goal as well as its more obvious meaning (see the following example).

EXAMPLE OF WORKING WITHIN THE PERSON'S RELIGIOUS BELIEFS

A man was very agitated because he believed he was possessed by an evil spirit. His evidence for this was the very strange visual, tactile and subjective experiences that he had had over the previous two weeks, some of which he could link to signs of spirit possession. He requested an exorcism. The hospital chaplain assessed the possibility of spirit possession and I carried out a psychological assessment, as a result of which we were confident that these symptoms were caused by schizophrenia.

Although exorcism was consistent with this man's religious beliefs, we were concerned that an exorcism service would provide evidence that other people believed he was, or could be, possessed. Therefore, although it would probably have provided comfort and support in the short term, a service of exorcism could have increased his fear of becoming possessed again in the future and made it more likely that the 'possession' explanation would be used if (as seemed quite likely) the psychotic experiences occurred again.

Our solution was to have a service of blessing and safe keeping for the future. This was consistent with our approach: 'We think that your experiences were due to psychosis, which means that your brain produced these dream-like experiences when you were awake, so we do not think that you were possessed by an evil spirit. But even if you had been possessed, the service has ensured that you are not possessed now and, furthermore, that you cannot ever be possessed in the future.'

This church service turned out to be the linchpin of his treatment. It provided immediate comfort, reassurance and the benefits from reduced arousal levels. Furthermore, it was an effective counter to the occasional recurrent doubts about possession, and when milder psychotic experiences occurred he *knew* that they could not be possession and therefore that they must be 'symptoms' produced by his brain. Because he knew that he could not be possessed, these latter incidents served to strengthen the replacement belief, namely that his brain was capable of producing these sorts of experiences without any outside influences being involved.

The guiding principle of setting the goals within the person's existing socio-cultural and religious beliefs is not an absolute one, though we should have very good reasons for breaking it, as in the following example. A young woman in hospital became very distressed whenever she was visited by members of a Christian evangelical sect with which she was associated. They prayed with her and then told her that if she was still ill it was because she was not praying hard enough. I do not doubt for one moment that this advice was lovingly given, that her visitors genuinely believed this to be the case and therefore that this advice was given entirely for her sake, but nevertheless it left her not only suffering from the very distressing symptoms of her illness but also with a feeling of guilt that it was her fault she felt this way because she did not love God enough. In this case, we did feel it was appropriate to modify these particular religious beliefs and to move her away from the sect towards a more liberal Christian group.

When the therapist's own beliefs intrude on goal setting

Religious and moral beliefs and values can be of fundamental importance to the therapist as well as to the client/patient, and for this reason delusions in these areas can present particular ethical difficulties when it comes to goal setting. For example, a man of Christian background has a terrifying delusional belief about eternal torture that is only possible because of his belief in hellfire: should his belief about the existence of hellfire be modified in order to reduce his distress, or does it reflect some fundamental religious truth that should not be ignored or denied however unpleasant and whatever the personal cost? Our own beliefs will affect what we consider to be the most functional goal in this type of circumstance, and to some extent I think that this is inevitable and unavoidable. For example, if I, the therapist, believe in hellfire as an afterlife punishment, then clearly it would be immoral for me to misguide someone else into ignoring this warning, however much false comfort it would give that person in the short term; equally, if I do not believe that hellfire exists, then my clear moral duty towards this person is to remove this cruel, destructive and distressing belief.

Ensuring that the goal chosen is the optimal one

The overarching aim of any CBT intervention is to be beneficial for the person receiving it, to reduce their distress and to improve their quality of life. The distress caused by a delusional belief and the extent to which it interferes with the person's life are not necessarily related to the conviction with which the delusional belief is held, so you should be careful to check that the goal chosen will target the *reason* for the distress and will help to reduce it. For example, if someone is distressed by the belief that their heart is rotten because this means their death is imminent, then removing this belief will reduce their distress; however, if the belief is distressing because it is just one sign of their being a thoroughly rotten person, then removing the belief about their heart will not remove the source of their distress, i.e. the belief that they are a rotten person. Similarly for auditory hallucinations, it is not the voices as such that cause distress but rather the beliefs about the voices and what they say. These issues are addressed in later chapters.

What is the belief being targeted for modification? What will the person end up believing if the modification is successful?

When we talk about goal setting for a belief modification, we are referring specifically to what the person will end up believing if the modification is successful.

The first step of goal setting is to *identify clearly and precisely the dysfunctional belief that you are intending to modify*. It is good practice to put this in writing. This may appear to be a rather obvious point but it is perhaps surprising how often a problem brought to clinical supervision originates in vagueness about which delusional belief, or which aspects of the delusional belief, are being affected by the treatment strategies used.

Having considered what changes might be beneficial (see below) the optimal goal for modification is set. There is a golden rule: *the goal **must** be clearly specified **before** you attempt any belief modification work.* If you are unable to put the goal into words and write it down, then this is a good indication that you need more information and/or understanding before you proceed.

There are two types of belief modification that can be used, a *total modification*, in which the delusional belief is rejected, and a *partial modification*, in which only certain aspects of the delusional belief are rejected.

TOTAL MODIFICATION OF THE DELUSIONAL BELIEF

Setting the goals for modification of delusional beliefs is not just a question of specifying what the person will stop believing; of equal importance is specifying what they will believe instead. We saw in Chapters 1 and 2 that a delusional belief is developed as the brain's best effort to make sense of the person's total subjective experience of what is going on in the world, so the delusional belief will not be abandoned until there is another interpretation or belief to replace it, i.e. one that explains the experiences and events that were previously explained by the delusion better than the delusion does. For example, if I believe that I was abducted by aliens, then I will only be able to change this belief if I can accept that the experiences I had were caused by something else. So, when seeking to modify a delusion, you must take care to set the most functional replacement belief and to use the appropriate strategies not only to disprove the delusional belief but also to shape up the new belief that will supersede it. If you fail to do this, you may find that the delusional belief is merely replaced by another delusional belief, and this new belief may be even more disruptive and harder to modify than the original one – definitely not a successful outcome for your intervention! In the example above, if you modify my belief about alien abduction without giving any attention to the replacement belief, then I may conclude that, as it was not alien abduction, my strange experiences must have been caused by the psychiatrist invading and manipulating my mind.

The goal for a total modification (referred to as a 'total goal') typically takes the form:

NEGATION OF THE DELUSIONAL BELIEF
+
REPLACEMENT BELIEF

In the example given above, the total goal might be:

'I have not been abducted by aliens.'
+
'The strange experiences I had were caused by the LSD that I took.'

The replacement belief that is used must be appropriate, functional and acceptable to the person. Setting the replacement belief and ensuring that it is acceptable can present a major challenge for the therapist, and it is not always possible to achieve in practice. *But unless and until the person is prepared for the replacement belief, a total modification should not be attempted.* For example, if I had never taken drugs and the only viable alternative explanation for my experiences of alien abduction was that these were symptoms of a psychotic illness, then it would not benefit me if I was so distressed when you brought me to this conclusion that I committed suicide.

Replacement beliefs for total modifications

There are two broad classes of replacement belief that you can use. Because they look at different levels of explanation for the delusional belief they are not mutually exclusive. The initial replacement belief you use will be the one that fits in best with the person's way of understanding things and that makes most sense to them. In some cases, as the person's understanding develops, it might be functional to develop the replacement belief accordingly, for example starting with the notion of 'oversensitivity of part of the brain' and then progressing to 'It's oversensitive because you have a mental illness, called psychosis'.

The replacement beliefs given below are described in detail in Chapter 6.

Biological explanations (medical model)
Explanations in terms of:

- mental illness/psychosis/schizophrenia, etc.
- oversensitivity/overactivity/dysfunction of part of the brain because ...
  - part of my brain sometimes acts as if it were asleep and dreaming, even though I am awake
  - the 2-route model
  - something happened to make it that way (e.g. LSD).

Psychological explanations
Explanations in terms of:

- how and why the delusional belief developed as it did and the cognitive-behavioural factors that maintain it
- 'I did not have enough information before, now I know better'
- 'I was mistaken'
- 'I've just changed my mind'.

(*Note*: These last three options are unlikely to be acceptable unless the delusional belief is of only minor importance to the person.)

PARTIAL MODIFICATION(S) OF THE DELUSIONAL BELIEF

The aim of CBT is not to get rid of a delusion just because it is a 'symptom' of an illness, it is not to modify a delusion just so that the belief is nearer to the 'truth' as other people see it, and it is not to make the delusional belief more socially acceptable or politically correct: the aim is to reduce the distress caused by the delusions. This being so, it is not always necessary to modify the core delusional belief to achieve therapeutic gain; indeed, in some cases modifying the core delusional belief might actually do more harm than good and cause the person more distress. In a partial modification only those parts of the delusional system causing problems for the person are targeted for modification; the core delusion is left intact. The goal of modification (i.e. the new belief) must be compatible with the parts of the delusional system that are left intact.

The goal for a partial modification (referred to as a 'partial goal') typically takes the form:

CORE DELUSION, **BUT .....**

Partial modifications can take many different forms including:

1. *Delusional belief* **but** ... *some aspect or implication of the delusional belief is not true*. For example, 'I was abducted by aliens, but they can't harm my family through me'.

This is the most common form of a partial goal.

2. *Delusional belief* **but** ... *it is not true now*. For example, 'I used to be possessed by the Devil, but I am not now'.

This form of partial modification can be particularly helpful where the person has invested so much in trying to convince other people that their delusion was true that they would suffer loss of face and self-esteem if they admitted they had been wrong (e.g. the man who had fought the mental health services for five years over whether his belief about being targeted by the Mafia was true or due to mental illness). It is also useful for long-standing delusions where the person would suffer by realizing what they had missed out on in life by believing the delusion to be true (e.g. the man who had been unable to go out for years because he believed gunmen were waiting for him outside), and where the delusion protects the person's self-esteem (e.g. the woman who attributed the fact she had no friends, family or nice home to the bone that grew in her throat when she was young and prevented her from going out).

3. *Delusional belief* **but** ... *it may not apply in all circumstances*. For example, 'The spirits protect me from harm, but I can't be absolutely sure that they will do it every time so throwing myself in front of a train is just too big a risk to take'.

4. *Delusional belief* **but** ... *other people genuinely do not believe or recognize it*. For example, 'I am inhabited by a ghost, but the doctors genuinely believe that this is part of a mental illness'.

Focusing on *what other people believe* can be a particularly useful partial modification for grandiose delusions because grandiose delusions often cause trouble not so much because of what people believe about themselves as what they believe other people believe about them. For example, a partial goal set for a young man who was detained because he hit strangers in the street was 'I am the reincarnation of the Emperor Claudius, but my reincarnated subjects do not recognize me when they see me in the street, and so I should not expect them to bow to me or try to punish them when they don't'.

When to use a partial goal

Typically, there are a number of possible partial goals for each core delusional belief that deal with its different aspects and negative consequences. As with a total goal, you must write down the whole of the partial goal(s), including the core belief that will be retained, to make sure you know exactly what the implications of the modification are and to highlight which parts, if any, need to be protected from a dysfunctional challenge (see point 1 below). Partial goals are used in the following situations.

1. As the goal of choice

If the delusional belief affords the believer some significant secondary gain that cannot be replaced from elsewhere, then a partial modification is often the modification of choice. For example, one young man believed he was the son of a royal prince. This caused problems at home because talking about this royal connection caused rows between him and his father. When asked what it would be like if he were not the son of royalty, he told us this would be terrible and that he would contemplate suicide. So, at least in the short term, a total modification of this belief was not acceptable. The goal of partial modification in this case was for him to change his beliefs about the old man he lived with, to recognize that the old man did not know he had royal blood but genuinely believed himself to be his father. With this part of the belief system modified, the young man spontaneously remarked that it would be unkind to the elderly man to talk about his 'real' father at home and so he refrained from doing so. In this way damaging conflicts between the man and his father were avoided but he retained the benefits from his belief about royal parentage.

Where a partial modification is the goal of choice because it would be detrimental to the person to modify their core delusional belief, then *you must protect the core belief from change* and be very careful that the new modified parts will not create a challenge to the parts you want to keep intact. For example, a man who believes he is an archangel (functional, because of its effect on self-esteem) hears the voice of God threatening him if he does not follow the tests that he is set to prove his obedience (dysfunctional, because of what he is told to do). The partial goal 'I am an archangel, but the voice is not from God, it is created in my own mind' would appear to retain the functional whist getting rid of the dysfunctional, but there is a very real risk that the work you do to prove that the voice does not come from God will cause his belief about being an archangel to collapse.

A partial modification may also threaten the core delusional belief if the situations involved are so similar that the work done to modify the unwanted part of the belief generalizes to the wanted part. For example, if a woman welcomed the voice of her dead mother but was upset by the threatening voice of her neighbour, then it would be almost impossible to change her belief about the origin of the neighbour's voice without this also changing her belief about the origin of her mother's voice. *If the core delusional belief needs to be retained* (even if this is only in the short term, before other therapy takes effect), *then you must not attempt a partial modification if there is a significant risk that this will threaten the core belief.*

2. Whilst the replacement belief is being 'prepared'
It is not uncommon when attempting to set a total goal to be unable to find a replacement belief that is immediately acceptable to the person. When this happens, you should still set what appears to be the most functional replacement belief, but you must not proceed with the total modification until you have done the necessary work to render the replacement acceptable (see Chapter 6). In these circumstances you could proceed with a partial modification(s) providing it did not threaten the core delusional belief.

Caution: A partial modification will weaken the core delusional belief if it removes an important aspect of that belief (e.g. 'I am the Queen but most people don't recognize me'), or removes evidence that supports the belief (e.g. 'I have special powers but I cannot foretell the future accurately'). Therefore, if you do a number of 'safe' partial modifications, this effect may be additive and cause the core belief to collapse.

3. As a stepping stone on the way to a total goal
A total modification is often proceeded by what is effectively a series of partial modifications. For example, 'I hear the voice of the Devil but (a) it cannot make other people do what it wants, (b) it cannot predict the future accurately, (c) it cannot carry out the harm it threatens, etc.' This is very similar to point 2, above, but you would not be proceeding with the total goal unless the identified replacement belief was acceptable, and so in these circumstances you do not have to worry about threatening the core belief; indeed, this is exactly what you want to achieve by the partial modifications.

4. Where the delusional system is too complex, extensive and/or flexible to be removed and replaced
Some people's delusional systems infiltrate every aspect of their lives, so even if it were possible in practice to change the entire system, the impact would be too great to be beneficial overall. In such cases, partial modifications may be appropriate to remove some unpleasant aspects of the beliefs. For example, one man had a complex belief system that included the belief he was an alien. This belief caused him no distress except that he also believed some people could see he was an alien, and, furthermore, that some of these people might themselves be aliens who would want to eat him. Two partial goals were set: 'I am an alien but . . .

(a) I look the same as everybody else so no one can see that I am an alien', and
(b) 'aliens would not want to eat one of their own kind even if they did recognize me'.

Some people's delusional systems seem quite vague and difficult to pin down, or they change fluidly when you talk about them. In these circumstances also, a partial modification may be useful if there is some stable, unpleasant aspect that you could change.

5. Where a total goal was set, but was not achievable in practice
It is not always possible to achieve the total modification that has been identified as the goal of choice, but you may be able to achieve and get positive therapeutic gain with a partial modification instead.

EXAMPLE OF USING A PARTIAL GOAL WHERE THE TOTAL GOAL WAS NOT ACHIEVABLE

A man had been referred to us from the courts after he had seized a policeman's walkie-talkie and smashed it to the ground. On a couple of occasions prior to this he had noticed that his eyesight and hearing were affected when he was near one of these sets in use, and as a result had developed the firmly held belief that some of the walkie-talkie sets used by traffic police are 'duff' and could affect his, and other people's, sight and hearing. According to his belief it was perfectly reasonable, and indeed even socially responsible, to approach a policeman using one of the duff sets and ask him politely to switch it off – and to smash the offending instrument to the ground when the policeman did not respond as requested. This was perfectly reasonable behaviour because it was the only way to protect his and other people's senses. The problem for the man now was that if he smashed another walkie-talkie after discharge, he would be returned to hospital or prison.

Since there were no positive gains to this delusional belief about the walkie-talkies we attempted a total modification, the goal of which was 'Walkie-talkies cannot affect anyone's sight or hearing; the odd experiences I had before were nothing to do with the walkie-talkie sets being used but were probably just minor sensations caused by my brain through anxiety or tiredness'. But despite trying many different approaches we had no success.[4] We discussed coping strategies to keep him away from the offending walkie-talkies but he did not feel these would be successful because he had a duty to protect other people's sight and hearing as well as his own.

This discussion was helpful because it suggested that a partial modification could be effective in controlling the unwanted behaviour, this modification being about the effects of the walkie-talkies on other people's sight and hearing. As he did not have the same sensory evidence to back up his belief about the adverse effects of the radio waves on other people, we were able to successfully modify this belief so that he ended up believing only his sight and hearing could be affected. Having achieved this

[4]I have noticed over the years that delusions based on people's sensory experiences are particularly difficult to modify, presumably because normally our senses are accurate and reliable sources of information and therefore to be trusted without question.

partial modification, we were then able to agree a set of coping strategies, such as moving away from the duff set as soon as he felt its adverse effects. Knowing that he had no responsibility for other people, that he only had to look after himself, meant that he was able to change his response, should he encounter a duff set in operation in the future.

DECIDING WHETHER TO GO FOR A TOTAL OR PARTIAL MODIFICATION

A total modification is the goal of choice when it is the core delusional belief that is dysfunctional and distressing. Partial modifications may still be helpful in these cases but, if possible, a total modification should be undertaken.

A total modification has the advantage over a partial modification in that it is more secure against future relapse. Once the delusional belief has been rejected, the replacement belief can be slotted into, and thereafter supported by, the person's network of rational, non-delusional beliefs; but if part of the delusional system is left intact, then there is always the potential for the remaining parts of the delusion to reactivate the parts that had been modified and overlaid by the new parts. For example, in the case described above, the partial modification allows for the possibility that humans can be affected by the walkie-talkies; so if the man should notice people looking perplexed or moving away from a policeman using a walkie-talkie, or rubbing their eyes or ears, then he may conclude that they, too, are vulnerable and therefore that he should 'protect' them by smashing the duff set.

A partial modification is much easier and quicker to achieve than a total modification. This is only partly because a partial modification is dealing with less of the delusional system than a total modification. A very significant factor is that a partial modification leaves the core delusion intact and as such does not require the identification and 'preparation' of a more functional, replacement belief. For this reason it is usually possible to start on a partial modification very early on in therapy, whereas this is only possible for a total goal if the identified replacement belief is already acceptable to the person. A partial modification runs less risk of inadvertently provoking an adverse reaction than a total modification because it leaves the core delusion in tact.

Setting the most appropriate goal(s)

When goal setting, you should set the ideal goal that affords the maximum overall gain for the person, even if you do not think that you will be able to achieve it in practice, and then set the sub-goals for along the way. Goal setting usually follows the steps described below.

1. What are the negative and positive aspects of the delusional belief?

Most of this information will come directly from the person themself, but you should also speculate about what these might be and then go back to the person to check them out, because people do not always report everything. They may not realize that something is relevant, or they may be reluctant to disclose something, especially if it is socially unacceptable. For example, one woman did not spontaneously report that there was one very positive aspect of having an evil spirit inside her, namely that it could destroy anyone who threatened her.

Consider the wider implications of the delusional system as well as the obvious ones. For example, the belief that I have a brain tumour may be distressing in itself but if it accounts for my doing poorly at school, not getting a job, partner, nice home, etc., then it is also protecting me from attributing my situation to some 'failure' within myself.

2. Consider the possibility of a total modification

The most important question is whether the person would *want* to end up no longer believing their core delusional belief. If there are some significant advantages for the person in holding an otherwise dysfunctional delusional belief, you should consider whether these advantages could be replaced from elsewhere. For example, in the situations just considered would it be possible to change my beliefs about not having a job, family, etc. so that I no longer saw this as failure? If this were possible, then the total modification could go ahead when this had been done.

3. What replacement beliefs are feasible?

The replacement belief must (a) make sense to the person concerned, and (b) be viable in fact, so that subsequent events and experiences do not undermine it but rather support and strengthen it. These will be crucial factors in determining what replacement belief(s) are feasible in the individual case, and in practice can mean that there is only one viable option.

4. Which is the most functional replacement belief?

If there is more than one possible replacement belief, or more than one way of presenting and describing it, consider the positive and negative aspects of each option. Consider the wider implications of the total goal under consideration, both positive and negative, and whether the positive effects of the total modification significantly outweigh the negative. Consider also any possible adverse knock-on effects from the modification. For example, you may have set the replacement belief for 'The voices come from my father' to 'The voices are my own thoughts, triggered by memories of my father' because a mental illness explanation is abhorrent to the person, but is it possible that they will go a step further and conclude that this must mean the doctor was right after all when he diagnosed schizophrenia?

5. Is the replacement belief available and acceptable to the person now? How long is the preparation work likely to take?

If the replacement belief is not acceptable, it may take a lot of work and time to make it acceptable: consider whether and how this would be done.

It is a reality of clinical practice that we do not have unlimited time to work with individual people. Therefore, an important decision to make when goal setting is 'Do I have the time to prepare the replacement for a total modification?' and 'Do the advantages of the total modification over a partial modification warrant the extra time needed to achieve it?'

6. Consider what possible partial modifications there are
At this stage you should consider all the partial modifications that are potentially possible before eliminating those that would clearly not be of benefit. Then consider in more detail the positives and negatives of each remaining option. You do not have to decide between partial goals. As you can proceed with more than one you just have to decide whether or not each partial modification would be beneficial.

7. Decide on the goals to be used
Bearing in mind the relative advantages and disadvantages of the total and partial goal options for this particular individual, and the different ways in which partial goals can be used (see above), you should specify what appear to be the most beneficial goals and a provisional order in which you would tackle them. The questions you are likely to be considering include: Would the total modification be the best modification, if it could be achieved? Which of the partial goals would be useful as stepping stones towards a total modification? If there are significant disadvantages for a total modification, would a partial modification be helpful? If a partial modification is being used, which bits of the delusional belief should stay intact? Are the new beliefs compatible with the parts of the belief system that are to be left intact? Could the modification have unwanted knock-on effects?

As the therapist, it is your job to consider and weigh up all these factors from the CBT perspective, but before making the final decision about which goal(s) to use you should check with the person themself, as far as is possible, using language that does not constitute a challenge to their beliefs.

CASE STUDY JANE

(See also pp. 76, 99, 136, 143, 188 and 277.)

Belief: *I am an evil witch.*

Immediate goal: *Reduce the distress caused by the belief using simple coping strategies.*

Possible goals for a total modification:

I am not an evil witch + these thoughts and feelings are due to my schizophrenia.

OR

I am not an evil witch + (explanation based on psychological case formulation).

A replacement belief in terms of being ill with schizophrenia was available and already acceptable to Jane, and therefore was considered to be the easiest one to use. Towards the very end of therapy, when the delusion had been removed, we did go on to explain at the cognitive level why her illness might have caused her to develop this particular delusional belief. This was done (a) to make the illness more understandable and as such less frightening, and (b) in the hope that this level of understanding would help her in the future, should similar symptoms recur.

If an illness-based replacement belief had been unacceptable, then we would have tried to develop an alternative one that linked the onset of her delusion to the feelings and stress she had had at that time, and used the cognitive model to explain why it had been maintained.

Possible goals for partial modification(s):
I am an evil witch **but** *I am not responsible for the war in Iraq.*
I am an evil witch **but** *I am not responsible for . . . (the other named world disasters)*
I am an evil witch **but** *I cannot change the weather.*
I am an evil witch **but** *other people cannot see that I am.*
I am a witch **but** *I am not evil.*

Being able to change the weather might have been a positive thing for Jane, but because it was secondary to the core belief 'I am a witch' it would not have been possible to set the partial goal 'I can change the weather *but* I am not a witch' even if we had wanted to, because eliminating the core belief would also have eliminated her belief about the weather.

In practice being able to change the weather was just something that Jane had noticed she could do 'sometimes'. Since she could not change it for the better, there were no positives for her in this.

TOTAL OR PARTIAL GOAL?

The following lines of questions were used to check out the acceptability of both the parts of the total goal:

What are the worst things about being a witch?
I feel so guilty about all the terrible things that are happening in the world – I don't want to cause people such unhappiness.

What was it like before you were a witch?
It was much better – I didn't have these awful feelings of guilt.

If you could go back to **not** *being a witch, would you want to do that?*
Yes, definitely.

I realize that it is mostly bad, but is there anything at all you would miss if you weren't a witch?
No, there's nothing at all.

What about being able to change the weather? That sounds as if it would be a nice thing to be able to do.

It would be nice if I could make the weather good, but I tried that and I can't do it, I only make it bad.

A lot of people might think that **having** *the special powers could feel quite good in a way, even if they didn't like what the powers were actually* **doing.** *What do you think?*
I don't like having these powers because they just do bad things – I dread hearing about what I've done.

I know that you've talked to Dr Smith about this; what does he say?
He says it's another symptom of my schizophrenia, but I know this is different because I'm taking my medication regularly so I'm not ill any more.

Do you wish he was right when he said that?
Yes, because then I'd know I wouldn't have to worry about the power, and people wouldn't dislike me and be rude to me any more.

Since the core belief about being a witch was very distressing and there were no positive gains from any aspect of the belief, the total goal was the goal of choice. We would only have considered a partial modification in this case if gains from the ability to change the weather and/or having the special status and power implied by the delusion had outweighed the negative aspects of the belief. In this case, the decision was an easy one because there were no positives aspects to any part of the belief.

If we had not been able to find or prepare an acceptable replacement belief, then we would have had to settle for a partial modification. Note that as each of the partial modifications identified in this case removes part of the evidence on which the core delusion is based, it would not have been safe to attempt them all if we had wanted to avoid bringing about a total modification. In this case, we would have gone only for the aspect that was the most distressing to her, namely that others were able to see she was a witch.

Goal selected (total modification):
I am not an evil witch + these thoughts and feelings are due to my schizophrenia

---

CASE STUDY STEPHEN

(See also pp. 78 and 192.)

Belief: *I get messages from a spirit guide via sounds in the environment.*[5]

Possible goals for a total modification:
I do not get messages from my spirit guide + replacement belief.

The main problem with a total goal in this case was that the delusional belief provided a lot of positives for Stephen and was generally very functional for him.

[5]Stephen was not distressed by his belief, so in this case it would have been inappropriate to consider controlling the effects of the belief using practical coping strategies.

Furthermore, the fact of getting the messages had been of central importance to his life for many years. A total modification was ruled out on these grounds, so it was not necessary to go on to consider possible replacement beliefs.

Possible partial goals:
I used to get messages from my spirit guide ***but*** *I no longer get them.*
I get messages from my spirit guide ***but*** *he can make mistakes.*
I get messages from my spirit guide ***but*** *I can make a mistake in interpreting them because . . .*

When the first possible partial goal was checked out with Stephen by asking him what it would be like for him if the spirit guide stopped sending him messages, he said that he would be devastated and life would not be worth living. This partial goal was immediately abandoned. Furthermore, we advised the rest of the care team of the potentially disastrous effects should a medication ever be found that removed this delusion.[6]

The notion of a mistake being made somewhere in the act of sending or receiving the messages was considered to be a functional modification in this case because if it was possible to introduce the possibility of some doubt about the messages' absolute authority, then it would be appropriate to suggest there could have been a mistake about a particular issue, for example the benefits of medication, and, therefore, that it was appropriate for Stephen to listen to other points of view as well.

When the possibility of the spirit guide making a mistake was floated to Stephen, he reacted very strongly, saying that his spirit guide could never make a mistake because of who he was. Therefore, this form of the partial goal was clearly unacceptable and was not pursued.

Stephen had already acknowledged that he could make mistakes in noisy surroundings, so the possibility of making mistakes was acceptable to him. The problem with this partial goal was the very real risk that when it was proved that he could get it wrong in quiet places as well as noisy ones, then Stephen would conclude that the only possible reason for this was that no messages were being sent. For many years he had been told by other people that they did not believe he was getting messages and so this 'no messages' explanation for being mistaken would have been readily available to him, as well as being very damaging.

The solution lay in finding a good reason why he could make mistakes sometimes, even in apparently quiet surroundings, which did not undermine the core delusional belief. One possibility was around the interval between the sounds, i.e. the difficulty in knowing whether two sounds comprised a single unit, meaning 'no', or were two separate 'yeses'. However, there was a potential weakness in using this reason as the basis of doubt because it would have been difficult to challenge a 'no' response based

[6]Over the years that I knew Stephen many different medications were tried and some proved very helpful, but this particular belief was never affected. Perhaps it was not delusional.

on two sounds occurring close together. Since Stephen freely acknowledged he could make mistakes when there were other noises around, another possible reason for doubt was that no place is entirely quiet so there must always be the possibility of other noises intruding, or perhaps going unnoticed by Stephen, and that this meant that he could never be 100% sure he had detected the answer accurately. When suggested, this was entirely acceptable to him and so this was the partial goal used in practice.

Goal selected: (partial modification)
I get messages from my spirit guide ***but*** *I can make a mistake in interpreting them because there are always faint noises around, even in quiet places, so I could miss one of these.*

IN WHAT ORDER SHOULD THE GOALS BE TACKLED?

Primary and secondary beliefs

Some aspects of a delusional belief or belief system may be more important than others. For example, I may believe that I am an archangel and *therefore* that I must have great spiritual powers, or I may believe that I have greater spiritual powers and *therefore* that I must be an archangel. The belief 'I am an archangel' is the primary or core belief in the first case but it is secondary to the belief about spiritual powers in the second case. Removing the primary belief removes the secondary beliefs; removing the secondary beliefs may weaken the primary belief but it does not necessarily eliminate it. Usually CBT proceeds by targeting the secondary beliefs before moving on to the primary belief. In some cases, removing the secondary beliefs weakens the primary belief so much that it collapses without any direct attack; it is not always necessary to remove all the secondary beliefs before this happens.

Some secondary beliefs will be more important to the integrity of the primary belief than others. For example, I may believe that I am an archangel and that this is why I have great spiritual powers and why I look so serene. Removing my belief that I look serene will have less impact on my core belief about being an archangel than removing my belief that I have great spiritual powers. This is because, according to my beliefs about them, archangels must have great spiritual powers in order to be archangels but they need not necessarily look serene all the time.

CASE STUDY **JANE**

(See also pp. 76, 95, 136, 143, 188 and 277.)

In this case, 'I am a witch' is the primary, core delusion because Jane could have been a witch *even if* she were not responsible for the war in Iraq and could not change the weather, and *even if* other people did not recognize her as a witch.

With respect to the relative importance of the secondary beliefs in providing support for the primary belief, perhaps somewhat surprisingly, being able to change the weather and other people recognizing her as a witch were at least as important as her being responsible for the atrocities in Iraq. This was probably because, although the war atrocities were more impressive features of being an evil witch, the evidence she had for the other two secondary beliefs seemed more convincing to her.

In practice it is usually apparent which the core delusional beliefs are without having to think of it in these terms. However, when planning the order of therapy it is important to consider the relative importance of the different aspects of a delusional belief.

It is also important for the overall treatment plan to consider whether hallucinations and/or other psychotic experiences are having an effect on the delusional belief and, if so, which parts are 'driving' which other parts. For example, a woman hears voices saying that the neighbour upstairs is practising voodoo on her. Are the voices no more than a statement of her delusional belief, or are the voices the *reason* why she believes the voodoo is taking place? Or is it a bit of both?

Where there are multiple delusional beliefs

When there is more than one core delusional belief or system, it makes sense to start with the less strongly held beliefs because these will be easier to work with, and the person will get experience of the CBT approach and strategies used before moving on to harder-to-shift beliefs. However, in practice this consideration is likely to be overridden by the need to focus on whatever the person themself wants to focus on, which is likely to be whatever is causing them most distress and difficulty.

ADAPTING THE GOAL AS TREATMENT PROGRESSES

Although you should not start to modify a delusion until you have specified the end goal towards which you are working, and any intermediate goals that you may need to reach in between, you may need to change these goals during therapy. We have seen above that it may be necessary to change from a total to a partial modification goal if it turns out not to be possible in practice to achieve the total modification. Another situation that may arise that makes it necessary to review the goal is where the person gives you some new information that suggests the 'ideal' goal is not ideal after all. For example, it may emerge that there are previously unsuspected advantages for the person in holding certain aspects of their belief, or that the new goal is incompatible with some deeply held, non-psychotic belief. In these circumstances you should not hesitate to change the goal of treatment to a more appropriate one.

6 Preparing for the belief modification

PREPARING FOR THE NEGATION OF THE DELUSIONAL BELIEF

Being convinced that something is so does not mean that it is so

We have already noted that an inherent problem with delusional beliefs as far as engaging in therapy is concerned is that they are experienced as being self-evidently true, and that as human beings we are predisposed not to doubt what we believe to be 'fact'. Therefore, an essential part of the preparation for a belief of modification is to establish that *it is possible to be wrong about something even though we are* ***certain*** *that it is correct*.

The second aspect of this line of preparation is to normalize (a) having inaccurate beliefs, and (b) changing beliefs in the light of new evidence. The main reason for doing this normalization work is to enable people to change their delusional beliefs without feeling that they must have been odd or stupid to have held these beliefs in the first place. As a general rule, the more important a belief is to us, the more firmly we hold on to it and the more vigorously we have defended it in the past, the harder it is for us to admit that we were wrong in that belief. Delusional beliefs are commonly of this type, so where the person has invested time and energy in maintaining and defending their delusional belief it is particularly necessary to ensure that they can change this belief without feeling loss of face or lowered self-esteem.

One or more of the following approaches may help to demonstrate and normalize the fact that being convinced that something is so does not necessarily mean that it is so, and that our brains can give us misleading information about how things really are. They also illustrate how common it is for all of us to change our minds about things.

Misinterpretation of everyday events

We all can and do misinterpret events that happen in our everyday lives. Misinterpretation can occur at a perceptual level, resulting in misperception, or further along in the processing, at the level of event evaluation, as the following examples show:

- I hear my next-door neighbours having a furious row but later discover it was a television programme they were watching.
- I overhear my friends criticizing my new hairstyle but later discover they were discussing someone else.

- I pull my hand away sharply as an insect lands on it, but it is only a leaf.
- I interpret the pain in my chest as a massive heart attack, but later realize it must have been indigestion.
- I am upset because my friend forgot to send me a birthday card, but I later discover that it was actually sitting in a postbox because of a strike.
- I think that my daughter has done very well to get a grade 1 in her maths exam, until she tells me that the usual way of marking is reversed and 9 is the top grade.
- I clearly remember putting my purse in my handbag, but it turns up on the kitchen table.

These examples may seem very obvious and unremarkable but this makes them all the more useful in demonstrating that it is really quite common for us to be misled in our interpretation of events and situations, and that believing something to be so does not necessarily mean that it is so. To destigmatize these 'errors' and make them relevant to the person you are working with, you should share any of your own experiences of this sort and also encourage them to recall any of theirs from everyday life.

Beliefs that are no longer held to be true

Discussing beliefs that have been held in the past but are no longer believed to be true is another way of demonstrating that believing something to be so does not guarantee that it is true. Furthermore, it normalizes the holding of inaccurate beliefs and the changing of beliefs.

1. Beliefs held in history

These beliefs are useful in demonstrating that a belief can be wrong even though large numbers of people believe it. There are very many examples you could use, including:

- The world is flat.
- A large number of illnesses can be cured by blood letting.
- If someone is thrown into a pond and floats, this proves they are a witch.
- Slavery is morally acceptable.
- Smoking is good for your health.

2. Beliefs held in everyday life

If you are comfortable with sharing some of your own former beliefs, then this will help to normalize not only holding inaccurate beliefs but also changing them in the light of new evidence or a different way of looking at them. Some examples from people attending CBT workshops are:

- Father Christmas visits each year with a sackful of toys.
- John Lennon was the most attractive man ever born.
- The Turin Shroud was Jesus' burial cloth.
- My partner will never leave me and go off with someone else.

- I will never feel happy again now that my partner has left me.
- I'm a better driver drunk than I am sober.
- You can pick up VD from lavatory seats.
- Argyll is in Northern Ireland.

3. Beliefs now recognized as 'delusions'
If someone with psychosis recognizes that a belief they held in the past was a delusion, then this will provide very useful evidence not only that their brain is capable of holding inaccurate beliefs but also that their sense of conviction in a belief can be totally misleading. Such recognition may also provide a rationale for suggesting that other currently held beliefs might also be delusional, and therefore that it could be worth checking them out, using rational reasoning rather than relying on strength of conviction.

Misperception at a physiological level

Sensory misperceptions are useful for demonstrating (a) that our brain is capable of misperceiving things and misleading us about how things really are in the world, and (b) that it can continue to do so even when we know rationally that it is not so. This strand of work is particularly pertinent to understanding the nature of hallucinations and so has been included in detail in Chapter 12 (see pp. 235–237).

Use of dream analogy

Dreams are totally convincing whilst they are happening and any inconsistencies, illogicalities, etc. are not appreciated until after waking. Therefore, this may be used to demonstrate that even if something *seems* to be obviously and evidently true, this does not necessarily mean that it *is* true. Furthermore, it is very rare for any of us to be aware that we are dreaming, or to question the bizarre things that are going on in the dream, but we do not think of ourselves as odd or stupid because of this – it is just how our brains work. So, similarly, people should not feel stupid because their brains[1] failed to detect at the time that their psychotic experiences were abnormal or that their thinking appeared to defy reason.

REPLACING THE POSITIVE ASPECTS OF THE DELUSIONAL BELIEF

In nearly all cases where the goal of choice is a total modification, the person themself would prefer their delusional belief *not* to be true, so in this respect it is not essential to prepare them for the negation of this belief. However, even if there is an overall gain associated with the modification, there may be some positive aspects of the delusional belief that will be lost. Where this is the case, you should consider whether you can replace these benefits from another source.

[1]Blaming 'the brain' for dysfunctional experiences, beliefs and thoughts can be a useful therapeutic strategy as it may help to prevent people blaming themselves for things that they cannot control and protect them from consequent feelings of stupidity, shame or guilt.

For example, a man was frightened by his belief that he was being targeted by the Mafia because of his artistic abilities and potential to make a lot of money from them, but the belief also gave him a sense of personal importance. Therefore, attempts were made to attach his sense of worth and importance to other of his attributes, and to modify his beliefs about what constitutes an 'important' person.

In the rare exception, the person themself may be quite happy with their delusional belief but it causes such problems for other people and indirectly for themself that a total modification is the goal of choice. For example, if someone believed they had the right to attack people in the street because they were an avenging angel sent by God, then the consequences for the person as well as for their innocent victims would be too great to allow the belief to remain unchanged, even if the person themself obtained a great sense of status and satisfaction from the belief. Ideally, in this sort of circumstance you should attempt to replace some of the positive aspects of the delusional belief before you start the modification. However, in practice, if you are involved with this sort of modification it is likely to be because there are significant risks associated with the behavioural consequences of the belief, for example risk of a serious assault, and so for this reason you may have to proceed quickly with the modification before this aspect of the preparation can be done. In that case you would work to re-establish the positives in some other way, as far as that were possible, whilst the modification work was in progress.

PREPARING FOR THE REPLACEMENT BELIEF OF A TOTAL GOAL

GENERAL CONSIDERATIONS

There are two principal aspects of working with replacement beliefs:

1 *To provide any information that is necessary in order for the person to understand the alternative explanation being offered.* This is most likely to apply to replacement beliefs expressed in terms of normal brain functioning and those expressed in terms of psychological factors.
2 *To ensure that the alternative explanation is acceptable to the person and more functional than the delusional explanation.* This is most likely to apply to replacement beliefs expressed in terms of mental illness.

Preparation for the replacement belief may require both, one or neither of these lines of work, depending on the replacement belief being used and the person's current level of knowledge and understanding.

When it is necessary to use an illness-based replacement belief with someone who rejects this as a possibility, then it may take months (and months) of work before the person finds this acceptable.[2] However, on a more positive note, once

[2]It is not always possible to achieve this goal.

a replacement belief is acceptable and preferred to the delusional belief, then the modification work as such is usually relatively quick and easy, especially if the delusional belief provides no or only minor benefit.

Introducing the replacement belief

The information that may be required for the different replacement beliefs is described in later sections of this chapter.

How you make the new information available to the person will depend on how welcome it is. Unwelcome information is usually associated with the illness explanations because of the stigma attached and the implications for the person's life. As we saw in Chapter 3, the gentlest and safest way of introducing new ideas is to float them, to see what reaction they provoke before making any suggestion that they might apply to the person's own case. The downside of this approach for giving information is that it can be very slow, not least because a key feature of floating ideas is not to dwell on the topic for any longer than would be appropriate for just a casual interest. If the new information constitutes a potential challenge to the delusional belief, then it is better if it can be given in small amounts, as and when the opportunity occurs during therapy, and going into only as much detail as the person wants or shows interest in.

If the information has only positives for the person, then there is no need to be reticent about proposing it. The only precaution you would need to take in this case would be to ensure that the person does not feel ignorant or stupid for not already knowing the facts you are describing. One way of doing this is to present the information as expert or technical knowledge, or as a recent discovery. Useful phrases include: 'A lot of people think ... though actually ...'; 'Doctors used to think ... but now ...'; 'One of the things psychology has recently discovered is that ...' , 'It's really interesting what scientists have found ...', 'Have you come across ...?', etc.

When giving information, it is advisable to check from time to time to make sure that the person has not picked up some distorted version of what you have tried to tell them. Some of the ideas are really quite complex; furthermore, it is easy to forget that we have become so familiar with words and ways of conceptualizing things through our professional training that what seems to us to be basic, shared human knowledge may well not be.

We also need to bear in mind that we are particularly likely to give confusing messages if we are not too sure of the facts ourselves. Because it is important that you do not convey a distorted or confused understanding of the alternative explanation for the delusional belief it is very important that you are clear in your own mind before you attempt to pass it on. If other members of the team are likely to discuss this with the person, then it is helpful if you brief them about the model or explanation you are using as well, to avoid confusion and ensure consistency.

When to introduce the replacement belief

It is a basic principle of CBT that it is better for someone to make the connections between facts for themself than to be told what these are. So where it is appropriate and possible, you would ensure that the person has the necessary information to come to the desired conclusion and then wait until they do so. However, it is often the case that you will not be able to make the information relevant to the person's particular situation without suggesting that this could or does explain what has been going on for them.

The approach of providing the information and waiting for the person themself to arrive at the desired conclusion is most likely to apply to the illness-based alternatives. The more closely you relate the information you give to the person's own situation, the more likely you are to cause them to conclude that you are suggesting or saying that this is what has been happening to them. Whether or not you wait until the illness-based alternative is fully accepted before you start on the strategies to modify the delusional belief itself is a matter of clinical judgement. It is quite common to be doing the general destigmatization work at the same time as starting to challenge the delusional belief, though you must be careful to ensure that the person is ready for the illness understanding before the modification programme causes the delusion to be negated. In clinical practice this timing is not such a difficult balancing act as it may sound, because while the alternative explanation is still an unattractive one it is unlikely that the person will be willing to engage in work that forces them to accept it.[3]

The non-stigmatizing replacement beliefs expressed in terms of oversensitive or overactive brain function are often introduced at the stage of the modification programme where the person is beginning to consider the possibility that their delusional belief might be wrong, and therefore is looking for other possible alternative explanations. But, as with illness-based alternatives, there is no firm guidance that can be given about this timing because it depends on the circumstances of the individual case and as such it must be a matter of clinical judgement.

The detailed psychological-based explanations are usually given in addition to one of the other replacement beliefs, in order to increase the person's understanding of what has happened in the past and what is happening now, so when used for this purpose, the information is typically given after the delusional belief has been negated. However, here also there is no hard and fast rule, because for some people it is the presentation of this possible alternative way of understanding things that brings about the negation of the delusional belief.

Fortunately, this is one aspect of the therapy that is much easier to do in practice than it is to describe in writing. The guiding principle to always keep in mind are the questions '*Will this person be better off if they accept this piece of information or explanation that I am offering?*' and '*Are they ready for this now, or would it be more acceptable if I said/did ... first?*'. The answers to these questions will help to guide you as to when to introduce and suggest the replacement belief.

[3]This is another example of when the 'be prepared to back off' maxim ensures safe practice.

Sharing the case formulation

The more someone understands about the development and maintenance of their delusional belief, the more stable the replacement belief will be and the better the chance that they will be able to recognize the delusional ideas or experiences and counter them should they recur in the future. After all if, for example, you feel that someone is trying to harm you, it is not unreasonable to suppose that the most likely explanation for this feeling is that someone really *is* trying to harm you. So when the feeling that someone wanted to harm you came on you again, you would need to have a very solid alternative explanation for feeling this way to outweigh the more obvious and straightforward interpretation, namely that it was true.

It is not necessary to present all of your case formulation, which may be very complex, just the relevant parts. Be careful not to overcomplicate it in your enthusiasm to be accurate and to include all the aspects. You can always expand and elaborate the explanations later, if the person wants that, once they have fully understood the simpler version. Remember that we use these concepts as second nature because we are so familiar with them, but other people will not be.

It is likely that your case formulation will contain parts that are speculation that you have not been able to confirm, so when offering an alternative explanation for a delusional belief, you should always make very clear that this is only one possible explanation of how the belief might have developed. If the person gives more information during your discussion of the case formulation, then you would, of course, change the formulation accordingly. Whether or not your speculation is correct in all particulars may not matter; the important thing is that it is reasonable, seems plausible to the person concerned, and is a helpful way of understanding things. A principal aim of this part of the work is to anchor the person in the objective, matter-of-fact world by showing them that it is perfectly possible to explain their beliefs and experiences in terms of the way they or their brains have misinterpreted ordinary events, that it is not necessary to resort to unlikely or esoteric explanations to account for them.

Moving from the intended replacement belief on to another replacement belief

Even if you are at pains to avoid using the labels 'psychosis', 'mania', 'schizophrenia', etc., you must consider the very real possibility that the person themself will conclude from the 'brain' explanation you are giving that this means they have psychosis, etc., especially as probably many people, including family and mental health professionals, will already have used these terms to describe their situation. Similarly, your case formulation may necessarily include or may imply the occurrence of abnormal subjective experiences, and this in turn may lead the person to question or conclude that they have something wrong with their brain and/or have a mental illness/psychosis. Where there is a significant risk that the person will move from the intended replacement belief to a psychiatric one you should prepare them for the possible illness/psychosis understanding as well. For example, if someone had the experience of thought withdrawal, you might set the replacement belief as 'mental illness', in which case you would have to change the person's negative views of mental illness. Alternatively, you might try to use something along the lines of 'Sometimes I lose the thread of my thoughts but my brain is not immediately aware of what has happened so it feels as if they have been taken away from outside', but in that case you would have to ensure that this explanation was a sensible and persuasive one for the person concerned, and that it did not have negative connotations for them. Furthermore, if there was a risk they would go on to ask 'But why does my brain do this?' or 'Does this mean that the doctor was right when she said I had schizophrenia?', then you would need to 'prepare' them in advance for the answers to these questions.

REPLACEMENT BELIEFS IN TERMS OF MENTAL ILLNESS/PSYCHOSIS/SCHIZOPHRENIA ('INSIGHT' PROMOTION)[4]

The person's psychotic subjective experiences will often be so abnormal that you cannot avoid using the notions of psychosis to explain them. Furthermore, the fact that other people have used the terminology of the medical model when talking to them about their experiences will increase the likelihood that this is the only viable replacement belief for a total modification. In practice, then, this is often the type of replacement belief that you will be trying to make acceptable. Unfortunately, doing this is a lot easier to describe on paper than it is to carry out in practice.

Decatastrophizing the diagnosis: destigmatizing and normalizing the symptoms and illness labels

Most of the general public have a poor understanding of mental illness in general, and of psychosis and schizophrenia in particular. Therefore, it should not be surprising if the people we are working with also hold some inaccurate or distorted beliefs, or fear the implications of such a diagnosis, so that they react adversely or even catastrophically to the suggestion that this diagnosis might apply to them. For example, one man claimed that he could not have schizophrenia because he did not think he was someone else, whilst another knew that he did not have schizophrenia because he did not hear voices. Someone else was terrified on being told she had schizophrenia because she thought this meant that she could go berserk at any time and kill someone without warning.

The CBT approach to altering this negative reaction involves correcting misunderstandings and increasing knowledge within a normalizing framework. 'Normalization' in this context means conceptualizing and understanding the psychotic beliefs and experiences as being similar to normal experiences, as differing from normal experiences in degree rather than type. The aim of this work is to help people to understand that having psychosis does not mean they

[4]The term *insight promotion* is used in this practice manual as a convenient shorthand for 'modifying the person's way of conceptualizing their experiences/illness so that it conforms to the medical model'. The word 'insight' is problematic if it is taken to imply that this is 'the truth': no such implication is intended when the term is used here.

are essentially different or set apart from 'normal' people, and furthermore that it is nothing to be ashamed or afraid of.

The stigma attached to the labels 'psychosis', 'mania' and 'schizophrenia' can be a difficult problem to deal with because it is unfortunately true that a large proportion of the general public does have inaccurate and negative views of what these terms mean, often fearing that they imply irrational behaviour and unprovoked violence, so there is very real prejudice against people who have these diagnoses. In these circumstances the destigmatizing work aims to correct, develop and strengthen the person's own awareness of what the term actually implies, with particular reference to their own case and symptoms, so that these more positive beliefs about themself are strong enough to counter and reject the misinformed beliefs of others. The work also aims to strengthen their understanding that the negative beliefs and attitudes of misinformed others are based on ignorance and are less accurate and knowledgeable than their own. Taking the role of 'expert' with respect to their own illness may help to protect the person's self-esteem against the prejudices of others, and to protect their own beliefs from being undermined by the inaccurate beliefs of others around them.

Although it is not possible to change the beliefs of the general public at large, it can be very helpful to work with the immediate family and/or carers in order to modify any misconceptions they may have about the person's diagnosis and what that implies for him or her and for them. Not only does this usually result in their adopting a more favourable attitude towards their family member but it also helps to reinforce and support the person's own knowledge about their illness.

Modifying people's attitudes to a psychotic illness is made harder by the fact that the end goal is for them to hold a different attitude and understanding about the illness from that held by the general public, so there is always the tendency for this latter to conflict with, or even to reverse, the beneficial changes being made. There is also the sad fact that even though the person themself and their carers may come to regard psychosis and schizophrenia as nothing to be ashamed or afraid of, they may still be subjected to the ignorance and prejudice of some people in the community and suffer accordingly.

The therapist's positive attitude towards the person, and his or her acceptance of them and their beliefs and experiences, can play a major part in destigmatizing the notion of 'psychosis/schizophrenia' and making it less dramatic and alarming. One or more of the following strategies for normalizing and destigmatizing the symptoms may be helpful.

Sharing experiences of 'odd ideas'

The main purpose of this exercise is for you to share with the other person any abnormal experiences you may have had in order to demonstrate that having 'strange' experiences and ideas is actually quite normal, and therefore that the person is not 'odd' or 'peculiar' because they have them. You should, of course, acknowledge that the psychotic person's experiences are probably more intense and disturbing than yours, but the point is that they are different in intensity and effect rather than in kind. Sharing experiences not only demonstrates that it is normal to get strange ideas or feelings from time to time but it also supports the key understanding that feeling something to be so does not necessarily mean that it is so. It may be helpful to share not only your own ideas and experiences but also those reported by other non-psychotic people. Given below are just some of the experiences reported by mental health workers on our CBT courses who have agreed that they may be shared with other people:

- Entering a party and thinking that people had stopped their conversation in order to look at me.
- A sudden panicky feeling that I was about to recover a 'lost memory' of having killed someone.
- A conviction that the woman on the other side of the street was my mother, who had died recently; it was so convincing that I followed her for several blocks.
- Feeling convinced that other people in the room could read my mind.
- Feeling sure that the plane would crash (which it didn't).
- Swimming in the sea and suddenly feeling that I could control the waves.
- Fearing that my partner had left me on my own in the house because he had arranged for me to be murdered by a 'burglar'.
- Thinking that the car behind must be following me.

Since you are attempting to destigmatize mental illness, ideally you would share your odd experiences without hastening to explain them away (e.g. 'I was very tired' or 'I hadn't eaten for 18 hours when that happened'); after all, the main purpose of the exercise is to demonstrate that the person with psychosis is not quintessentially different from you because they have strange ideas and experiences. And bearing the purpose of the exercise in mind, the more psychotic-like the experiences that you share the better! Whilst you should not feel under pressure to share a personal experience if you would feel uncomfortable in doing so, it may shed some light on your own beliefs about the stigma of psychosis if you consider why you feel uncomfortable in doing so. Are you ashamed or worried about having had the experiences? Do you think, perhaps, that others would look down on you, or think you were odd or peculiar? Are you concerned that other people might think this was a sign of madness? Or tell others behind your back? And if they did, why would that matter?

Discussing the factors that increase vulnerability to 'odd ideas'

Discussing the circumstances in which delusions or odd ideas are more likely to occur in non-psychotic people helps to normalize the phenomenon by showing that, given the necessary conditions, anyone's brain can produce these psychotic-type experiences. Put another way, it demonstrates that anyone can get psychotic-type experiences as a result of their brain not functioning properly.

People with psychosis are often able to make a connection between the factors that increase the brain's tendency to produce odd ideas and the circumstances in their own lives when they were experiencing the strange feelings, happenings and thoughts. For example, they may recall being unable to sleep or eat properly, or being agitated or under stress, before their strange experience, or before their relative called the doctor and they were admitted to hospital. Although attributing the symptoms to tiredness or stress is not entirely accurate, since it is probable that the tiredness and stress are caused by the same illness that also causes the delusions, nevertheless it can be a very helpful intermediate step on the way to insight (see 'Partial insight', p. 128) as it does enable the person to recognize their experiences as abnormal, and also to explain them in terms of some physiological cause.

In non-psychotic people delusions and hallucinations are more likely to occur:

- in traumatic situations, for example being held hostage
- where there is sensory deprivation, for example solitary confinement
- when deprived of sleep, food or water
- when physically ill with a high temperature
- in circumstances of high or prolonged anxiety or stress
- when under the influence of street drugs or alcohol
- when depressed.

In conditions of extreme sensory deprivation, where the body is suspended in water at body temperature, unable to see or hear anything except white light and white noise, and unable to touch anything, the brain can produce full-blown psychotic experiences, including hallucinations and delusional ideas, within the first few hours. Most people's brains will produce psychotic symptoms if they are completely deprived of sleep for several days. These are useful illustrations to indicate that it is really quite easy to tip the brain into this state. Indeed, our brains produce psychotic-type experiences every night, when we dream.

Delusions as intuitive thinking

When talking with people about their delusions, it can be very helpful to liken their delusional beliefs to intuitions, because intuitions are very normal occurrences that can and do happen to all of us. Intuitions are very similar to delusional ideas in that they can be based on very little, or no, objective evidence and yet they carry with them their own sense of conviction and certainty. Intuitions are also very similar to delusions in that, although they can be accurate representations of reality, they are more often inaccurate and can be completely wrong, despite their feeling of absolute correctness.

Discussing the meaning and implications of the terms 'psychosis', 'schizophrenia', 'delusions', 'hallucinations', etc.[5]

The information that you give about psychosis and/or schizophrenia, and the way that you give it, will depend on the person's present level of understanding about

[5]Whether you discuss and use the terms 'psychosis' and/or 'schizophrenia' will depend on how the diagnosis has been expressed and how this has been conveyed to the person concerned. For example, if someone who meets

their psychotic experiences; as a general rule, the better the level of insight, the more direct you can be in your discussions. It is important, therefore, that you ask questions to ascertain the person's knowledge of, and attitude towards, mental illness and psychosis/schizophrenia in general, as well as assessing level of insight about their own particular psychotic experiences. Some of the questions you could ask include:

- 'Why are you in hospital?' or 'Why has your doctor/nurse asked you to come to see me?', 'What does your doctor/nurse think is the problem?', 'Does he or she say you have an illness?', 'What is it called?', 'What does that mean?' 'Why does he or she say that?'
- 'How do you feel about that?, 'Would it be awful if you had ...? Why?', 'What would be the worst thing about that?'
- 'Do you know anyone with (psychosis/schizophrenia)?', 'How do you know he or she's got that?', 'Why does he or she (or the doctor) say that's what they've got?', 'How does he or she feel about that? Why do you think that is?'

Note that even if people are fluent in their use of psychiatric terminology to describe their situation, you cannot assume from this that they are using the words in exactly the same way you do, so you should be careful to check this out. For example, one woman talked freely about her schizophrenia but was shocked by the suggestion that this meant anything other than her being tired and unable to work. In another example, I had been working for over a year with a man who vehemently denied any mental illness despite having a long history of detention in hospital. When he started talking to other team members about his paranoid psychosis, we thought that my months of gentle destigmatization had paid off. However, when I checked out this most welcome insight, he told me the term meant that he was being persecuted by particular people.

Neutral questions of the type given above can also be used as a natural way of introducing the topic of psychosis into a session when you want to start the work of information giving and destigmatization.

If the person has an antagonistic attitude to the possibility of psychosis, then you should be prepared for this work to take many (many) sessions. As a general guide, introduce only one or two ideas at a time and only as much information as feels comfortable and natural as part of a topic of conversation that the other person may feel is of little interest or relevance for them. If they turn the conversation along a different tack, then go with this rather than persisting with your own agenda; you can always return to the topic on a future occasion. The art is to introduce the information as part of a general conversation and exchange of ideas about a topic of general interest. In the early stages it may be important not

the criteria for schizophrenia accepts the diagnosis of psychosis that they have been given but dislikes the term 'schizophrenia', then there is nothing to be gained by insisting they view their illness in terms of schizophrenia. On the other hand, if the person has been told they have schizophrenia, then it is the meaning and implications of this particular diagnosis that will have to be discussed. (See also Preface p. viii for note on terminology.)

to imply to the person that you believe they could have this illness, though later on in therapy you hope to be able to discuss what this would and does mean for them.

The information given

The model of psychosis that we use is the *stress-vulnerability model*, which says that psychosis occurs because of a vulnerability to develop the illness plus the stress from environmental factors that trigger the illness. According to this model, people differ in their vulnerability to psychosis because of innate biological differences in their brains. At one end of the continuum are those people who require little or no stress to set the illness off, whilst at the other end are those who would require very high levels to produce just some of the symptoms, with most people falling somewhere in between. The stress can be either mental (e.g. with major life events such as bereavement, divorce, new home and job) or physical (e.g. illness, drugs, isolation). This model provides a framework within which the brain can be seen to be responsible for producing the symptoms of the illness, and also prepares the way for the notion that medication may help by correcting the biochemical imbalances involved.

It is important to point out in your discussions that *psychosis is not a single illness* but is a general term used to cover a wide range of possible symptoms and severity levels, so that no two people with psychosis will be affected in exactly the same way. Indeed, it is possible to have two people with a diagnosis of schizophrenia or psychosis who have completely different sets of symptoms, and in one person the symptoms may be so mild that they do not interfere with everyday life at all whereas in another they may be persistent and disabling and require frequent hospital admissions.

When talking about psychosis, it will probably be helpful to concentrate on the person's own particular symptoms, taking care to point out that for them the diagnosis does not imply anything more than their particular experiences and symptoms. It does not mean that they will develop any of the other possible symptoms given in the textbooks or that other people with this diagnosis may have. You can give the reassurance that although their illness may recur in the future *the typical course of these illnesses is a fluctuating one rather than a progressive, worsening one*.

If the person holds prejudiced beliefs about psychosis, or has been the victim of prejudice in others, it may be worth making explicit that *psychosis is not a character or personality defect or weakness*, and furthermore, that this diagnosis does not mean the person concerned is 'mad' or 'weird', and it does not imply they may suddenly behave in a peculiar way or go berserk and make a violent attack on someone. *Unprovoked violence towards others is rare in psychosis*: the very large majority of early deaths associated with this group are the result of suicide, not murder or manslaughter. Non-psychotic young men between the ages of 18 and 26 are more likely to be physically violent towards someone else than someone with a diagnosis of schizophrenia or psychosis.

Anyone might go on to develop psychosis in the future, including the therapist and other members of the mental health team. If you take as an example someone that the person respects and admires now, then you can reason that their respect and admiration for this other person would be just as applicable *after* the other person developed psychosis as it is now, because they would still be the same essential person. It may be helpful to focus on particular people known to the person in this way because most people with psychosis seem to find it easier to see that developing psychosis would not demean someone they like and respect than to apply this to themselves.

Many people seem to treat the diagnosis of psychosis as if it described some core, essential part of the person concerned, as if the illness invaded and affected every part of that person. Because of this widely held attitude it may be reassuring to point out to the person that most of their brain and body still works perfectly normally, and it may be helpful to go through all the things that they still do just like everyone else. It may also be helpful to point out that, even though the effects on the person themself may be anything but minor, it is only a *relatively very small part* of their overall brain functioning that *sometimes* works inappropriately. As with all aspects of this work, you must be sensitive to whether this approach would be helpful for the individual concerned. For example, if their illness makes the person feel very different from how they were before, or if they are grieving for the loss of life's opportunities that the illness represents, then reassurance about what may, to them, seem unimportant areas of preserved functioning may be experienced as unempathic rather than reassuring. If the implication of having the illness is a significant source of distress, then CBT should be used to address these issues directly; this applies whether the perceived implications are accurate or whether they are exaggerated and catastrophized.

Seeing the positive side of psychosis

There are some potential positive aspects of the psychotic illness, including a depth and range of subjective experiences that most people will never know, and that can lead to artistic creativity and innovative, lateral thinking. Manic depression is particularly associated with creativity (see 'Famous people who have had psychosis', below). Some people with psychosis may also have a heightened sensitivity to, and awareness of, spiritual and mystical feelings and insights, which enriches their life.[6]

Although you should be sensitive not to imply 'It's really not that bad – look on the bright side', noting any positive aspects that may apply for the individual person can help to reduce their negative view of the illness and improve self-esteem. One woman I worked with had short periods each day when her psychosis became very active, producing some very strange experiences and ways of thinking about things. These periods were dominating her life and preventing her from getting out and continuing with her studies because she spent most of the time waiting for the next episode to occur. As she came to appreciate that

[6] The suggestion has been made that psychosis is the price we pay, as a species, for the evolutionary development of the parts of our brain that mediate our awareness of the spiritual side of life.

these were richly creative experiences, she lost her fear of them, and although she would have preferred not to have them, she was able to learn to live in the present moment, to experience the episodes for what they were and nothing more, and to carry on successfully with the rest of her life in between.

Famous people who have had psychosis
There are a number of web sites that have been set up to provide information for people with psychosis: the following names are just some of those reported on these sites.[7]

- John Nash (Nobel Prize winner, who was the subject of the film *A Beautiful Mind*)
- Vaslov Nijinsky (ballet dancer)
- Andy Goram (Scottish soccer player)
- Peter Green (guitarist for Fleetwood Mac)
- Syd Barrett (Pink Floyd)
- Mary Todd Lincoln (wife of the American president)
- Vincent van Gogh (artist)
- Virginia Woolf (novelist)
- Ludwig van Beethoven (music composer)
- Robert Schumann (poet)
- Isaac Newton (scientist).

REPLACEMENT BELIEFS IN TERMS OF 'MY BRAIN PRODUCES THESE EXPERIENCES' AND OVERSENSITIVITY/OVERACTIVITY OF THE BRAIN

If you are seeking to avoid psychiatric terminology and are going for a replacement belief couched in terms of 'brain function' instead, it is important to explain and normalize these explanations as far as possible in order to make them acceptable. Three possible replacement beliefs of this type are described below.

1. 'Part of my brain sometimes acts as if it were dreaming, even though I am awake'

Some people use the dream analogy to make sense of their psychotic experiences. 'Dreaming' is a very useful analogy for clinical work because everybody has experienced abnormal or bizarre events, perceptions, feelings, etc. in dreams, and so they are a very useful 'normal' equivalent of psychotic experiences. For example, one man used 'The dreaming part of my brain sometimes works when I am awake' as the replacement belief to account for the 'ghosts' that he saw. In another example, a woman who had very intense and convincing delusional memories learnt to recognize and label these as 'one of my waking dream experiences'.

[7] In some cases the diagnosis has been assumed from the symptoms displayed.

The 'dream' interpretation emphasizes the essential normality of these experiences because although it is not normal to experience such things when awake it is certainly normal to experience them whilst the brain is in sleep. Therefore, the person's brain is not weird or essentially different from other people's brains in being able to produce these strange experiences.

Another aspect of the dream analogy is that it can be used to reinforce the understanding that it is inappropriate to feel guilty or ashamed because of the delusional ideas or what the voices say. Almost without exception, the people we have worked with do not feel guilty about the content of their dreams, and so it can be argued that just as they are not responsible for the material produced by their brain during dreaming, neither are they responsible for what it produces during hallucinations or for the delusional ideas that come unbidden to their mind.[8]

2. The 2-route model

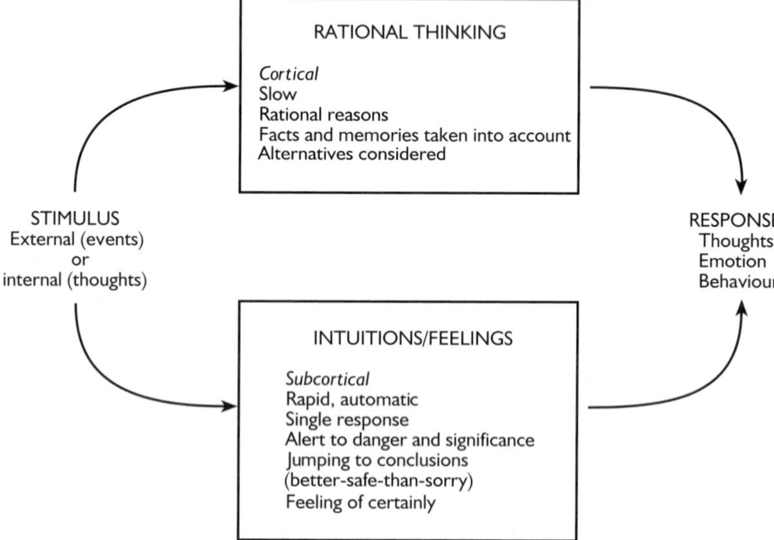

Figure 6.1 The 2-route model of responding.

The verbal explanation that you give to explain the diagram illustrated in Figure 6.1 can be adapted from the following:

'Our brain has two ways of responding to a situation. The lower route corresponds to the lower level, automatic responses that come from the parts of our

[8]Of course, if the person did believe their dreams reflected their inner thoughts and desires, then you could not use this particular line of argument unless and until you were able to modify this belief about dreams. The theory of dreams that we usually promulgate is that dreaming is the brain's way of clearing out all the remnants of the previous day's unwanted thoughts and perceptions, so although they are likely to reflect the person's interests and concerns they do not necessarily do so in any accurate way.

brain that are concerned with our more basic needs, including the detection of danger and significance. It is literally the 'lower' route since it involves the more primitive subcortical areas that sit in the centre of the brain. Because this route is concerned with our survival and well-being it has to be capable of responding quickly and so it is characterized by a single, rapid, all-or-nothing type of response. For this route, jumping to conclusions is a virtue, not a vice, because it enables fast, decisive conclusions to be drawn and action to be taken. Furthermore, it is geared to operate on a 'better-safe-than-sorry' principle since it is better to take protective action when there is no threat than to fail to take such action when a threat exists. In order to prompt rapid action the conclusion reached must feel as if it is absolutely correct; we cannot afford to dither about this sort of thing and so the conclusion is accompanied by a sense of certainty. If this sense of certainty is very strong, then the conclusion, reached without any conscious thought or awareness on the part of the person concerned, may be experienced subjectively as an intuition or 'gut feeling'.

The higher level route of responding uses the rational thinking abilities of the more advanced parts of our brain, situated in the cortex, which lies above the subcortex. Previous memories may be tapped as alternative interpretations are considered, and as alternative courses of action and the possible consequences of those actions are thought through. This route is able to handle probabilities and to weigh up the different options before coming to a final conclusion. Because of the greater range and depth of the thinking via this route it takes longer to respond but it will be more accurate in its reasoned analysis of the situation. We are consciously aware of much of the thinking that goes on in this route, and to a large extent we are able to control the direction it takes. It rarely comes to absolute conclusions so it does not give us a feeling of certainty about the conclusions it reaches.

In normal situations both routes of responding operate, the subcortical route producing a rapid response, which can be an action, thought and/or feeling, that is then tempered and modified by the slower rational thinking of the cortical route. An example to illustrate the use of the two routes of responding in everyday life is that of a woman who is walking along the road when she hears a loud bang from somewhere behind her. Her immediate response is to duck her head, put her arms up protectively and turn round – the rapid, immediate response of the subcortical route which has jumped to the conclusion that this may be a sign of danger. The slower but more thorough reasoning route will then evaluate the situation and consider possible options. For example, if the bang had come from an out-of-control car hitting a lamp post, then her likely considered response would be to take more effective protective action against the possible danger of being hit, perhaps by diving into a nearby garden, whereas if the bang had come from a workman knocking out the window of a house under repair, then her likely considered response would be to straighten up and carry on walking.'

This illustrative example can also be used to show how the person's beliefs, environment and innate instincts can influence the relative strengths of these two routes. For example, if the woman is walking through an area of town she believes to be dangerous because it is used by drug dealers, then she is likely to be more anxious and this will make her immediate 'danger response' stronger. Similarly, if the same incident happens on a lonely street after dark, when she is likely to be more vigilant, then here, too, her automatic danger response is likely to be stronger and she may consider more sinister explanations for the sound.

Use of the model in clinical practice

The 2-route model is a general model to describe how different parts of the brain are involved in determining responses to situations, and so when it is used to explain a symptom of psychosis it is non-stigmatizing and does not require the person to accept they have a mental illness. The model is not an alternative to the medical or stress-vulnerability models of psychosis because it focuses on only one aspect of the illness, but it can explain to people why they might *feel* convinced that something is true even though they have no apparent evidence to back it up, and why those feelings of certainty *could be incorrect*.

It also explains how CBT can help, namely by developing strategies to check whether the 'feelings' are accurate or not, i.e. whether they are an appropriate response to the external situation or the result of overactivity/oversensitivity of part of the brain. The strategies used for this purpose are very similar to those used for CBT with non-psychotic disorders, such as depression and anxiety, and essentially rely on the test *'If I cannot find any hard evidence to support my conclusion then it must [or 'might', or 'probably', etc.] have come from my brain rather than something that is actually happening'*.

The notion of hypersensitivity (some people use the terms 'supersensitivity' or 'oversensitivity') of the lower route may also provide a *rationale for taking medication* that does not require the person to accept they have a mental illness, for example 'The medication stops that part of my brain being oversensitive' or 'It brings the overactivity back to normal'. An example of this from clinical practice was a young man with whom I worked who vehemently denied he had an illness and had spent several years fighting against enforced medication. Having discussed the 2-route model and how that could apply to him, he agreed that his lower route must be hypersensitive, especially in alerting him to the possibility of danger even when there was none. He concluded that medication might be helpful in calming this route down and so willingly tried it for this purpose.

The 2-route model is particularly suitable and useful for *paranoid feelings and thoughts*. In this case, the explanation used is that the part of the lower route responsible for the person's safety and detection of danger has become relatively hypersensitive so that even neutral events are 'alerted' as being potentially dangerous. Whilst this means that the person will never 'miss' a potentially dangerous situation, the better-safe-than-sorry tendency has gone too far and is now counterproductive.

The subcortical areas of our brain are also responsible for our sense of position within the social hierarchy, so the 2-route model can be adapted to explain *grand-*

iose delusions. In this case, it is the person's sense of being very important that has been overactivated, which affects their subjective experience of the world and consequently distorts the way external events and situations are evaluated.

Some people with psychosis get the feeling that events, gestures, words, etc. carry a *special* or *mystical significance*. In these cases, the part of the brain that would normally only respond in this way to things that *were* of great significance is triggered by non-significant events as well – the notion of 'oversensitivity', again. Although it is not known which part of the brain is responsible for producing this sense of significance, there are good reasons to suppose that the subcortical areas are involved, so the 2-route model could be adapted and used to explain this phenomenon as well.

3. 'Something happened to make my brain this way'

An explanation for the brain dysfunction in terms of *the effects of illicit drugs*, taken either in the past or in the present, is not stigmatizing and so, in this respect, requires little in the way of preparation. Where it applies, this alternative explanation is generally preferred to that of psychosis or mental illness, especially amongst younger people. However, if the brain dysfunction is a permanent effect of earlier drug abuse, then there may be regret and grief over past actions that cannot be undone, in which case this would be an important aspect to address.

Where explanations for the brain dysfunction and consequent symptoms are related to present drug abuse, then this will also provide a strong reason for avoiding these drugs in the future.

Replacement beliefs in terms of *poor diet, lack of sleep*, etc. tend to be used as interim explanations on the way to a fuller illness explanation because for most people they do not provide a solid, sustainable explanation for their experiences, not least because some of their symptoms may remain despite improvements in diet, sleep, etc. However, some people prefer to stay at this level of explanation because it avoids the notion of mental illness. Whilst it is not normal practice to suggest one of these explanations, because they are both flimsy and inaccurate, if the person themself has settled on it, then it can be helpful in making some sort of link between physiological factors and the subjective experiences they can produce.

Factors such as poor diet and lack of sleep may have a role in exacerbating someone's symptoms, so where they apply it is appropriate to explain why they produce the effects they do.

REPLACEMENT BELIEFS IN TERMS OF PSYCHOLOGICAL FACTORS

Explaining and normalizing automatic thoughts and the psychological processes involved in belief formation and maintenance

The amount of information you give and the detail you go into will depend on the complexity of your psychological explanation and the person's interest and ability to understand. Unless you are asked, you would normally only cover those areas relevant to the replacement belief that you are preparing to use. It is recommended that you do not attempt to cover more than one aspect of the explanation at any one time as it is easy for the person to become overwhelmed, especially if they have not come across these concepts before.

Automatic thoughts

You should share whatever information about automatic thoughts (see pp. 4–5) you think would be useful, and you should be careful to present it in a way that makes sense to the person concerned. The facts about automatic thoughts that are likely to be particularly pertinent for this aspect of the preparation work are as follows:

1 Automatic thoughts are not the same as deliberate, purposeful thinking. Our brains are throwing up automatic thoughts and ideas all the time, though we are not consciously aware of most of them.
2 It is functional for our brains to do this because it enables us to consider a whole range of possibilities, including possible interpretations of the present situation, possible responses and also the possible consequences of those responses.
3 Part of our brain selects the most useful ideas and brings them into conscious awareness so that we can think about them more carefully.
4 Because our brains are throwing up these different ideas so rapidly it is not surprising that some of them are poorly formed, nonsensical or even completely wrong.
5 The unhelpful and poorly formed ideas normally drop out of our thought system straight away before we have become consciously aware of them, but occasionally our brain will latch on to one of them and give it more credence than it is worth.
6 Our automatic thoughts often reflect our worries, hopes and concerns, but not necessarily so – they can be about anything at all, anything we have ever seen, heard or learnt about, anything we know about from any source at all.
7 We cannot control our automatic thoughts and therefore cannot be held responsible for them; nor is it appropriate to feel guilt or shame.
8 Our automatic thoughts are 'pre-moral', i.e. they occur at a very basic level of brain functioning that is not influenced by our moral beliefs and standards. Having had the automatic thought we can then apply our moral code to it. Therefore, we are not 'moral' or 'immoral' for having a particular automatic thought – it is how we act on it that is moral or immoral.
9 Trying not to think a particular thought may, paradoxically, increase the probability of thinking it.

Responsibility for automatic thoughts: implications for guilt and shame

A very important aspect for CBT with delusions and hallucinations is the understanding that we cannot control the occurrence or content of our automatic thoughts and therefore cannot be held responsible or guilty for them. This follows directly from the more general argument that *we cannot be guilty for what we cannot control*. Most people readily accept the truth of this general proposition but if the person you are working with has any doubts about it, as may occur if they are subject to magical thinking, then you should establish it by using scenarios from everyday life in which the person can see they have no responsibility for what is going on because they cannot influence it and have no control over it. It is often helpful to include a friend in the scenarios because most people find it easier to absolve a friend of responsibility and guilt than themselves. Events from history (e.g. 'Were you responsible for the execution of Anne Boleyn? Why not?') also make very clear the need to be able to control a situation in order to be responsible for it.

Having established the general principle that we cannot be responsible or guilty for what we cannot control, it is easy to demonstrate that our automatic thoughts are not under our control by one or more of the following experiments. It is recommended that you also take part in the test so that when you discuss the results afterwards you can share the fact that you 'failed' as well.

1 'Try to think of nothing at all for 30 seconds. (Having the thought "I'm thinking of nothing" does not count as success!')
2 'Try not to think about the pressure of the chair on your legs; you can think about anything else, but *not* that, for 30 seconds.'
3 'Try *not* to think of chocolate for 30 seconds.' (This works particularly well just before mealtimes.)
4 'Try to think *only* of chocolate for 30 seconds.'

People enjoy trying out these simple tests and they clearly demonstrate the point you are trying to make, namely that we cannot control our thoughts at this level. It is interesting that even very experienced meditators are only able to control their thoughts and 'stop' thinking by concentrating on a specific something, for example a mantra or their breathing, which is still thinking in its broadest sense. It may be helpful to point out that we are no more able to control our automatic thoughts than we are to control the sensation of pain when our hand is pricked, or to control the messages our brain sends to our heart to keep it beating; our brain does all these things automatically and we just experience the results. Indeed, it is functional for us that we are *not* able to consciously override these automatic systems, including our thoughts, because they are important for our survival.

Sometimes, having gained understanding about the nature of their psychosis, people feel this means they ought then to be able to control their paranoid feelings, or suspicious thoughts, or hallucinatory experiences, etc. If this happens, you can remind them that these are produced directly by the brain and use the analogy of not being able to control the pain of an injection, even though we know exactly what is causing it; nor has anyone ever succeeded in stopping a toothache by telling the tooth that they have booked an appointment at the dentist next day and so there is no need for it to carry on hurting! There are many other automatic functions that you can use to reinforce this point, if necessary.

The exercise in trying to ignore the feel of the chair is particularly useful in demonstrating that trying *not* to think of something actually increases the likelihood of that thought coming to mind. Indeed, it is worth pointing out to the person that they were probably completely unaware of the physical sensations from the chair until these particular instructions were given. The reason for this is that by trying to stop it we are inadvertently priming our brains to think about it. This paradoxical effect is one reason why unwanted ideas or hallucinations may recur despite the person's best efforts to keep them at bay. It is interesting to note that meditators are taught that the best way to reduce stray thoughts is not to try to stop them but rather to accept them as 'just thoughts' with as little emotional response as possible, letting them come and go like clouds across the sky.

Another factor that may cause thoughts and voices to recur is if they produce a strong emotional response. This effect applies to all beliefs and experiences, not just psychotic ones: anything that produces a strong emotional response in us is likely to be potentially important for us and so our brain is likely to bring it back to mind from time to time. Unfortunately, even when the person has a good understanding about their delusional thoughts and hallucinations, the unpleasant or distressing material they contain can still trigger a strong emotional response, and so they are still likely to occur for this reason. Modifying the beliefs associated with the material contained in the delusions and hallucinations is a major way of reducing the emotional response that they can cause (see Chapters 8 and 11), and this in turn can have a major effect on the actual occurrence of the delusional ideas and voices.

One of the main reasons why people feel guilty and ashamed about their ideas and voices is the widely held belief, probably stemming from misunderstood psychoanalytic theory, that our thoughts always reflect something about ourselves, so that even if they seem alien to us, nevertheless they must be the product of our innermost longings and desires. It is worth exploring this issue in case the person has some underlying belief along these lines. You should point out that this popularly held belief is not accurate and that our automatic thoughts can reflect anything in our memories or knowledge systems, and as such do not necessarily imply anything about ourselves, our wishes or our moral codes and standards. Indeed, as we have just seen, thoughts can recur for the very reason that they are *not* consistent with our desires, or because we feel guilty or ashamed about having them.

Another factor that may influence the person's sense of responsibility for what is going through their mind is the fact that most of the thinking of which they are consciously aware will be under their conscious control and so they may assume that they must be responsible for *all* their thinking. If this is the case it may be helpful to clarify the difference between purposeful thinking and automatic thoughts, perhaps describing the automatic thoughts as the building blocks produced by the brain that can then be used or rejected by our more conscious and purposeful trains of thought. Whilst the latter is generally under the control of the person concerned, the former is not.

It may also be helpful if you draw a distinction between thoughts, the function of which is to suggest possibilities and offer options, and the actions that the person actually takes as a result of these thoughts. Thus, whilst we have control over our actions, and as such are responsible for them, we do not have control over many of the thoughts that go through our minds. If someone is worried about having had a thought or feeling, it may be helpful to ask whether or not they would put the thought into action if they had the chance – the 'real' them is the person who chooses between the options, not the brain that just recognizes what these options are. For example, if someone had the thought of driving their car into a bus queue, do they think they would choose to do this if they had the chance? This often helps people to recognize the distinction between an automatic thought (neither moral nor immoral) and a deliberate thought (moral) that produces action. The same strategy can be extended to emotions. For example, if someone was feeling guilty because they were more upset and worried when their cat went missing than when a child was reported missing, the question 'If you had the choice, who would you make turn up safe and well, your cat or the child?' may help to distinguish between what they 'really' want and their emotional responses.

A useful way of reassuring people about the occurrence of their antisocial and 'shameful' thoughts is to normalize them by discussing the prevalence of such thoughts in the general population. For example, well over 50% of the population who have stood on a railway platform have had the thought of pushing a fellow traveller onto the rails, and it is quite common for car drivers to have the thought of driving onto a pavement and mowing down the pedestrians. You should point out that it is actually functional for people to have these 'antisocial' thoughts because they warn us of what *could* happen. The fact that our platforms and pavements are demonstrably safe places to be indicates that thoughts are very different things from desires to act! (If you are one of the minority of people who have not had the thought of pushing someone off a railway platform, do not be surprised if you have it next time you travel by train – it does not mean you have become more antisocial, it is just an example of how knowing about something can cause the thought to occur.)

Whilst on the topic of antisocial thoughts in ordinary people, it may be helpful to consider what can happen when a mother has the thought of deliberately harming her own child, as an example of what can happen if there is a strong adverse reaction to an automatic thought. Most mothers will have had the thought at one time or another of deliberately harming their child, though very few ever carry it out in practice. Most women are able just to disregard the thought, without worrying about it, but a few feel so guilty and upset at having had such a thought that they keep thinking about it, leading to more emotional distress, leading to more thoughts about it, and so on into a vicious cycle. This example may serve as a useful analogy to the recurrence of emotionally provocative thoughts and hallucinations that the person is trying to suppress.

Belief formation and the confirmation cycles, and the symptom maintenance triad

It is helpful if you can adapt the models described in Chapter 1 in order to make whichever parts of them you are using relevant for the particular person with whom you are working. The psychological processes involved can be explained and normalized by using everyday events and examples to illustrate them.[9]

Using the model for the formation and maintenance of delusional beliefs

There will be many factors involved in the development and maintenance of a particular delusional belief and an even larger number of potential ones to consider. As your assessment delves deeper the complexity can seem overwhelming, so it is very important to have a structure within which to think and speculate about the individual case. The model described in Chapter 2 includes the major factors and processes that are likely to be involved, so even if you do not intend to share your diagram with the person themself it is recommended that you try to formulate your own ideas in this way (a) because it may help to clarify your thinking about the relevant factors involved, and (b) equally importantly it may help to expose gaps in that thinking and suggest factors you have not considered. As noted in Chapter 2, this model is a relatively simple one, so for your particular patient you may want to add factors from the general models described in Chapter 1.

If you are using a diagram based on this model, only include those parts that are relevant for the alternative explanation you are giving. It may be better to use several simpler diagrams to cover the different aspects of the case formulation rather than putting them altogether on a single, complicated one.

EXAMPLE OF SHARING THE CASE FORMULATION[10]

A young woman asked me why she would think that people were insulting her when they used the 'ė' vowel sound if they were not really doing so. This belief caused her a lot of distress in everyday life. It was also having an adverse effect on other aspects of our therapy because I would use the 'ė' sound many times during our sessions and, despite my efforts to consciously control them, I would inevitably stress a number of these (e.g. I discovered that it is particularly easy to emphasize the 'ė' when replying 'Yes' to a question). So we frequently had to stop what we were doing to challenge this interpretation of my speech each time it occurred. We had used several different ways to challenge the validity of her underlying belief, and these were sufficiently successful in instilling doubt in her mind to enable her to ask me what other explanation there could be for her feelings of being insulted other than the obvious

[9]It is recommended that you work these out ahead of your session. Real life situations are complicated and it is likely to be confusing for the other person if you find that you have to make corrections whilst in the middle of your explanation.

[10]In the first edition of this practice manual the model used to structure this case was the one in use at that time. The same clinical case has been used to illustrate the use of the updated model in order to show how similar this is in practice. The verbal explanation has not needed any alteration.

one that people were really insulting her. She was already aware that she had schizophrenia and that this made her feel paranoid, though like many people with otherwise good insight into their illness she denied this particular belief could be part of that illness. But the fact that she knew she had a paranoid illness meant this could be incorporated into our suggested model of how this particular belief could have arisen, a model that was able to account for her belief without needing to include the factor of people really trying to insult her. She found diagrams helpful, so an adaptation of the general model was given.

USING THE MODEL FOR THE FORMATION AND MAINTENANCE OF DELUSIONAL BELIEFS

Figure 6.2 represents the adaptation of the model given in Chapter 2 for the case formulation used.

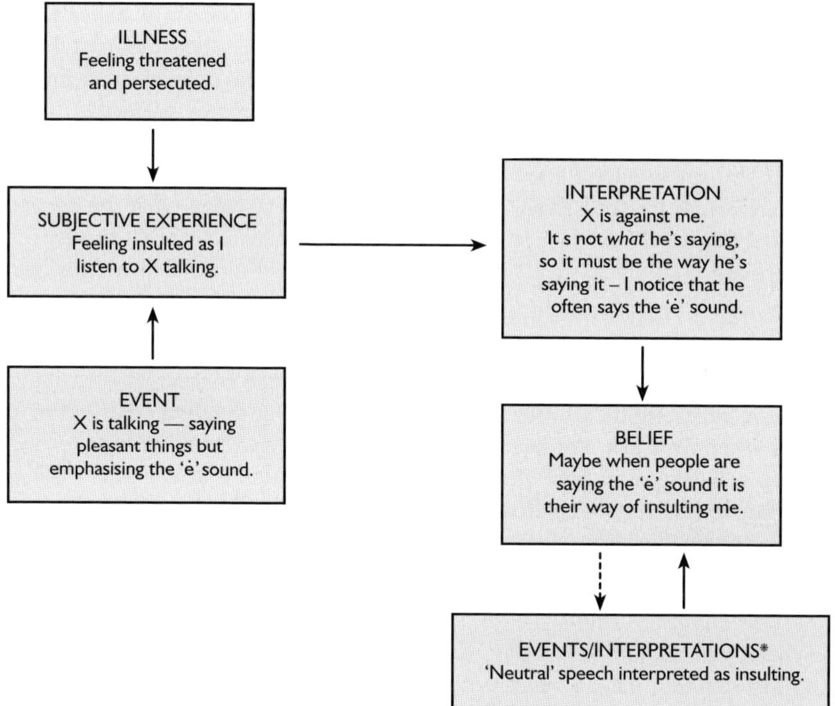
ILLNESS
Feeling threatened and persecuted.
SUBJECTIVE EXPERIENCE
Feeling insulted as I listen to X talking.
EVENT
X is talking — saying pleasant things but emphasising the 'ė' sound.
INTERPRETATION
X is against me.
It s not *what* he's saying, so it must be the way he's saying it – I notice that he often says the 'ė' sound.
BELIEF
Maybe when people are saying the 'ė' sound it is their way of insulting me.
EVENTS/INTERPRETATIONS*
'Neutral' speech interpreted as insulting.

*NOTE

The more this happens, the more likely you are to jump to the conclusion that you feel threathened and insulted because people are using the 'ė' sound. In this way the belief is built up and strengthened.

Now that you have the belief that people using the 'ė' sound is their way of putting you down, this will confirm your belief that emphasizing these sounds is a way people use to insult you: so just hearing those sounds may be enough to make you feel threatened.

Figure 6.2 Possible explanation of why the woman would develop the belief that using the 'ė' sound meant that people were trying to insult her.

The explanation accompanying the presentation of this model would run along the following lines:

'You have an illness that makes you feel threatened and persecuted. That's what you take your medication for, but, as you know, unfortunately this doesn't completely control your illness so there will be times when you feel threatened and persecuted, not because anything threatening or dangerous has actually happened, but just because that's the way your illness makes you feel.

'Once the danger-warning system in your brain has been alerted, then it looks to see what might have caused it to be alerted, and since danger normally does come from outside of us, it is perfectly reasonable for the brain to look to the outside world for the source of that danger. It doesn't do this consciously, of course; it's at a much more basic, instinctive level than that. So at this basic, automatic level your brain is trying to work out who or what is posing the threat, and how this is being done. Suppose all this happened at some time when you were sitting in a room talking to somebody. Now our brains are biased towards interpreting people or animals as more likely sources of threat than things like tables and chairs, because in real life people are indeed more potentially dangerous than inanimate objects, so in this case if there was one other person in the room, then it would be perfectly reasonable for your brain to fix on that person as being the most likely source of threat. But you still wouldn't know how this threat was being signalled and it could be important for your brain to know that in order to judge what the danger was. Again, in these circumstances it is not unreasonable for your brain to suspect that if there are no physical signs of threat, then the threat must lie in what is being said.

'Suppose, when all this happens, that the person you are talking to is saying pleasant things. If they are saying pleasant things, then it can't be the content of what they are saying that is indicating threat. But perhaps you notice that they are emphasizing the 'ė' sounds when they talk. We have already seen, when we looked at tape recordings of our own conversations, how often people emphasize the 'ė' sound when talking to one another, so it is very likely that the person you were talking to at that time was emphasizing some 'ė' sounds. So maybe in this situation, the best explanation your brain can come up with as to why you have been 'threatened' is that it must be in the way the other person stresses the 'ė' sounds.

'Once your brain has jumped to this conclusion, it is not unreasonable for you to develop the idea that maybe when people are saying the 'ė' sound it is a sign that they are trying to put you down. If this feeling occurs again when you are in a social situation, then you have an immediate explanation for it, i.e. the idea that when people stress the 'ė' sound it's a sign that they are insulting you. Once this belief has been established, then even neutral speech containing the 'e' sound is likely to be interpreted as being insulting or threatening, and this interpretation will serve to strengthen the belief about the 'ė' sound. It's perfectly normal for people to interpret a situation in terms of their existing beliefs, so once your brain had assumed that people stressing the 'ė' sound was a sign they were insulting you, then it was perfectly understandable why you interpreted subsequent situations according to this belief. But, unfortunately, these misinterpretations will have reinforced the incorrect belief, and so it got stronger rather than weaker.'

The diagram was also used to explain how CBT could help the woman combat these unpleasant feelings, and the role that medication has in controlling them. Medication was shown to act on the 'illness' part of the model and this explained why it could help stop the feelings of persecution that were caused by the illness, whilst CBT was shown to act on the maintaining belief/interpretation cycle and this explained why it could help stop the feelings of persecution caused by the inaccurate/delusional belief. The model was also used to explain why we thought it would not be a good idea for her to attempt to control her symptoms by CBT alone, because although CBT could combat the unpleasant feelings produced by the delusional beliefs and misinterpretations, it could not get rid of those feelings that were caused directly by the biological activity of the illness. Only some biological intervention, such as medication, could do that.

USING THE 2-ROUTE MODEL

Although the 2-route model was not used with this woman, the following description illustrates how it might deal with the same material. The basic diagram would have been shown and explained as given in Appendix 2.

'As we've seen, the lower route works on a better-safe-than-sorry principle, so all of us tend to see potential dangers even when none exist. I think that what could be happening in your case is that your lower route sometimes gets particularly active and oversensitive, which results in your getting an absolutely convincing feeling that you are in danger, that people are getting at you even when they are not. This feeling feels so certain, so quickly, that the rational route never gets a chance to come in to check it out.

[The explanation for why the lower route has fixed on the 'ė' sound as the source of threat is the same as that given in the previous model, except that the lower route is identified as the part of the brain responsible for the feelings and for the jumping to conclusions.]

'If this is right, then I think there are two things that might help. Firstly, the medication you take should help to make the lower route less sensitive so that it doesn't keep going into 'danger alert' all the time. Secondly, we can try to work out some strategies to make sure that the more accurate, rational route *does* get involved when the lower route jumps to conclusions. One possible strategy might be to practise questioning every time you get the feeling people are getting at you by the way they are talking. Use your rational route to ask 'Is there any hard evidence that people are getting at me?'. If the only evidence you have is the *feeling of certainty*, then this is a very good indication it is just your lower route being oversensitive – because if people were really getting at you, then your rational route would be able to produce some hard evidence of how this was happening. Remember we agreed that people stressing the 'ė' sound was *not* hard evidence on its own, because no one else would interpret this in that way.

'Unfortunately, your lower route will continue to give you this *feeling*, even when your rational route has worked out that it is not accurate in fact; but with practice, your rational route should be able to provide you with some reassurance when this happens and this in turn may help to calm down the overactivity in your lower route.'

REPLACEMENT BELIEFS IN TERMS OF 'I MADE A MISTAKE – I KNOW BETTER NOW'

The 'I've changed my mind' type of replacement belief is undoubtedly the easiest to prepare because it does not include any notion of abnormal functioning or illness. Unfortunately it is rarely a valid option because it is only appropriate as a replacement belief in those circumstances where psychotic factors do not play an obvious part in the development of the delusional belief. For example, 'I thought the drug dealers were trying to kill me because I had underpaid them on a cannabis deal 10 years ago – but now I realize they would not still be worried about £5' would be possible, but 'I thought I was the head of MI5 because I was convinced that car number plates carried secret messages to me about terrorist threats – but I could just have been mistaken about that' is not really plausible because the events are too abnormal to explain away like this.

You are more likely to be able to use this type of replacement where the delusional belief is of little significance or interest for the person. Where it does apply, the only preparation needed is to ensure that the person will not feel stupid because they made a mistake and came to the wrong conclusion. This would usually be done by establishing that it is normal for everyone to make mistakes from time to time, and normal for people to change their belief when they realize their mistake (see pp. 101–103).

PARTIAL INSIGHT/UNDERSTANDING

Subjective experiences, particularly those involving the senses, may be imbued with their own assurance of truth and reality that is just too convincing to be countered by arguments or apparently conflicting evidence. In some cases, therefore, it may not be possible for the person to achieve full insight about their symptoms or illness even though this was included in the treatment goal of choice; in these cases, significant gains may still be possible if a partial insight can be achieved. In other cases there may be good reasons to suppose that full insight would not be functional, but in these cases, also, it is worth considering whether partial insight, about just certain aspects of the illness or symptoms, would be beneficial. There are two broad types of partial insight or understanding.

Using an intermediary concept

The first type of partial insight is where the person has made some movement away from believing their experiences are entirely accurate indications of what is going on in the outside world, but where the cause of those experiences is still given as something other than illness or the brain not functioning properly. This sort of partial insight is usually more vulnerable to subsequent loss than full insight but, nevertheless, these partial, alternative explanations for the symptoms can function as a proxy for the full illness explanation, and as such can enable the person to put into effect some appropriate coping strategies that would not have been possible if they had had no insight at all. The following three cases illustrate this point.

1 A man concluded that being in hospital helped to get rid of the evil spirits that invaded his mind because they could only get to him when he was not sleeping properly, and when he was in hospital he was able to relax and take 'sleeping' tablets to help him sleep through the night.
2 Another man came to the understanding that when he went through periods of being up all night, chain smoking and drinking heavily, periods that he called 'high spirits', then he was likely to have paranoid ideas. This was a therapeutic gain for him because it meant that when he was going through one of these 'high' periods, he would use cognitive strategies to test whether his ideas about having the phone tapped, etc. were accurate, or whether they were caused by the high spirits.
3 A woman came to the conclusion after some weeks of CBT that there was dust in the air that could make her 'imagine' she heard things. This was an important step forward for her as it meant she could recognize that the voices she heard came from her own imagination and therefore did not indicate that what they said was true, namely that other people really thought badly of her. The 'dust' explanation was also useful because she came to the conclusion that the medication that she had previously blamed for making her feel unwell could actually help to control the dust and therefore that it was worth taking for this reason. Interestingly, this young woman was contacted in the community a year later, in connection with a CBT research project, and at this time it was found that she accepted she had a mental illness and that this was what caused her to imagine her voices. It was as if she had needed to modify her beliefs in stages, first by recognizing that her voices did not come from a real person and only later being able to recognize that the cause of this false perception was internal (the illness) rather than external (the dust).

This latter case raises the question of whether one is colluding with a delusional explanation by helping the person to use it to trigger appropriate coping strategies and, if so, whether this is acceptable practice from an ethical point of view. Individual therapists are likely to differ in where they draw the line. My own position in such cases is that whilst I would not suggest a partial insight explanation that I believed to be frankly untrue, I certainly would not seek to disprove any explanation that the person had arrived at themself if it had beneficial effects for them, not least because this alternative explanation might be a stepping stone for them on the way to full understanding.

In general, alternatives to the delusional belief that are untrue in fact are potentially vulnerable because there is always the risk that they will be shown to be wrong by subsequent events, so factually accurate alternatives are to be preferred for practical as well as ethical reasons. However, in seeking to achieve a robust, factually accurate alternative belief, you should be careful not to risk dislodging an inaccurate but functional alternative until you are sure that the more factually accurate one is the one that the person will adopt in its place.

When dealing with inaccurate but functional explanations and beliefs, it is recommended you adopt a position of neutrality or ignorance about the person's views if you do not want to challenge them, and in some cases even indifference to the explanation may be appropriate. For instance, in the 'dust' example given above I took a stance along the lines 'I really don't know whether your voices are caused by the dust or not; I've never heard of that happening before but people can react differently to things, so who knows? I agree that the work we've done certainly indicates that the voices are not coming from the people whose voices they appear to be. But I don't suppose it really matters what's causing the voices; the only things that are really important are (a) that they are not telling the truth, and (b) to try to find ways to stop them when they are having a go at you.'

If you are working towards a total modification that has an illness-based replacement belief but the person seems to be more comfortable with an intermediary concept that attributes the symptoms to some other external cause rather than to something within themself, then you should be alert to the possibility/probability that the illness-based alternative is not yet acceptable, and that more work needs to be done to make it acceptable before you press on to establish it as the replacement belief.

Acceptance that other people genuinely believe the 'illness' explanation

The second broad class of partial insight or understanding occurs when people deny having an illness but accept that other people genuinely believe they are ill. In most cases the person believes that the other people are wrong but, nevertheless, this level of insight allows them to accept that other people have good intent towards them when they treat them as if they were ill.

Holding incompatible beliefs about the 'illness' explanation

A rather peculiar variant of the above class of partial insight may occur, especially in those with long-standing illnesses, where the person seems to accept the truth of both their own belief that they are not ill and other people's belief that they are. It seems they can move flexibly from one apparently conflicting belief to the other and to act in accordance with both the beliefs without being affected by the incongruity. It is unusual for two significant and incompatible beliefs to be held together, without one being modified, but it may be that in these cases the evidence that the person has to substantiate each of the beliefs is so convincing that neither can be rejected, and so neither is able to take permanent precedence over the other. The maintenance of both beliefs may be enhanced by the fact that both can be functional for the person in different contexts. Be that as it may, this type of partial insight is useful in that it allows the person to use coping strategies despite their denial of illness. For example, the person may continue to take their medication reliably, even when they are out of hospital and self-medicating, despite denying any need to do so or that they derive any benefit from it. When I first encountered this presentation, I thought that the most likely explanation for the treatment compliance was the power of the patient role in making them submissive to authority, but I no longer believe this to be so, certainly not in all cases. In some cases people seem genuinely able to behave according to two apparently directly opposing beliefs, without being aware of the incompatibility of those beliefs.

PREPARING FOR A PARTIAL MODIFICATION

The core delusional belief is left intact with a partial modification and so, as a general rule, no replacement belief has to be identified or prepared. However, partial modifications do actually involve a type of replacement belief, because partial modifications can be regarded as total modifications of one small part of the delusional system. For example, in the illustration of goal setting given on p. 96, the partial modification 'I am a witch but other people cannot see that I am' could be treated as a total modification of the sub-belief 'People can see that I am a witch', the total goal being 'People cannot see that I am a witch' plus a replacement belief explaining why the woman thought in the past that they could. It is not normally necessary to specify the replacement belief used in partial modifications because they do not cause widespread disruption of the person's belief system, and the implicit explanation for having got it wrong is the very common, normal and non-stigmatizing one of 'Now I've got more information I'm changing my mind about . . .'.

However, even with a partial goal you should be careful to consider the possible implications and consequences for the person should the goal be achieved. This is likely to be especially important where the secondary belief that is being targeted for modification is an important part of the primary delusional belief or if it is important to the person in its own right. Two key points to consider are (a) 'Will modification of this part of the core belief bring about an unwanted modification of the core belief itself?' (see Chapter 5, pp. 90–91, 99), and (b) 'Is the significance of the part being modified such that an explanation other than "I was mistaken" is needed to account for it?'. As an example of this latter situation, a man believes that for the past 20 years there has been a conspiracy to defraud him of a rich inheritance and that the doctors are part of this conspiracy. Suppose a total modification is not possible for some reason, in which case the partial goal 'There is a conspiracy to defraud me but the doctors are not part of the conspiracy' looks as if it would be a positive and helpful one. However, if the man has blamed his doctors for wrongful detention in hospital for 20 years, then the implications of the doctors *not* being part of the conspiracy would be too great for him to be able to attribute his earlier belief to 'a mistake'.

If you think there is a risk that a partial modification could have significant, wider implications, then it is safer to treat the modification as a total modification of the secondary belief and formally consider whether another, more functional replacement belief should be set and prepared.

Destigmatizing and normalizing the symptoms and illness labels when a partial modification is being used

Even when the goal of modification is a partial one, destigmatizing the psychiatric terminology and concepts is likely to be beneficial, providing you can do it without upsetting or antagonizing the person. The aims are (a) to protect the person from distress when health professionals, family and friends talk to them in these terms, and (b) to protect the person from the impact of sudden insight should medication and/or time bring this about in the future.

The strategies used are the same as those used for preparing an illness-based replacement belief. The difference is that if you are using a partial goal as the goal of choice, then this means that you are not aiming for the person to understand their delusional belief in terms of mental illness, and therefore you would be particularly careful not to relate the symptoms being discussed to the person themself. In these circumstances the best strategy is usually to keep alert to whatever opportunities arise naturally in the course of conversation or therapy rather than drawing attention to this work by focusing on it. Do not spoil the opportunities that arise by concentrating too much or for too long on them.

7 MODIFYING THE BELIEFS THAT INFLUENCE AND UNDERLIE THE DELUSIONAL BELIEF

DEEP AND SURFACE MEANINGS OF A DELUSIONAL BELIEF

A delusional belief develops within the context and constraints of the person's existing belief and knowledge systems. The 'surface' meaning of the belief is its obvious, literal meaning; for example, 'I am visited by the spirits of my dead ancestors, they come to stand by my bed' means just that. The surface meaning is influenced and constrained by the person's belief/knowledge system; for example, someone would not interpret their experiences in terms of a visitation from dead ancestors unless that latter notion or possibility was already present within their belief system.

The delusional belief may also incorporate and reflect non-psychotic beliefs that are of particular significance and importance for the person; this is sometimes called the 'deep' meaning of the delusional belief. Indeed, in some cases the delusional belief may be regarded as a symbolic representation of these underlying, non-psychotic beliefs. For example, a man believed his heart and blood were black and that this meant he would contaminate those he loved with the same disease. This man had suffered prolonged emotional abuse as a child and as a result had core beliefs that he was unacceptable to other people, and that he would bring them bad luck. When he became psychotic, these core beliefs took on a concrete form and became a 'delusional' belief.

Delusional beliefs do not always have a deep meaning. Whether or not a delusion has a deep meaning as well as the obvious, surface meaning will depend on why and how the delusion developed. For example, a man experiences pain and other sensations in his stomach area, he gets hallucinatory tastes and smells of rotting flesh, and he has read in the newspapers about a flesh-eating bacterial disease; this is sufficient for him to develop the belief 'I am rotting away inside'. No other beliefs are involved and in this case the belief does not have a deep meaning beyond its obvious, literal meaning. In contrast, a woman develops the belief 'I am rotting away inside' without having any physical signs of an internal problem; it is the result of the overwhelming influence of her strongly held belief that she is a bad and rotten person. In this latter case, the deep meaning of the delusion is more important for the woman's well-being than the surface one.

When there is a significant, deep meaning(s), then working on the non-psychotic beliefs that underlie it may be as or more important than working on the literal meaning of the presenting delusion. For example, in the cases given above, modifying the delusional belief about their insides being rotten would effectively remove the source of the man's distress, but it would be of little benefit to the woman because she would still believe she was a thoroughly bad, nasty person.

Although the deep meaning may be of more significance for the person than the surface meaning, nevertheless it is often helpful to modify the surface meaning as well, because it is likely that this will be reinforcing the underlying non-psychotic belief. For example, a woman believed that people despised her because she had fleas. Although the most important aspect of this work was to modify her underlying beliefs about her unworthiness and unacceptability to others, nevertheless, her belief about having fleas exacerbated her fears of rejection, and so removing the delusion was an important part of the overall treatment programme.

MODIFYING THE BELIEFS UNDERLYING THE DEEP MEANING OF THE DELUSION

The main reason for targeting an underlying dysfunctional belief that is incorporated into the delusional belief is because that belief is dysfunctional for the person. If the modification is successful then this is likely to weaken the delusional belief as well, and may even cause it to collapse, but this is usually the secondary rather than primary purpose of this aspect of the therapy.

The steps involved in identifying and modifying 'deep' underlying beliefs

1. What non-psychotic beliefs might be influencing the content and/or form of the delusional belief?

The underlying beliefs that are influencing the delusional belief(s) may be apparent and readily expressed, but in many cases they are not immediately obvious and so you should always be alert for clues as to their presence and content. One useful indicator is if there is a persistent theme running through the delusion(s) and/or voices, for example other people being critical and judgemental, or particular types or groups of people being involved.

If the associated beliefs are not apparent, you may be able to elicit them by asking more about the delusion. For example, if the delusional belief involves other people, you might ask the person how they know that *these particular* people are involved, why *they* would be involved rather than other people, and *why* they should want to act in that way. This simple approach was useful for our treatment of a young man who had a record of occasional violence towards other residents for which there was no apparent reason. During therapy he complained that one of his fellow residents was deliberately trying to provoke him and that if he carried on then he would have to hit him. When asked why this particular man would want to do this, he explained that it was because this resident was an Irish Catholic. When asked about Irish Catholics, a number of dysfunctional beliefs were revealed, including that they were jealous of Ulster Protestants (the group to which the man belonged) and that they wanted to take the material wealth that the Protestants were entitled to. On going back over his history, it was found that most of the people who had been hit by this man were of Irish descent. It was not expected that modifying this man's beliefs about people with Irish accents would weaken his feelings of paranoia per se, but it was effective in removing a factor that predisposed and sensitized him to see Irish people as a source of threat.

Where they are not obvious, the therapist *speculates* about what underlying beliefs *might* be relevant. Indeed, even when you are aware of some underlying beliefs it is still important to speculate about the possible presence of others because the most significant underlying beliefs may not be the most obvious ones. (See also 'Concealed beliefs' pp. 138–140.) At this early stage, even unlikely beliefs should be considered: as a general rule, it is better to consider and reject a 'possible' underlying belief than to miss a potentially significant one.

2. Check out which, if any, of the possible underlying beliefs are relevant
This is done primarily through discussion with the person themself, but useful information may also be obtained from the case history. Checking out your speculations should be done *very* gently and carefully, for the following reasons. Firstly, you may be eliciting core beliefs that the person themself is not aware of holding, and/or that they are not ready or willing to acknowledge and talk about. Secondly, there may be reasons why the person does not want you to know or talk about the belief, for example shame, guilt or fear. Thirdly, by asking questions about an issue it is easy to imply that you think it *is* relevant, even though you are only checking out a remote possibility. If the speculation is wide of the mark, this may cause irritation, indignation, confusion and distress, or may suggest to the person that you really do not know them at all if you could make such a suggestion.

3. Set a goal(s) for each relevant underlying belief
Goal setting for non-psychotic beliefs that underlie a delusion follows the same format as goal setting for a delusional belief, namely: (a) What would the *goal* of modification be? (b) Would it be more *functional* than the present belief? (c) What are the *wider implications* of changing this belief? (d) Would the modification be *acceptable* to the person?

4. Attempt to modify the dysfunctional underlying beliefs
Where it has been possible to set a goal that will be both functional and acceptable to the person, it is usual practice to start working on these beliefs at the same time as working on the delusional belief itself. The CBT strategies used to modify the underlying beliefs are essentially the same as those used to modify the delusional belief itself (see Chapter 8).

Caution: Going deep into someone's belief system to identify the belief(s) that predispose them to their delusional belief may uncover dysfunctional core beliefs that they hold about themself and the world (what are sometimes called *schema* or *schemata* in personality change work). This is particularly likely to occur in people with psychosis who also have features of so-called personality disorder, or who have the sort of traumatic personal histories that can lead to a personality disorder. Core schemata are expressed in global terms and refer to fundamental aspects of the person and their views of other people. Some examples of negative core schemata are: 'I am bad/unlovable/incompetent' and 'Other people are untrustworthy/critical/dominating'. It is strongly advised that you do not attempt to modify core schemata in such cases unless you have the necessary training, or have access to a supervisor who can guide you through this difficult work.

EXAMPLE OF IDENTIFYING BELIEFS UNDERLYING A DELUSIONAL BELIEF

A young man reported that he sometimes hit strangers that passed by in the street because they were secretly mocking him and trying to take away his sexuality. It was noticed that the strangers he hit were all young adult females. This suggested that one or more of the following beliefs *might* underlie the delusion:

1 I am sexually unattractive to young women.
2 I look ugly/unattractive.
3 I ought to find women sexually attractive.
4 There is something different/wrong with my sexuality.
5 Women do not respect men.
6 Women try to belittle men sexually.

Gently exploring these issues with him enabled beliefs 1, 3 and 4 to be identified as the relevant ones. The man believed that women did not generally lack respect for men or try to mock them, but rather that this behaviour was directed only at him. His belief that he was sexually unattractive to the opposite sex was distorting his perception of events and fuelling his delusional belief. The goal set for modification of this belief was 'Young women do not find me unattractive; they do not think I look different from other young men'. Identifying beliefs 3 and 4 led on to work with his underlying concerns about his sexual preferences and identity.

CASE STUDY JANE

(See also pp. 76, 95, 99, 143, 188 and 277.)

Belief: *I am an evil witch.*

Some of the possible 'deep' underlying beliefs that *might* have been relevant included:

1 I am different from other people.
2 I look odd/peculiar/different.
3 I am a special person: I have always had special powers.
4 I am an evil person.
5 I am awful/bad inside.

6 Bad things happen to people when I am around.
7 I have done something(s) bad/evil in the past.
8 I come from an evil family.
9 Other people think I am different, or look odd.
10 Other people don't like me.
11 Other people reject me, don't want to be my friend.
12 Other people are frightened of me.

Exploring these possibilities with Jane indicated that beliefs 1, 2, 9, 10 and 12 applied but the others did not.

Beliefs 4, 5 and 7. It is unusual to have a delusion about being evil without some underlying belief about self being bad or unworthy, etc., or some guilt about things done in the past, but careful assessment indicated that this was not the case with Jane.[1] Prior to the onset of her present psychotic experiences and the subsequent development of this particular delusional belief, Jane had felt herself to be part of her community and well liked, and viewed herself as a kind, thoughtful person. Furthermore, she could not recall doing anything that could be described as evil before she became a witch, and neither was there any indication of such an event(s) in her medical history or from people who knew her well. Although she appeared to have no relevant underlying beliefs about being bad or evil, nevertheless some CBT work was done to elicit and reinforce the reasons she already had for knowing she was a kind and thoughtful person (apart from the unintentional things she did as a witch!), and this was reinforced by examples of her generous and helpful actions. This was done as a precautionary measure, just in case there was a hidden belief that we had not detected, and also to protect her against the ongoing 'evidence' of being evil that came from the daily war atrocities.[2] In any case, it never does any harm to do work that reinforces someone's self-esteem and sense of value.

Beliefs 1, 2 and 9. Jane's belief that she looked odd and different from other people only developed as a result of her believing she was a witch, i.e. it was not a stable, underlying, non-psychotic belief that was being incorporated into the delusional belief.

[1]When the delusional belief is based on guilt about some relatively minor action or event in the past, then the CBT approach would be to change the person's understanding and judgement of that action/event to bring it in line with a more normally accepted evaluation (e.g. the married woman who felt 'evil' because she had kissed another man during an office party). One way of doing this might be to construct an 'evil/badness scale', with specific actions and events of differing evil/badness at set points from 0–9 so that the person can rate their previous and present actions against this objective scale.

However, sometimes the action/event would be regarded by most people as 'bad' (e.g. a frenzied knife attack) and therefore this normalizing strategy would not be appropriate in these circumstances. In such cases, the approach would be to promote the person's understanding of why the event happened in order to reduce the notion of blame (e.g. 'I tried to kill the man because I genuinely believed at the time that he was a terrorist agent planning to blow up the crowd of people').

[2]Jane relapsed some two years after this episode and on this occasion believed that she had special powers because she was an archangel. This was harder to manage clinically because she liked the belief and therefore refused to engage in treatment of any kind, but it was much less distressing for her. We did wonder whether the work we had done to improve her self-esteem and self-image had been a significant factor in the different way the delusion presented.

Therefore, we predicted this belief would disappear once the delusional system had been successfully modified, without the need for extra work on it. This turned out to be the case.

Beliefs 10 and 12. The beliefs that some people did not like her and were frightened of her were also a direct result of Jane's belief that she was an evil witch, and therefore did not represent an underlying negative belief about herself that required a separate treatment plan. Whilst we were collecting evidence of the nice things she had done (see above), we took the opportunity to point out to her that these were good reasons why people would like her, and reminded her that the people who knew her both liked and respected her.

Concealed beliefs

Delusional ideas may be associated with underlying beliefs that are not immediately apparent and only emerge during therapy. You should consider the possibility of an undetected underlying belief in the following situations:

1 If there are aspects of the delusional belief you cannot account for in your case formulation about why the delusion might have developed in the way that it has.
2 If the delusion seems to be more strongly held or to provoke more emotion than you would expect from the person's circumstances and from your discussions about their delusion.
3 If the delusional belief is retained despite covering the appropriate areas of CBT that one would expect, theoretically, to be sufficient to have modified it.

As described above, if you think there could be a significant underlying belief(s) then you should speculate about what this might be and then carefully check out your speculations with the person concerned.

EXAMPLE OF A CONCEALED BELIEF

Martin was a middle-aged man who believed that two particular nurses on the ward wanted to put him in a coffin and cremate him alive. The reason he gave for this was that they knew about a crime he had committed some years ago. We were successful in modifying his beliefs about the crime, so that he accepted this would not be a sufficient reason for anybody to want to kill him, and we were able to show to his satisfaction that the two nurses concerned felt kindly towards him. He was able to use this information successfully to combat the fearful thoughts when they arose, but we were puzzled as to why the thoughts continued and why the CBT appeared not to have modified the underlying beliefs but only allowed them to be successfully countered when they occurred. We also wondered why these two particular nurses were seen as the potential killers, as other members of staff also knew of his prison record, but we were unable to come up with any convincing explanations. The man did have a racial prejudice, but one nurse was black and one was white and the rest of the team was multiracial, so this did not seem to be a relevant underlying belief. Similarly, he did feel more confident with female staff, but one of the potential 'murderers' was female, so his generally negative view of male staff did not seem to be relevant either.

It was not until many months later, when another member of staff joined the ranks of potential murderers, that we suspected a previously undetected but very influential belief. A few days earlier Martin had hit the nurse badly enough for her to be off work for several days. He was adamant that he had not hit her because she had been trying to harm him in any way but because she would not give him his money out of hours so that he could go to buy cigarettes. If this incident was not a response to the delusion, could it have triggered it in some way, and, if so, why? When asked if he thought the nurse would want to kill him because he had hit her, Martin looked slightly alarmed before admitting that he thought she might well do. This seemed to be a gross exaggeration of the nurse's likely reaction to the incident so we asked him why he thought the nurse would react in such an extreme way: what evidence did he have that people would respond to being assaulted by plotting murder? He was visibly agitated and discomfited by the questions but he was unable to come up with any supporting evidence or possible explanation as to why he made this assumption.

Reviewing what we knew about Martin, and bearing in mind his reaction to the questions, we came up with a possible hypothesis. We knew he found it difficult to put himself in other people's positions and would assume that they felt exactly as he would in the same situation, so we postulated that perhaps Martin believed the nurse wanted to kill him because that was how *he* felt when people behaved aggressively towards him. If this hypothesis were true, the fact that he was not spontaneously admitting to it suggested he might be ashamed of it, so we prepared the way by doing some normalizing/destigmatizing work around automatic thoughts, noting that it was not uncommon to get aggressive and even violent thoughts towards people, but that thinking and doing were quite different things morally. Having done this, we gently broached the question of how he felt towards people who were aggressive towards him, and in response to direct questioning he admitted that when this happened to him, he would wish the other person were dead and sometimes even think about killing them.

Having elicited Martin's own response to these situations, and agreed that despite his thoughts he never had and never would kill anyone, we then referred back to the nurse's reactions. We agreed that the nurse had probably felt pretty negative towards him and that her immediate reaction may well have been an urge to hit him back, but we noted that, nevertheless, she had not done so. We argued that since she had not hit him, even in the heat of the moment, it would not be reasonable to suppose that she would attempt to retaliate more violently after the heat of the moment had faded.

We asked Martin why *he* had never killed anyone when that thought went through his mind and noted that it was because of the penalty he would have to pay. (We took the opportunity of reinforcing the negative outcome, to help him resist turning his thoughts into actions in the future.) We then looked at the penalty that the nurse would have to pay for harming or attempting to kill him, namely loss of job, loss of profession, time in prison, separation from family, etc., to show that this would far outweigh any fleeting satisfaction she might receive from revenge.

Although we had normalized the occurrence of violent thoughts with Martin, and shown why the nurse would not act in a violent manner towards him however badly she might feel, we were reluctant to leave him believing that the nurse did or had hated him so much as to want to kill him because of this incident. We noted that psychiatric nurses working on this particular ward must realize there was a fair chance of being hit by a disturbed patient at some time or another and so the nurse concerned would not have asked to work on the ward if she felt so strongly about being hit that she would want to murder the patient later. It was suggested, therefore, that although it had no doubt been very unpleasant for the nurse to be hit, and although she had no doubt felt fairly negative about Martin for a while afterwards, she would also be understanding about the incident, especially as he had since expressed his regret for his action. Having considered these other possible ways of viewing and reacting to the situation from the nurse's point of view, Martin felt able to check it out with the nurse concerned and she confirmed and reassured him that the incident was now in the past as far as she was concerned, and that she did not want to hurt him in any way for what had happened.

Subsequent enquiry revealed that Martin had hit the other two potential murderers in the past, but so many years ago that the nurses themselves had, to all intents and purposes, forgotten about it. But having uncovered this, we were then able to use the same arguments as we had used with the third nurse to show that these two nurses would not be trying to kill him because they had been hit by him years before. They, too, were able to reassure him that they did not want to do him any harm, and indeed that they liked him.

MODIFYING THE BELIEFS THAT ARE NECESSARY FOR THE SURFACE MEANING OF THE DELUSION

Experiences are interpreted in terms of the person's beliefs and knowledge about the world, so these latter are *necessary* in order for the delusional belief to be held in the form that it is. For example, I could not blame the death of my cat on the magical powers of my neighbour unless I believed that people could kill using magic.

The reason for identifying and attempting to modify these non-psychotic beliefs or knowledge is that the delusional belief will no longer be valid if one or more of the necessary, underlying beliefs is no longer held to be true. For example, I cannot blame my neighbour for my cat's death if I no longer believe that magic can bring about an animal's death. Similarly, I cannot continue to believe that the man upstairs is influencing me with crystals if I no longer believe that crystals can have any power; I cannot continue to believe that spy satellites are burning my skin with lasers if I learn that lasers cannot travel through buildings; I cannot continue to believe that I sometimes turn into a werewolf if I come to understand that werewolves are only fictional creations. The sole purpose of modifying underlying beliefs in this aspect of the therapy is to undermine and modify the delusional belief (cf. the purpose of modifying the beliefs underlying the deep meaning, which is to reduce the distress caused by those underlying beliefs).

The steps involved in identifying and modifying 'necessary' underlying beliefs

1. What beliefs are necessary in order for this delusional belief to be held?
The therapist can *deduce* what these underlying beliefs/factors must be by using logical reasoning. For example, in order to hold the delusional belief 'I was abducted by Martians and taken to their planet, where I walked around with them' the person must believe:

(a) that Martians exist
(b) that Martians can and do visit the earth
(c) that Martians can and do take people on their spaceships to their planet
(d) that they have developed some way of overcoming the problems of travelling at the speed required to get the person back within hours of leaving
(e) that they can launch their spaceship back to Mars without requiring any launch pad and without leaving any rockets behind (cf. human space travel)
(f) that humans can survive on Mars without special breathing apparatus, pressure suits, etc.

If you could prove to the person that any one of these beliefs was not valid, then the abduction, as reported, would not have been possible.

2. Set the ideal goal for each necessary belief and consider whether modification would be possible in practice
Goal setting follows the basic format of (a) specifying in detail what the person would end up believing, (b) considering the wider implications of changing the belief, and (c) ensuring that the new belief is more functional and acceptable to the person, before going ahead with it. The requirement of keeping the goal consistent with the person's wider socio-cultural and religious beliefs is likely to be an important consideration in this area of work.

In practice it is often impossible even to attempt to modify many of the necessary underlying beliefs identified. After all, these are non-psychotic beliefs and as such are likely to be commonly held in the person's socio-cultural group, and it is likely that the factual knowledge on which a delusional belief is based is essentially correct. Even where the beliefs or knowledge represent a minority view (e.g. belief in alien abduction) there may be enough 'normal' people in the person's peer group to make the belief effectively impossible to challenge. This is one reason why it is important to identify as many 'necessary' underlying beliefs as possible, because it may be one of the less obvious ones that can be successfully challenged with CBT. For example, in the case of abduction by Martians, the existence of Martians may seem the most obvious underlying belief to tackle but this would probably be a difficult modification to achieve in practice: firstly, because there are a number of people who believe in Martians and there are books on the subject, and secondly because the non-existence of something is very hard to prove (especially when it is so far away!). It is the perhaps less obvious belief about walking on Mars without breathing apparatus, etc. that will be the most susceptible to CBT strategies and as such the best prospect for modification.

3. Attempt to modify any underlying, necessary beliefs for which a functional goal has been identified

Although, according to the rules of formal logic, eliminating just one of the logically 'necessary' beliefs should make the delusional belief untenable, in practice it seems to be more effective if you can eliminate as many as possible.

Even if you cannot completely eliminate a necessary belief, if you can introduce some possibility of doubt, then this may help to weaken the delusional belief that is based on it.

In some cases, modification of a dysfunctional underlying belief may be the only way of ensuring a stable and permanent change to the delusional belief itself. In the example used above, if the possibility of abduction by Martians is left intact, then even though the person may realize now that they were mistaken in thinking they had been abducted in the past, the 'Martian' explanation is still available for them to use if they have similar subjective experiences again in the future.

The CBT strategies used to modify the necessary underlying beliefs are the same as those used to modify the delusional belief itself (see Chapter 8). This work would be undertaken as part of the delusional belief modification programme.

EXAMPLE OF MODIFYING A DELUSIONAL BELIEF BY MODIFYING A BELIEF THAT IS NECESSARY IN ORDER FOR THE DELUSION TO BE POSSIBLE

A woman believed that she was going to die because the woman living upstairs had put a voodoo spell on her. Underlying her delusion were the beliefs (a) that people cast voodoo spells, and (b) that voodoo spells can produce death.

It was not feasible to attempt to modify the first underlying belief, namely that some people are involved in a religion called voodoo that can involve casting spells on people, since there is much evidence to suggest that this practice is still carried out today. However, as there was no good reason why she would need to retain her belief in the power of voodoo (she was attached to a Christian church), the second belief about spells being able to produce death could be targeted for modification. The goal of this modification was 'Even if a voodoo spell is cast, it cannot actually affect the person it is directed at'.

Although it was not considered feasible to attempt to modify the general belief that some people in the world go through the rituals of casting voodoo spells, the specific belief relating to the woman upstairs was targeted for modification because there was absolutely no evidence or reason to suggest she was a member of the voodoo cult. The goal for this modification was 'A few people may be involved in voodoo but, if it happens at all in this country, it is very rare indeed, and the woman upstairs is not one of them'.

EXAMPLE OF GOAL SETTING FOR NECESSARY BELIEFS

A woman believed that she ought to be living in Buckingham Palace because she was the rightful Queen of England. The beliefs that were necessary for this delusion to be held were (a) that Buckingham Palace exists, (b) that there is a Queen of England, and (c) that Buckingham Palace is the home of the Queen of England. The Queen of England and Buckingham Palace both exist, and if the woman were the rightful Queen of England, then it would be appropriate for her to be living in Buckingham Palace, so this delusional belief could not be undermined by targeting any of the necessary underlying beliefs.

CASE STUDY JANE

(See also pp. 76, 95, 99, 136, 188 and 277.)

Belief: *I am an evil witch.*

The following beliefs would be necessary in order for Jane to believe she had become an evil witch some three months previously:

(a) Witches exist, i.e. people exist who call themselves witches and claim supernatural powers.
(b) Some people have special powers and can do supernatural things.
(c) It is possible to become a witch without knowing about it or attending any special ceremony.

An important part of the assessment was to clarify exactly what Jane meant by the term 'witch' because this might have furnished other necessary beliefs that could be open to challenge. For example, if she had believed that witches always carried a secret mark on their bodies, then the fact that she had no mark could have been used as contradictory evidence, or if she had believed that witches always belong to a coven, then the fact that she did not do so could have been used in the same way. In practice Jane believed that witches were women who had supernatural powers, like the ones from history, but otherwise she held no firm beliefs about them.

Necessary belief (a). It was not possible to modify the beliefs about the existence of people who call themselves witches and who claim to be able to make bad things happen, because such people do exist.

Necessary belief (b). Theoretically, modifying Jane's belief that some people can have special powers would have helped to undermine the delusional belief about herself, but as this belief in its most general form was compatible with her religious beliefs about miracles and saints it was not considered appropriate to target it for modification. (The belief as it relates to saints would, in any case, have been very difficult, if not impossible, to modify in practice because so many people hold the belief in this form.)

However, the belief in special powers as it relates to witches was not a functional one for Jane to have, and modification of it would not impact on her belief about saints. Therefore, an attempt was made to modify her belief in the power of witches, using a combination of logical reasoning and evidence evaluation. It was argued that historical belief in witches was based on superstition and fear, and that modern science had shown that supernatural powers are not possible. It was noted that witches in history did not have the power to protect themselves against persecution and death at the hands of ordinary people, and that modern day witches reported in the newspapers do not seem to have a lifestyle that would suggest they can change things supernaturally.

We did not suggest looking for evidence from the so-called experts in this area because it is likely that a good proportion of books written about witches will be by people who are interested enough to write about the subject, i.e. those who believe in their existence and power. However, if Jane herself had been using information from books as evidence for the existence of witches' power, then they would have been challenged, and 'expert' books written to contradict this position would have been introduced.

Necessary belief (c). Although at first sight this looked a promising line of work, because it would probably have been easy to establish from books about witchcraft that a 'witch' has to undergo certain trainings and initiation ceremonies before she can become a witch, in practice this line was not pursued. Firstly, Jane's knowledge of witchcraft was vague and sketchy and it was considered that it would be unhelpful to bring her into contact with writings that would confirm their existence and special powers and that would provide her with more 'supporting' information and evidence on the topic. Secondly, Jane did not know where her powers had suddenly come from but there was a suggestion in some of her answers that, if pressed for details, she might conclude that if they did not come from witchcraft, then they must come from the Devil. This would not have been a helpful modification.

BELIEFS NOT DIRECTLY ASSOCIATED WITH THE DELUSIONS OR HALLUCINATIONS

CBT treats the person as a whole, not just their symptoms, so it may well be appropriate to undertake modification of dysfunctional beliefs that play no part in the delusions or hallucinations as such. Where this applies, it would be carried out at the same time as the work on the delusions and hallucinations, using the appropriate CBT strategies.

Self-esteem

A common consequence of developing psychosis is poor self-esteem. If someone has low self-esteem because they have failed to achieve academic or occupational success, have no job, no partner, no family, etc., then a distinction should be made between what these things can bring to the person in the way of comfort and happiness and what they mean in terms of the person's value; commonly, these two aspects are confused. Whilst acknowledging the real loss and impact of the consequences of psychosis for the person concerned, the modification undertaken would be to change their beliefs about self-worth so that these beliefs become linked to the person's intrinsic value as a unique individual, and/or to characteristics that they possess (e.g. kindness and generosity) rather than to the acquisition of 'things', including the things valued by other members of society. At the end of the day, acquisitions, be they of material goods, money, knowledge, skills, social status, friends or family, are only of value if they bring the person fulfilment and happiness; acquisitions have nothing to do with the value of the person as a person.

Caution: When working with people who have had to drop out of education or who have failed to obtain employment at the expected level, a common mistake is to attempt to reassure them that of course they would have done well if it had not been for their illness, or that, in the circumstances, they are doing very well to attempt training for an unskilled job.[3] The problem with this approach is that emphasizing their previous academic achievements will covertly indicate to them that you, too, believe academic success is important and to be sought after, and therefore, by implication, that they have 'failed'. Similarly, enthusiastically praising any occupational efforts will signal your approval of having a job and job success, which will not be helpful when the person's job potential is severely limited. It is generally safer in such cases to adopt from the start an attitude of general indifference to educational achievement or occupational success as such, noting that these things have no fundamental value in themselves, other than their enjoyment value (if there is one), and that they do not indicate personal worth. This latter point may be reinforced by asking the person to describe what they like about a particular friend and noting if, as is likely, worldly success is *not* one of the characteristics mentioned. More likely to

[3]As an analogy, if you had been badly burned by a fire, how comforting would it be for someone to reassure you that of course you *would* have looked attractive, if your face hadn't been so awfully scarred?

be mentioned are factors such as friendliness, generosity, independence, sense of humour, courage, etc., some at least of which are likely to apply also to the person with whom you are working.

8 Modifying the delusional belief

Introduction

Once the ground work for the belief change has been carried out, including setting the most functional goal and ensuring that it is acceptable to the person, the modification work can begin. Although the word 'challenge' is often used to describe this part of the therapy, this work is rarely ever done as a direct challenge. It is probably more accurate to think of it as 'nibbling at the edges' of the delusion, making little forays of attack and retreat to determine the effective lines of work and best strategies to use. As many different approaches as possible are used to build up the onslaught, until the delusion crumbles and modification becomes inevitable.

The interrelationship between evidence evaluation, logical reasoning and reality testing

Although these core CBT strategies are described separately in this chapter, in practice they are closely interrelated. For example, logical reasoning is used to evaluate the evidence for and against the delusion and also the results of any reality tests carried out, whilst reality testing is one way of re-evaluating evidence supporting the delusion and of providing evidence that contradicts it.

The order in which the strategies are used

There is no fixed or 'correct' order for using these modification strategies, but it is nearly always necessary to eliminate, or at least substantially undermine, any evidence from the past that supports the delusion, and so this is usually a sensible starting point. For example, a woman believes that her next-door neighbour tortures and murders women and that she is at risk: she has heard their screams and heard him making threats directed at her. If this 'evidence' is left intact, then it will be impossible to establish that the neighbour has no bad intent towards her.

Although it is usual to start by considering the evidence supporting the delusion, in some cases, notably where the delusion is based on a feeling of certainty rather than actual events, it may be appropriate to start by using logical reasoning. This will also be appropriate in cases where the delusional belief is so strongly held that it is necessary to use logical reasoning to instil some doubt before the person will consider it sensible or worthwhile to review the evidence. For example, a man who visited our department became upset when he heard noises from the offices upstairs because he interpreted this as a sign that the people there were reading his mind. He would not consider discussing the evidence, because it was so obvious to him that it was happening, until the therapist argued that it seemed to her that since the people upstairs had not seen him arrive (a fact that he readily accepted) they would not know to read his mind, even if they could do so.

In contrast, in some other cases it may be necessary for some contradictory evidence to occur before the person considers it worthwhile to engage in logical reasoning. For example, a man was so sure he knew in advance what people were going to say or do that he was not willing to entertain any doubts or questions about it, until he was faced with the unexpected and therefore disconfirming evidence of being hit by a fellow resident.

A well-constructed reality test of the delusional belief can provide irrefutable evidence against it and as such may be sufficient to cause it to collapse. Although reality testing the evidence supporting the delusion may occur from the earliest stages of therapy, reality testing the core delusional belief itself usually occurs towards the end. There are a number of reasons for this. Firstly, because of the power of a direct reality test of the core belief it must not be undertaken until the goal of modification has been fully prepared. Secondly, it may be necessary to instil some doubt about the belief using evidence evaluation and logical reasoning before the believer will consider it worthwhile to put it to the test. Thirdly, where the delusion involves potential danger the person will, understandably, be unwilling to risk a reality test until they are pretty certain that their belief is not true and therefore that the reality test is safe. For example, if a man believes that if he cuts his hair something terrible will happen to him, the ultimate reality test of that belief would be for him to have his hair cut – but the arguments as to why no harm could befall him as a result of the haircut would need to be very persuasive if they were to give him the confidence to carry it out. Lastly, reality testing the core delusional belief may be the final strategy of this part of the therapy because the evidence it produces is so unambiguous that it cannot be ignored or explained away and, therefore, forces the belief to change.

EVIDENCE EVALUATION

There are two aspects to evidence evaluation: eliminating or undermining the evidence that the person has to support their delusional belief, and building up evidence that contradicts it.

ELIMINATING THE EVIDENCE SUPPORTING THE DELUSIONAL BELIEF

As we saw in Chapter 2, delusional beliefs are always based on *something*; the person (mis)interprets their internal experiences and external events and this then becomes the evidence that supports their belief. Therefore, an essential part of the modification process is to identify the evidence supporting the delusion and to eliminate it, i.e. change the person's interpretations so they no longer provide support for the delusional belief.

In practice it is not always possible to completely eliminate a piece of supporting evidence by re-evaluating it, but even if you are only able to instil some doubt, then this may be sufficient to lead on to other aspects of treatment that can complete the re-evaluation. Nor is it always possible to target all the evidence for re-evaluation. For example, there may be too much evidence from the past, or new confirmatory evidence may occur faster than it can be re-evaluated, or the evidence may have happened so long ago that it is no longer possible to get any independent information. Fortunately, removing key pieces of supportive evidence, or weakening it by introducing doubt, is often all that is required.

Eliminating evidence that supports defining or otherwise important features of the delusional belief is more likely to bring about the required modification than eliminating more peripheral evidence. For example, a woman believes she is the Virgin Mary. The evidence she has for this belief is (a) she hears messages from God telling her that this is so, and (b) a friend told her that she looked like a picture of the Virgin Mary by Raphael. Changing her understanding about the nature of the voice, so that she no longer believes it come from God, is likely to have a much greater effect on her core belief than convincing her that she does not resemble this particular picture, or reasoning that resembling a picture of someone does not mean that you are that someone. Whether you choose to target the more or less important evidence first will depend on your overall treatment plan and the need to do preparation work. As a general rule, working on the less important evidence will be easier and safer but the speed of treatment will be slower.

The evidence to be eliminated or undermined includes both evidence from the past and evidence from ongoing events and experiences. These latter are usually easier to work with because they are more available for discussion, exploration and challenge, but for a total modification significant evidence from the past will also have to be removed.

The evidence supporting a delusional belief will fall into one or more of the broad, overlapping categories described below. The ways of re-evaluating these different types of evidence so that they no longer support the delusional belief are presented as a *solution*.

A1 The evidence is true and accurately recalled, but has been misinterpreted

Solution: Provide and strengthen an alternative explanation(s).

Examples:

- 'I know that I own Buckingham Palace because the policemen there admitted it to me.' *The alternative explanation was that the policemen had agreed with her to stop her getting angry and upset.*
- 'The spirits are putting drops of poison in my mouth: I can sometimes taste it at the back of my mouth.' *The alternative explanation for this taste was dental decay.*

A2 The interpretation is an exaggeration of the truth

Solution: Suggest and strengthen a more moderate, normal interpretation.

Examples:

- 'My neighbours want to kill me: they told me I was a nuisance and said they wished I'd never come to live here.' *The alternative explanation was that the neighbours had become irritated by the person's behaviour but that this was very different from them wanting him dead, which in turn was very different from them actually attempting murder.*
- 'The doctors don't want me to get better and get a job: they said I would be useless if I went back to college.' *The alternative explanation was that the doctors did not think college was advisable at this time because of the person's difficulty in concentrating.*

A3 The interpretation and/or recall of an event is inaccurate or distorted

Solution: Find out what actually happened from an independent source, or speculate about what might have actually happened from the person's own account, and use this as the basis for an alternative interpretation.

Examples:

- 'The shop assistant sneered at me to show that she thought I was ugly.' *The alternative explanation was that the man was afraid the shop assistant would think he was ugly and was expecting her to sneer at him, so when she did not smile he interpreted this as a sneer.*
- 'The foreigners were out to get me: they put a ladder up against the wall in the night and tried to climb in through my window.' *The alternative explanation was that the woman was frightened, agitated and had not slept properly for days, so in this tired, confused state she misinterpreted the sounds from the street below.*

Generating the alternative explanation(s) for the re-evaluations of A1–A3

Following the general CBT principle that it is better if the patient/client comes up with the ideas rather than the therapist, ideally you would encourage the person themself to suggest possible alternative explanations for the evidence they have. However, in practice it is often very difficult or impossible for people to stand outside their strongly held beliefs and experiences in this way, so when this is the case it is the therapist's task to generate and suggest the alternatives.

Whether you offer one or more alternative explanations depends on what you are hoping to achieve by this exercise. If, for example in the early stages of therapy, you are only wanting the person to accept that there are possible alternative explanations for most situations, without suggesting that any of these alternatives is more appropriate than their delusional one, then you would offer as many alternatives as possible, including some with a low probability of being correct. (Needless to say, you should be careful not to suggest anything dysfunctional or that would feed into other delusional beliefs.) Floating a number of alternatives not only makes the point more forcibly that other possibilities exist but also avoids any suggestion that you are pushing a particular alternative in preference to the delusional one. If, on the other hand, you are at the stage of wanting to establish one particular alternative explanation to replace the delusional one, then you should go for just the one most likely to actually apply.

The 'true' explanation for what happened may not seem the most persuasive alternative to the person themself, particularly in the early stages, but it will certainly be the most resilient to logical reasoning and testing, and it is the one most likely to be confirmed by subsequent events in the person's life, so this is usually the one you would try to establish. This means that you will often be in the position of trying to work out 'what is *really* going on here?'. Is the evidence accurately described but wrongly interpreted? Or is what is being described an exaggeration or gross distortion of what happened in fact? Asking the person about specific details will often provide the clues you need to answer these questions.

In some cases it may be difficult to ascertain which of a number of possible alternative explanations is the true one, or there may be more than one true explanation (see case example 1, below). When this occurs, you should float the likely alternatives and discuss them to see which the person feels are the most likely to be true, and work from there.

EXAMPLES OF GENERATING ALTERNATIVE EXPLANATIONS

Delusion 1: *People know I'm not really human.*

Evidence: *People were looking at me in a strange way when I went into Epsom* [the local town].

Possible alternative explanations:

(a) People are looking at you in a normal way but you feel uneasy and self-conscious and so you are oversensitive to them looking at you.
(b) It is because you stare at them when you are trying to check out their response to you; they notice you staring at them and are worried why that might be, so they look at you.
(c) It is because people in Epsom are not used to people who dress like you; people wouldn't take any notice in London but this is conservative suburbia.
(d) It is because you mutter under your breath, which is unusual, so people are worried that you might be very upset about something.

Delusion 2: *There are insects under my skin.*

Evidence: *I can feel them crawling around.*

Possible alternative explanations:[1]

(a) It is the tiny nerves just under your skin that are firing off for no particular reason, a bit like when you suddenly get an itch, but more so.

(b) It is a skin disorder.
(c) It is irritation from your clothing and/or bedding.

Note: When this delusion occurred in clinical practice, only (a) was considered to be a viable alternative explanation because there was no evidence of a skin disorder, and the possibility of irritation from clothing or bedding was too unlikely and easily disproved.

Presenting the alternative explanation(s)

In general, it is harder to generate and discuss alternative explanations for internal, subjective experiences than for external events. Partly this is because subjective experiences, including perceptions and misperceptions coming from our five senses, come imbued with their own sense of certainty. However, another important factor is that we all, understandably, think we are in the uniquely best position to interpret our own subjective experiences because we are the only ones directly aware of them, and therefore we do not take kindly to having our experiences queried by other people. For example, I may disagree with you about whether or not the ball was out during a game of tennis but I will admit that you have as much right to form an opinion about the event as I do; however, I would think you had overstepped the mark if you told me that, in your opinion, I did not really have the toothache that I told you I had. Therefore, if you are suggesting an alternative explanation for a subjective experience, you should make it very clear to the person that you do not for one moment doubt their experience, and that the alternative you are suggesting is for what *caused* the experience and not for the experience itself.

One way of introducing an alternative explanation is by using a phrase such as 'I've been thinking about what you were saying the other day ... and it occurred to me that ...' , or '... and I was wondering if ... What do you think?'. (See also p. 51.)

Another way is to ask the person how other people interpret what has happened to them, and then go on to discuss and explore why they think these other people might see things in the way they do. (See also p. 52.) Note that if the person is sensitive about your disbelieving their point of view, then you need to pursue this line gently and slowly, making clear that you are not judging the other peoples' views one way or another but are just curious as to why they have come to the conclusions that they have. Even if the person concludes that the other people have no very good reasons for coming to their different conclusions, it can be important and helpful for them to understand that different people can genuinely and honestly see and interpret things quite differently, even though not all the interpretations can be correct in fact.

The way in which you respond to the evidence when you are given it may also be important because of what this can imply covertly. For example, in the case of the man who believed the noises from the rooms above indicated that the occupants were reading his mind (see p. 147), the therapist's immediate response was to express surprise on the grounds that she had assumed the murmur of talking and scraping of chairs meant the same as they did on every other day of the week, namely that they were people in a meeting discussing some management issue about the wards. By expressing surprise and using the word 'assumed' for her own interpretation of events, the therapist was able to put forward an alternative explanation without implying she was dismissing the man's interpretation. This led naturally to a discussion about his suggestion and hence to the first tentative piece of logical reasoning to question it. If the therapist had responded in a neutral way, then the man might have interpreted this as confirmation that she, too, thought this was the most reasonable explanation.

B1 The evidence comes from a misunderstanding of what is possible in reality

Solution: Change/correct the misunderstanding by giving more information and discussion.

Examples:

- 'The spy satellites are burning my skin with lasers.' *Information about the inability of lasers to pass through solid buildings and pinpoint an individual was given and discussed.*
- 'I turn into a werewolf for brief periods.' *Information about the inability of solid matter to change form and to increase or decrease by large amounts was given and discussed.*[1]

B2 The evidence comes from something read, seen or heard, or from someone else's opinion/belief

Solution: Obtain information about the source of the evidence and 'challenge' it accordingly, for example on the grounds that it is fictional; or that the 'expert opinion' is not authoritative and/or correct; or that the person has misread, misunderstood or misremembered it.

Examples:

- 'I know that dinosaurs exist because I have seen them on TV.' *Information about how these programmes are made using computerized images was given and discussed.*
- 'Schizophrenia is caused when the spiritual awakening is blocked by medication.' *The therapist read the book in which this claim was made, and on the basis of this was able to challenge the author's authority on schizophrenia.*

[1] In practice, eliminating this type of evidence often involves more than one type of 'solution'. For example, in this case the therapist also identified the film the man had seen in which this had happened and then explained, in detail, how the film studios would have produced these effects.

Identifying the source of the inaccurate 'knowledge' that is the basis for B1 and B2

It is a great advantage if you can identify the source of this type of evidence because this gives you the best chance for launching an appropriate and detailed, targeted challenge. For example, if you know which book is involved, then you can read it; this will enable you to check the person has not misunderstood what was written and to check the basis for the author's claims (which may be open to challenge) and the authority of the author to make them.

Ideas depicted in science fiction and fantasy range from the scientifically possible (e.g. life on another planet) to the frankly absurd (e.g. becoming very small and travelling round someone else's bloodstream). The problem with this area of fiction is that often it does not discriminate for the reader or watcher what is feasible and what is not, and with the development of sophisticated computerized animation the 'evidence' can look very convincing. Without explicit guidance, and without a solid scientific understanding of the world on which to judge the ideas portrayed, it is easy to see how people could conclude that even the most fantastic things are at least possible.

There has also been an unfortunate trend (unfortunate from the point of view of developing delusional beliefs) in recent times to deliberately blur the distinction between fiction and fact, so it is not surprising if some of these ideas find their way into people's belief/knowledge systems. For example, the popular *X-Files* series on TV implied that it *could* be depicting real events, and a number of novels about secret, covert operations have been presented as 'true' diaries of actual events.

Another problem is that some magazines that purport to be serious journalism present fictional stories as if they were real events. In the UK, one newspaper is particularly notorious for doing this, so if the person gives as evidence that they 'read it in a newspaper', it is worth asking which one.

It will often be the case that you are not able to identify a specific source for the person's 'knowledge'. In these circumstances the re-evaluation will have to be based on obtaining and giving more accurate information about the 'fact' that is given as evidence, together with logical reasoning and, if appropriate, reality testing.

C The evidence is another delusion or hallucination

Solution: CBT to modify the delusion or hallucination.

Examples:

- 'My husband wants me dead because he is having an affair with Madonna.' *Modifying the delusion about her husband having an affair with Madonna eliminated one reason why he might want her dead.*
- 'I overheard the nurses saying that they wanted me dead.' *Understanding that what the person had heard were voices reflecting his own fear removed this powerful evidence for his delusion about the nurses.*

In people with complex delusional systems one delusion may support another, and so on. This is not surprising, of course, given that delusional beliefs, once established, act like any other underlying belief in that they can influence the development of new delusional beliefs and become incorporated into them. Where this has happened, there may be no alternative to painstakingly tackling one delusion after another (see p. 99 for discussion of the relative importance of delusions in a delusional system).

Voices can provide very definite, positive evidence to support the delusion. Again, this is not surprising, given that voices are the thoughts of the person heard out loud. Although it may be possible to weaken the impact of the voices by working on their content (see Chapter 11), in many cases it will also be necessary to change the belief about the origin of the voices. Once the voices are understood to come from within oneself, then they will have no more authority or power than one's own thoughts (see Chapter 12).

D The evidence is a feeling of conviction ('I just know it's true')

Solution: Establish that 'feeling something to be true does not mean that it is true'. Establish that if there is no 'hard' evidence, for example that which would permissible in a court of law, then the feeling of certainty could be wrong and needs to be checked out.

Examples:

- 'I just know that when the woman ahead picked up the jar of Tesco's marmalade she did this in order to insult me.' *It was possible to show that this feeling of certainty had been wrong in the past, and therefore that it could have been wrong here as well; plus, there was no hard evidence that the stranger had wanted to insult her.*
- 'I just knew when the aeroplane passed overhead at that moment that it was very significant.' *The general principle 'Feeling something to be significant does not mean that it has significance' was established, together with the recognition that 'My brain is oversensitive in this respect and so if, when I check out the feeling, I can find no hard evidence to corroborate it, then I know it is most likely to be a feeling and not a genuine response to an externally significant event'.*

Establishing that feelings are not the same as facts

The ways of establishing that 'feelings' are not the same as 'facts' are essentially the same as those used in the insight promotion work (see Chapter 6) to demonstrate that 'Believing something to be true does not mean that it is true', but they focus specifically on feelings of certainty. The strategies are summarized below.

1. Use common examples from everyday life to establish the general principle that all of us can be sure that something is true even when it is not. These examples can be obtained from your own experiences and from the experiences of the person you are working with and/or other people, and may include:

- misinterpretations of everyday events
- beliefs held in the past but no longer held

- intuitions that turned out to be wrong
- dreams.

2. Use explanations that are generally applicable to explain *why* we can feel sure that something is true even though it is not, for example:

- the brain jumps to conclusions on insufficient evidence
- the 'Feeling Brain⟷Logical Brain' model (see below and Appendix 2).

3. Use explanations that are specific to the individual to explain *why* he or she can sometimes feel sure that something is true even though it is not, for example:

- overactivity/oversensitivity of part of the brain
  - for example, the part that decides that something is *definitely* rather than probably true
  - the part that recognizes significance/importance
- the 2-route model (particularly useful for feelings of paranoia).

The 'Feeling Brain⟷Logical Brain' model (see Appendix 2)

This model can be used to explain why it is that we can feel something to be true even when it is not, and also why we can continue to feel something is true even when we know it is not. It is a general model to describe how these different aspects of thinking function and interact, and can be used with a wide range of disorders, including anxiety and depression, as well as psychosis.

In clinical practice this model has proved easy to understand and acceptable to people with psychosis. One of its big advantages is that it describes how we all think in normal life and so it is a non-stigmatizing way of explaining what might be happening in psychosis and is suitable for people who deny having a mental illness.

BUILDING UP THE EVIDENCE AGAINST THE DELUSIONAL BELIEF

Evidence against the delusional belief comes from the past, from ongoing events during the course of therapy and from reality testing (see later in this chapter). The evidence against the delusional belief should also support the replacement belief being used, so building up the evidence against the delusion and in favour of the replacement belief are two sides of the same coin.

As a general rule, evidence that contradicts key aspects of the delusional belief will be more powerful than evidence that contradicts unimportant, peripheral aspects. For example, with the belief 'I am the reincarnation of Marilyn Monroe', the fact that Marilyn Monroe died 10 years after the person was born is likely to be a more powerful piece of evidence against the belief than the fact that she does not look or sound like Marilyn Monroe. Nevertheless, there seems to be something persuasive about sheer quantity of evidence when it is amassed, so it is worth collecting as much as possible. One of the advantages of starting with the less significant pieces of disconfirming evidence, i.e. evidence that suggests the delusion *may* not be true but that cannot say more than that, is that you can gauge the other person's response to it before going on to the more powerful evidence. This can be useful if, for some reason, you are progressing cautiously with the belief modification.

Events recalled from the past are likely to be biased in favour of the delusion because, like any other strongly held belief, the delusional belief will not only have distorted the way the events were interpreted but will also have biased the attention paid to them and the likelihood that they will be remembered. Asking directly for disconfirming evidence (e.g. 'Do you have any reasons for believing that ... is not true?') is likely to be a fruitless exercise because had the person been aware that something contradicted their belief, then they would either have modified their interpretation of it at the time, so that it was no longer contradictory, or they would have modified the delusional belief to accommodate it. Furthermore, such direct questioning is likely to imply that you have some doubt about the other person's view of things, which may lead to loss of rapport and adversely affect engagement in therapy. Nevertheless, you should be on constant alert for anything you are told about the past that might run contrary to the delusional belief. If this information is given freely, in the early stages of therapy, then it is likely that the contradiction is not appreciated and so you should be careful not to point it out at this stage but just to make a note of it for later consideration and use. For example, a man believed he could read minds, but was very angry because his social worker had deceived him by not telling him that the phone call she made had been to his psychiatrist. At that particular time, it would have been confrontational and unhelpful to point out this apparent inconsistency.

It is usually easier to spot contradictory evidence when it occurs during ongoing therapy because the memory of the incident will be stronger and in this respect less likely to be forgotten or to be distorted as it is recalled. Gathering this information is one reason why it is often helpful to start CBT sessions with a general enquiry about how things have gone for the person during the period between sessions. As with events from the past, in the early stages of therapy it will probably be appropriate to just make a note of any incidents that seem to contradict the delusion rather than trying to use them then and there to challenge the belief (see 'Exposing the contradictory evidence', below).

Reality testing can provide powerful evidence against the delusional belief and, because of the open, cooperative way in which it is set up, the person is immediately aware of the full implications of the results.

Evidence and logical reasoning based on what the delusion implies

In some cases it is relatively easy, at least in principle, to see what evidence would be needed to disprove the delusion, for example with the man who believed he owned houses in Kent and Cornwall, or with the woman who believed she passed only a few drops of urine every day. In other cases, however, it may be difficult to see what evidence could disprove the delusion in the form it takes, for example in the case of the man who believed his son intended to poison him in order to inherit his money, or the woman who believed God would be angry if she stopped fasting. In these latter cases, where it is difficult or impossible to collect evidence directly related to the delusion itself, it may be possible to collect evidence about some implication of the delusion, i.e. about something that would necessarily follow if the delusion were true. The line of logical reasoning behind this approach is:

If the delusion is true, then X follows.
Therefore, if X is not true, then the delusion cannot be true either.

For example, in the case above, the only way of directly testing whether the man's son intended to poison him would be to ask the son; but in the circumstances the father is unlikely to be convinced by his denial. However, the implications of this delusion, namely (a) that his son does not love or care for him, (b) that the man has enough money to make murder worthwhile, and (c) that the son would be prepared to risk prison and losing everything for the sake of the money, are potentially more easy to contradict.

In the second example given above, there is no way of knowing in advance whether God would be angry or not if the woman stopped her fast because there is absolutely no way of checking out how God might feel about something. However, one of the implications of this delusional belief is that God requires people in hospital to starve themselves for no apparent reason, so you might be able to counter this implication by seeking the views of the acknowledged experts from the person's own religious group.

Before you can collect evidence that contradicts the implication of the delusion (i.e. evidence that X is not true) you have to work out what these implications are, using logical reasoning. Useful questions to ask yourself are: 'What would it be like if the delusion were true? What else would have happened in the past, or would be happening now? What would be different?'. The things that would be different are the things that you might be able to use as indirect evidence against the delusion. For example, a man believed his father had been replaced by a double. If the delusion were true, then this would mean, amongst other things, that the double would not have any memories of the man's childhood except what he had learnt from other people. So you might ask questions like: 'What does your father's double talk about? Does he talk much about when you were a child?' If his father talks about his childhood and knows in detail about their shared experiences from those days, then this is good evidence that he cannot be a double. As with all logical reasoning and evidence evaluation work, if you are not ready to expose the inconsistent information obtained, then it can just be noted for future use, when the time is appropriate.

Evidence and logical reasoning to cast doubt on the delusion rather than disprove it

As a general principle, whilst it is possible to collect evidence about present situations, no direct evidence can exist about future events. For example, a man believed that self-castration would guarantee him eternal life in this world. There is no direct evidence that can be collected to refute this belief, and it cannot be reality tested (even if it were ethical to do so!) because only death will disprove the belief, and it will be too late then for the results to be beneficial. In this sort of case, the best therapeutic goal you can hope for is to instil sufficient doubt in the delusional belief for the person to consider it would be too big a risk to act on it. In this particular case, all the evidence to date, from history, indicates that people who have been castrated do die in the normal way, so although this does not absolutely prove the same would happen to this man, nevertheless it was argued that he would need some good, solid proof that such an extraordinary claim were true before risking such an irrevocable step.

In another case, a man believed he had a special relationship with God so that God would protect him whatever he did: he was keen to prove this by throwing himself in front of a bus. It was suggested to him that God might not like being tested in this way. This was backed up by arguing that such evidence as exists, for example from the Bible and the lives of the saints, suggests that God does not seek to 'prove' things by dramatic, showy displays of power. When asked if he could think of any other possible reasons why God might not intervene, the man thought it might just be possible that God would not want to reveal their special relationship in this way. The therapist suggested he should not take the risk of doing something that could go so disastrously wrong until he was absolutely certain he would be safe.

USING THE CONTRADICTORY EVIDENCE TO MODIFY THE DELUSION

When contradictory evidence is 'exposed', i.e. brought to the person's notice for consideration and discussion, one of four things can happen.

1 Their interpretation of the contradictory evidence stays intact and the delusional belief is modified accordingly. (This is the desired outcome.)
2 Their interpretation of the contradictory evidence is re-evaluated and distorted so that it becomes consistent with the delusional belief, which stays intact.
3 An additional factor is brought in to explain the conflicting evidence, so that the interpretation of the contradictory evidence remains intact but it no longer contradicts the delusional belief. This is sometimes called 'finding an escape route'.
4 There is a compromise between 1 and 2 above, so that the delusional belief is only partially changed. This partial change may or may not be a helpful step towards the goal of modification.

EXAMPLE OF POSSIBLE WAYS THAT SOMEONE MIGHT INTERPRET CONTRADICTORY EVIDENCE

Belief: *I have no brain; my head is completely empty.*

Contradictory evidence: *X-ray of the person's head showing a normal skull with a brain inside.*

A woman believes that she has no brain. When shown the X-ray of her head, the desired result for this woman is for her to conclude that the X-ray shows a brain and therefore that she must have a brain.

However, if the delusional belief is very strong, when faced with the apparent contradiction she may conclude that her immediate interpretation of the X-ray must be wrong (this is not as unreasonable as it may sound because she knows for certain that she has no brain) and therefore that what the X-ray actually shows is mostly empty space with just a few lines caused by the X-rays as they passed through the skull. This sort of distortion tends to occur when the person's delusional belief is very strong and the contradictory evidence is relatively weak and can be easily reinterpreted in line with the delusion.

Alternatively, this woman may find the escape route of concluding that the X-ray is not of her head but of someone else's. This allows her to keep her delusion about her own head whilst not denying that the X-ray shows a brain within the skull. As a general rule, escape routes tend to occur when both the delusional belief and the contradictory evidence are very strong so that neither can give way to the other.

Another possibility is that this woman will conclude that the X-ray shows there is something inside her skull but that it is a small or malformed brain. In this particular case this is unlikely to be a helpful change in the delusional belief, not least because it is potentially easier to disprove 'no brain' than to disprove a small, malformed brain. As a general rule, this sort of distortion to the delusional belief occurs when the person cannot refute or escape from the contradictory evidence but on the other hand holds the delusional belief too strongly to let it go, perhaps because they still have too much other convincing evidence of its truth.

Strengthening the contradictory evidence

In order to help protect the contradictory evidence from being re-evaluated it may be possible to strengthen it before it is exposed. For example, in the case above, the woman's interpretation of her X-ray could be strengthened by showing her X-rays of other people's heads beforehand so that both she and the therapist were in agreement about how these should be interpreted.

Another way of strengthening a piece of evidence is to collect other evidence that supports it, because multiple pieces of evidence are harder to dispute and distort than a single piece. For example, in the case of the man who believed that two nurses wanted to kill him, one of the strands of work was to collect evidence that they liked and cared for him. As many incidents as possible were collected, mostly from ongoing events during the course of therapy.

If the interpretation of the contradictory evidence can be firmly established and fixed in the person's memory, then it is less likely to be distorted when it is set against the delusional belief. For example, in the case of the man who believed his father had been replaced by a double, the conversations he had with his father about his childhood experiences were discussed at some length so that the memory of these conversations was clear and definite *before* the therapist suggested that they contradicted his delusional belief.

For similar reasons, if you are noting contradictory evidence before you are ready to use it, then it is advisable to make the written notes clear and accurate so that you can remind the person of what they said at the time, before they realized that it contradicted their belief. This will help to protect the memories from being distorted when the inconsistencies are exposed.

Exposing the contradictory evidence

When to expose a piece of contradictory evidence is a matter of clinical judgment. As a general rule, if it is early in the course of treatment when other lines of CBT have not been developed and the delusion is still held very strongly, then it is advisable to proceed slowly and with caution. If a piece of contradictory evidence is distorted as a result of being exposed too soon, then this may have no more serious consequences than your losing a potentially useful line of treatment, and even this may be reversible in the future. But if you press someone too strongly to confront a contradiction, then you may force them down a very unhelpful escape route, or it may force a very unhelpful change to the delusional belief. A particularly pernicious escape route would be for the person to conclude that somehow you must have manipulated or falsified the evidence you are presenting. For example, in the case above it would not be a good outcome if the man concluded that the only explanation for the 'double' having this information about his childhood must be that you must have passed it on to him, and that you did this in order to protect the double and to convince other people that he was lying or mad!

In order to avoid revealing the contradictory evidence too soon, you may have to ask the questions about the potentially disconfirming evidence at a different time or in a different session from questions directly related to the delusional belief. For example, in the case where a man's delusional belief about being taken over by another resident is supported by the warnings he gets from the newscaster, you would not ask him whether or not the newscaster knows him personally immediately after discussing the personal information that the newscaster had given him. Nor should you attempt to elicit too many pieces of contradictory evidence at one time. If the person is very sensitive about having their delusional belief doubted, then you might have to separate all of these questions by general conversation about neutral or unrelated issues.

However careful you are to separate your questions about the contradictory evidence, the person may make the connection between the information you are asking about and their belief and become suddenly aware of the contradiction. Some of the signs to look out for are appearing suddenly puzzled or disconcerted or becoming suspicious, or restating the delusional belief. If this occurs at an early stage, before it is safe to expose the contradiction, you should back off rapidly by showing little interest in the answer to your question or by covering the other person's inability to respond by changing the topic or the direction of the conversation.

When you consider the contradictory evidence is secure against reinterpretation, and the person has been otherwise prepared for the belief modification, then you may gently introduce the contradiction and set it against the delusion.

One way of doing this is to ask questions about the contradictory evidence and the delusion close together, so that the person becomes aware of the contradiction without it being specifically pointed out to them. The advantage of doing it this way, if it is possible, is that the person discovers the contradiction for themself and so avoids the situation of being proved wrong by someone else. This latter is a situation that most of us dislike, particularly if it involves something that we have argued for in public.

Alternatively, you may float the contradiction. For example, in the case of the man who believed his father was a double you might float one of the inconsistencies thus: 'I've been thinking about what you've told me about your real father and about his double. You were telling me a couple of weeks ago that the double had been talking at dinner about an incident that happened with your real father when you were on a fishing trip together, how he had given you a can of beer and made you promise not to tell your mother because you were only eight and she would have been very cross with him – do you remember? And both of you must have kept that secret because it was the first time your mother had ever heard the tale? Well, it occurred to me that only your real father could have known of this incident, because it was a secret between the two of you, so it seems strange that the double could have talked about it ... if he really were just a double.' The advantage of floating ideas rather than making the contradictions explicit is that it gives you better control over how thoroughly or sharply you expose the contradictions, and also enables you to reiterate all the support you have for the contradictory evidence in order to protect it against reinterpretation when it has been set against the delusional belief. Furthermore, it may give you the opportunity to see how the person is going to react. If it looks as if the reaction is not going to be favourable, then you can back off and keep the contradictory evidence for use at a more suitable time.

If there appears to be no shift in the delusional belief when the contradictory evidence is exposed, then it is better to withdraw rapidly to a position of puzzlement, reinforcing if you can the desired part of the contradiction as you do so. For example, 'It's a bit puzzling, that, isn't it, because the double can't possibly have learnt about that incident from anyone and yet somehow he was able to talk about it. Oh well, it's not important, what I really wanted to talk to you about is ...'.

Avoiding escape routes and unhelpful belief changes

Where it is possible to anticipate that a particular escape route might be used, it may be possible to 'seal it off', i.e. to work on it before the contradiction is exposed so that it is no longer available as an escape route.

In the example above, the use of the shared experience that no one else had known about as the contradictory evidence, namely the beer on the fishing trip, helps to prevent the use of the escape route 'Someone else told the double about it' and this is why this point was restated as a fact by the therapist in her lead-up to exposing the contradiction.

If the therapist had been worried that the man might use the escape route 'My therapist told the double about it', then before exposing the contradiction she would have made explicit (a) that she had never met the double (providing this was correct), (b) that she had never met the 'real' father, i.e. someone other than the double, and (c) that she had not known, and could not have known, about this particular incident before being told it by the man himself.

An unhelpful delusional belief adaptation would be if the man concluded that the double must be able to read his mind and that this was how he knew about their shared past.[2] Unless you had reason to suppose that he might use 'mind reading' as an escape route (for example if this was another of his delusional beliefs), then there is no reason why you might anticipate this happening and so you would have to tackle the belief about mind reading after it had arisen.

In the example given on p. 159 of the woman who believed her head was empty, it was suggested that she might use 'It's not my X-ray' as an escape route. This escape route could be sealed off by asking her to sign her X-ray immediately it had been taken so that she had 'proof' after it had been developed that it was the right one.

Even if you think you have successfully sealed off an escape route, if the delusional belief is very strong, then this may just result in another escape route being used. For example, in the case above, presenting the woman with the signed X-ray might force her to conclude that someone must have forged her signature on someone else's X-ray.

In this same example, it was suggested that one of the possible outcomes of presenting the contradictory X-ray was that it might distort her interpretation of the X-ray to 'It shows a brain but it is small and deformed'. One way of protecting against this would be to agree with her to first see and interpret her X-ray whilst it was one amongst several other unnamed ones. If her interpretations were recorded at this time, then this would help to remind her of her unbiased evaluation, and would help to prevent it being distorted subsequently after the X-ray had been identified as hers.

In practice you will not be able to predict every possible escape route (or even most of them!) so a common feature of this part of therapy is 'challenging' and sealing off an unexpected escape route after it has been used, i.e. showing why this particular explanation for the apparent contradiction between the evidence and belief is not a valid one. Fortunately, escape routes can usually be closed off even after they have been used, but it is harder to do it then because the apparent contradiction between the delusional belief and the contradictory evidence constitutes confirming evidence for the escape route.

If you have presented the contradictory evidence too early or too forcefully and the person appears to be at risk of going down a dysfunctional escape route, then you should try to divert them down a more functional one as quickly as possible. This is one of the few situations where a rapid intervention is required

[2]Fortunately, these unhelpful adaptations to the delusional belief occur less often in clinical practice than one might suppose or fear, especially if you go cautiously and sensitively and are prepared to back off.

and so you should not take your time to go away and think about it. For example, in the case of the double that we have been considering, it is much safer for the man to conclude that he himself had given the information about his childhood to the double than that you had. So if he were to start to consider the possibility of your duplicity, it would be safer to state very firmly that you had not spoken to the double and suggest that perhaps he had inadvertently given the double this information himself during one of their many conversations together.

SUMMARIZING THE EVIDENCE ON CARDS

Once the person has agreed that it is possible their belief may not be entirely correct, for example as the result of logical reasoning or a particularly impressive piece of evidence, then it may be appropriate to engage them in an evidence collection exercise. This may extend over several weeks. The aim is to build up a collection of evidence 'against' the delusional belief and 'for' the alternative, replacement belief. If any evidence should come up that appears to support the delusion, then this is eliminated by re-evaluation, using the CBT strategies described above.

The evidence against the delusion and for the replacement belief is essentially the same but, since most people find it more pleasing to prove that they are right than that they have been wrong about something, where it is appropriate it is preferable to check out the alternative belief rather than the delusional one.

When collecting evidence around the delusional belief, it is often helpful to have an agreement that only solid, objective evidence of the sort that would be acceptable in a court of law is permissible. For example, you would accept that the person has a 'feeling' that something is so, but you would not accept this feeling as 'hard evidence' because unsubstantiated feelings or intuitions are not accepted in courts of law and that is because they are known to be unreliable and misleading.

Needless to say, you do not need to cast the same critical eye over the evidence against their delusional belief that someone gives you as you would over the evidence they give in support of it, and nor do you need to point out what might seem to you to be weaknesses in the logic involved. Nevertheless, although you would accept it without challenge, it is better not to stress any weak or inappropriate evidence because the person may later come to reject it themself. For example, a woman argued that she could not be subnormal because she was able to look after her personal hygiene. We accepted this piece of evidence and refrained from pointing out that subnormal people can have perfectly good personal hygiene, but we took care to find more solid evidence to support her conclusion, not least because there was the risk that in the future she would meet someone with learning difficulties who was clean and well presented (see p. 220 for more details of this case).

Delusional beliefs do not suddenly disappear, and the conviction with which they are held and the distress that they can cause can vary according to the person's situation. In particular, they are more likely to be troublesome when the person does not have the immediate support of the therapist and the therapeutic situation; so many people find it helpful to have the contradictory evidence and any supporting reasoning written on a card so that they can use it to counter the delusional ideas as and when they occur. The card is usually written jointly by the person and their therapist, and as far as possible it should use the person's own ideas and words.

EXAMPLE OF A CARD USED TO REMIND A WOMAN OF KEY EVIDENCE AGAINST HER DELUSIONAL BELIEF

The example given below is a card developed for a young woman who believed she was evil. Note that the card does not gloss over the 'real' piece of evidence she produced to support the belief, namely that she would physically attack people when angry, but rather seeks to re-evaluate it. Since it was more than possible that she would attack someone in the future, it was important that the modified interpretation of this behaviour be included on the card in order to protect her from exaggerated interpretation if and when this happened again.

I KNOW I'M NOT EVIL BECAUSE:

An EVIL person is someone who deliberately wants to make people suffer and who enjoys seeing them suffer. An evil person doesn't do nice things.

1 I don't do things deliberately to hurt people. Even when I do things when I'm angry I'm sorry later and try to put things right. Everyone is unpleasant sometimes during their lives but that doesn't make them evil.
2 If I see others suffering, I try to comfort them if they want that. I don't enjoy seeing people suffering.
3 I get pleasure from seeing other people happy – it makes me feel more cheerful when other people are cheerful.

Some of the nice things I've done recently:

1 I swapped a meal with another patient so she wouldn't go hungry.
2 I let my room-mate listen to her Hindi music before she goes off to sleep even though I don't enjoy it.
3 I chatted to a new patient on the ward to make him feel at home.
4 I helped Wendy cook some pancakes.

Note that in the above card the term 'evil' is clearly defined, an example of making a general concept more specific so that it can be challenged and contradicted by evidence.

Beliefs about being evil or the Devil are unfortunately not uncommon, and in these cases we find it useful to agree with the person some definition of evil that specifies that the harm or suffering inflicted on others is (a) deliberate, and (b) a source of pleasure. For the young woman above, specifying that the essential characteristic of evil was that of gaining pleasure from deliberately inflicting harm on others was sufficient to allow her to see that the delusion was not true.

However, if in a case like this the person had intended to harm someone else and had got some satisfaction from doing so, then the definition of evil would have to be made more extreme to ensure that they did not meet any of the criteria. This might mean extending the definition of evil to include doing harm *all the time*, or *to everyone*, and to include *never* doing anything nice for anyone. In this sort of situation, in order to get an appropriately worded definition you have to do the exploratory work first to ensure that the person concerned will not fit the final definition in any way. This is just another example of the therapist doing preparatory work before proceeding formally with a challenge in order to ensure that the challenge, when made, has the best chance of a successful outcome.

LOGICAL REASONING

As we have already noted, logical reasoning is an integral part of evidence evaluation. This relationship is not one-way. Logical reasoning is always reasoning about *something*, and as such, some sort of fact or evidence is always involved. However, the relative importance of the evidence and the logical reasoning does vary from case to case, so that in some cases it may be the quality of the evidence that is the most important factor in determining its effect on the delusional belief, whereas in other cases it is the quality of the reasoning used, and this is why these two aspects of CBT are considered separately in this manual.

Logical reasoning can be used in three, overlapping ways: (a) to argue about the evidence for and against the delusion, (b) to link indirect evidence to the delusional belief, and (c) to explore the implications of the delusional belief, to make them explicit and to argue for their relevance.

The line of logical reasoning used may be conclusive or only suggestive, depending on the nature of the logical connections being made. For example, in the case described above, implicit in the young woman's understanding of 'evil' was that the person got pleasure from being evil, so pointing out that she was upset by the thought of being evil was conclusive proof that she could not be evil.[3] In another case, a man believed he would go to hell when he died; the only evidence he had for this was a strong feeling of certainty. He also had a strong feeling of certainty that he would die before he was 50 years old, so when he

[3]This was an example of logical reasoning being used to make explicit some contradictory aspect of the delusional belief of which the person was not aware.

passed his 50th birthday the therapist was able to use this to argue that his 'strong feeling of certainty' could be wrong. If it could be wrong then it was not valid evidence for his belief about going to hell, which meant that he had no evidence this would happen. And if he had no evidence that he would go to hell, then this indicated it was an ungrounded fear only. In this latter case the logical argument is a less powerful one because it does not prove that the delusional belief is wrong but only argues that the evidence on which it is based could be faulty.

Although the lines of argument that can be developed will depend on the individual person and their particular delusion, using logical reasoning to expose inconsistencies and contradictions in the belief is not as difficult as it might sound. For the most part, beliefs are only described as 'delusional' because they are considered by other people to be unreasonable, so other people must have reasons for coming to this decision. Logical reasoning is a way of making use of these reasons in order to challenge the feasibility and truth of the delusion. It is almost certain that by the time you see the person for CBT they will already have heard the arguments of other people telling them why their delusion is not true, without any positive effect. The skill in using the logical reasoning approach as part of your CBT programme is to develop a line of argument that moves in small steps, involving facts and arguments that have been well prepared to protect them against distortion, and that takes the person inexorably from one step to another so the final step which challenges the delusion cannot be ignored or denied.

STAGES IN THE USE OF LOGICAL REASONING

1. Determine what inconsistencies and contradictions exist

If you consider the belief you are working on to be delusional, then you must have one or more reasons for believing this to be so: these reasons may relate directly to the delusional belief and/or to some implication(s) of the delusional belief. Therefore, a very simple way of starting to identify possible inconsistencies and contradictions in the delusional belief is to ask yourself the questions:

- *'Why do I think this belief is delusional; why do I think it is not true?'*
- *'If this delusion were true in fact, what would follow from that? 'What would be different from how things actually are?'*

Thinking about the implications of the delusion in this way may expose inconsistencies in the belief or contradictions between the belief and reality. For example, a man believed that his next-door neighbour had magical powers and could see into the future. But if this were true, surely the neighbour would have been able to see the winning lottery prize numbers and become a millionaire, and would not be living in the run-down council house next door? As with all logical reasoning, a line of argument can only be used to challenge the delusional belief if the person themself agrees with each of the key steps. For example, in the case above, the man would have to agree that the magical powers would allow his neighbour to predict lottery numbers and also that a millionaire would not continue to live in an old council house.

Making the general specific

We saw in Chapter 5 that asking for details about a delusion that the person cannot give may, in some circumstances, act as a challenge to the delusion. We can see, now, why that is. The logical reasoning runs 'If this is really happening, then I would be able to give more details: I cannot give more details, therefore it cannot really be happening'. Or, for evidence reported from the past, the reasoning runs 'If this had really happened, then I would be able to remember more details: I cannot remember more details, therefore it cannot have happened'.

Although it is appropriate to go cautiously during the assessment phase in order to avoid the risk of inadvertently presenting the person with this challenge, later on in therapy this line of reasoning can be used deliberately to counter the delusional belief. For example, in one case a woman believed one of the other residents was trying to harm her. It was argued that since she did not know who was trying to harm her this suggested no one had actually done anything to indicate that they wanted to harm her (she agreed that this was so), and that this, in turn, indicated that the belief must be based on a feeling since it was not based on a fact. It had not been possible to challenge the supporting evidence whilst the person(s), motives and modus operandi were unknown, but having established that the only supporting evidence was a *feeling*, then it was possible to remove this evidence by using the 'feeling is not the same as fact' work. In another example, a man thought he had killed some women a few years ago and put them under the floorboards. One of the main ways used to counter this memory was the argument that his inability to recall any details about the victims or where it took place indicated that this was the memory of some dream-like experience rather than an actual event.

Deciding which lines of reasoning are the most suitable to use

It will often be the case that the main reasons that *you* have for thinking the belief is delusional will be too difficult to establish and therefore cannot be used to counter the delusional belief. When this happens, you may find you have to rely on less significant but more easily used factors. For example, suppose a man believes that he is the reincarnation of Jesus Christ. Depending on your own beliefs, it is likely that your main reasons[4] for believing this to be untrue will be around reincarnation in general, or about the spiritual uniqueness of Jesus which would rule out another incarnation as a man, etc. These are powerful reasons but very difficult to establish in practice. Therefore, you might have to use a much less significant implication of the delusion, if this is more easily tested. For

[4]i.e. apart from 'I just know it's not true', which, as we have seen, would not be acceptable in a court of law and is not considered to be a valid reason in CBT!

example, if the man knew he was a reincarnation of Jesus, then you could argue that he ought to be able to remember the things that Jesus said, or perhaps be able to do some of the things that Jesus did. These lines would be potentially easier to argue and test than notions of reincarnation.

As with evidence evaluation, what you think are good solid reasons why the delusional belief cannot be true may not be the reasons that impress the person themself, and vice versa. Needless to say, you should concentrate on developing the lines of counter-argument that the person finds persuasive, though you would probably try to establish the other reasons as well, at some later stage, in order to provide more support for the modification and to strengthen it against future relapse.

Having identified a potential line of logical reasoning, you must find out whether the person themself agrees with the arguments and facts that form each of the key steps. Suppose, for example, that a man believes he has ants living under his skin. A potential line of argument to counter this belief is that ants need to breathe oxygen in order to live and there is no oxygen under the skin. But this argument will only be effective if the man agrees both (a) that ants need oxygen to live and, (b) that there is no oxygen under the skin. Therefore, you would have to find out if he knows that insects have to breathe air and also what he understands about the construction of a human limb and how tightly the skin is attached.

When you are still at the stage of assessing whether a particular line of argument will be viable, you should be careful to put the questions in a neutral, conversational way so that the inconsistency with respect to the delusion is not obvious. This is particularly important if the person is not ready for a challenge to their belief at this stage. For example, in the case just described, the man is unlikely to have considered the question of how the ants breathe and so asking this question baldly might force him to reason that they *must* be breathing air from under his skin, somehow (perhaps through the hair follicles?), thereby establishing a dysfunctional belief that will effectively undermine this particular line of reasoning.

It is likely that it will be important to strengthen the constituent parts of the logical argument before it is used to counter the delusional belief, and so for this reason it is usual to work on establishing these constituent parts at times that are well separated from any discussion you may have about the delusional belief itself. Ideally you would do this work in separate sessions, but if you are pressed for time and want to use a single session, then you should ensure that something else is discussed in between. Certainly you should not move immediately from discussing the delusion to discussing the things that are going to be used as the basis for logical reasoning against it, or move immediately between key elements of the logical argument, until the person is ready for these connections to be made and for the logical argument to be put. As with the work on contradictory evidence, if you suspect that the person is becoming aware of a challenging line of logical reasoning before they are ready for it, then you should back off rapidly and turn to another topic of conversation.

2. Strengthen the functional part(s) of the inconsistency and the logical reasoning used

As with contradictory evidence, described earlier in this chapter, exposing a line of logical reasoning that contradicts the delusion too soon may cause the logical reasoning to be distorted and changed rather than the delusional belief. Therefore, an important aspect of this line of therapy is to establish and strengthen the logical arguments *before* they are set against the delusional belief.

The more secure the constituent parts of the argument, the less likely it is that the chain of logical reasoning will be rejected or distorted when its conclusion is set against the contradictory delusional belief. Knowledge and beliefs that are held already are the most secure against change, so wherever possible you would try to use lines of argument that rely on already accepted points. However, where the person does not have the necessary knowledge it may be possible for this to be provided as part of the therapy. As a general rule, adding compatible information to an existing body of knowledge is likely to be more effective and more resistant to change than information about something completely new.

Where the person holds an inaccurate belief or has incorrect knowledge about a key element required for the argument, then it may be possible to change this during therapy. As a general rule, knowledge that has had to be corrected is much less likely to stand firm against the delusion than knowledge that is already well established and accepted, and so the former would only be used if more effective lines of argument were not available, or as an extra line once the delusion had been seriously undermined.

The case of the man who believes he has ants living under his skin can be used to illustrate these differences. (a) If the man were a biology student and already knew that all living things need oxygen to live and that the skin on an arm is firmly attached to the flesh underneath, then this line of argument would be difficult for him to dispute. (b) If he knew little about biology, then it would be possible to explain to him why all living things, including insects, need to breathe to live, and also why living skin must be attached firmly to the underlying flesh. But when the inconsistency with his delusion was made explicit he might start to doubt whether *all* living creatures need to breathe, or whether *all* skin needs to be firmly attached. (c) If the man thought there was a layer of air between skin and flesh, then it might be possible to correct this belief by discussion, referring him to experts and/or consulting textbooks. But when confronted with the fact that ants need oxygen to live, then he is likely to revert to his former position and conclude that this proves he must have been correct all along in saying that his skin is not joined to the flesh beneath.

One way of protecting a line of logical reasoning against subsequent distortion is to make it explicit and agree it with the person before it is set against their delusional belief. For example, a man believed his sister wanted him dead, but she visited him regularly and brought him cigarettes. In order to counter the delusion about his sister the therapist first talked with him about hospital visitors and how visiting was one way of showing that people cared about their relatives in hospital, and they agreed that he was lucky to get so many visits and to be kept supplied with expensive cigarettes. This work was repeated casually, on several occasions, before this 'evidence' and line of reasoning was considered robust enough to set against the delusional belief. As recommended, these discussions took place at different times from our discussions about the events from his past that had led him to believe his sister wanted him dead so as to avoid bringing the inconsistency to his notice too soon, before the functional part about his sister caring for him had been strengthened.

When seeking to establish and strengthen the constituent parts of the logical argument, it may be necessary to establish the required facts about people or things in general before attempting to establish the same facts as they affect the person themself. Questions relating to other people and their situations are less likely to be perceived as being relevant to the person's own situation and therefore are less likely to be distorted by the delusional belief or to be perceived as a challenge to it. For example, with the man who fears he has ants living under his skin, the reason why ants need oxygen to live would be established first in terms of living things in general and then moving to insects. Only when that belief is secure would this be extended to ants in particular, because as soon as ants are mentioned the man is likely to make a connection with his delusional belief.

Once established, it may be helpful to remove any potential for flexibility that there may be in the facts that will be used in the steps of the logical argument – this is one area of CBT where black and white thinking is more functional than allowing for variations of grey. For example, in the case above, the therapist might explain why living things in general, and ants in particular, *could not possibly* live without oxygen, and why it is *impossible* for living skin to exist separate from the flesh beneath.

The constituent elements of the argument will be more secure against subsequent change if they are supported and strengthened by evidence that is easy to confirm and that is not open to alternative interpretations. For this reason, objective evidence obtained from events and situations is preferable to evidence based on subjective factors such as attitudes and feelings. For example, in the case of the man who thought his sister wanted him dead, the evidence collected to support the conclusion that she cared for him focused on the journeys and the time these took and on the cigarettes and the money that these cost, rather than on the fact that she had smiled at him and seemed interested in what he said, because these latter would have been easier to re-evaluate when set against the delusion (e.g. 'I thought she had smiled at me but now I think perhaps it was more of a sly smirk').

Seal off any potential 'escape routes'

The same considerations with respect to escape routes apply to setting a line of logical reasoning against the delusional belief as apply to using contradictory evidence. Before you expose the chain of logical reasoning you should think ahead as to whether there is any other way that the person might resolve the apparent contradiction other than realizing that their delusional belief seems to be in error. If other possible resolutions do exist then you should remove them or effectively counter them before you expose the logical argument. For example, in the case of the man who believes he has ants under his skin there is the potential risk that, when faced with the logical argument that contradicts his delusion, he might conclude that although the ants need oxygen to live they are getting it from his bloodstream, or that although the skin is normally attached to the flesh in his case the ants have eaten away a space in between that is now filled with air. In order to ensure he does not come to either of these unhelpful conclusions the therapist would need to establish (a) that only specially adapted water creatures can get oxygen from a liquid, that all land creatures, including ants, need to get oxygen in a gaseous form, and (b) that skin cannot live if cut from the flesh beneath, and that one way of testing whether the skin is living or not is to see if it can feel a pinprick.

Of course, there will be occasions when the person you are working with will use an escape route you have not anticipated. For example, in the case above, when faced with the apparent conflict between the established facts of the argument and his strongly held delusion, the man might conclude that the ants are not ordinary ants but must be a special sort of swimming ant, previously unknown to science, that can get their oxygen from liquids like blood. If this happens then you have to challenge the escape route in the same way you would challenge any other delusional idea or belief. The reason for trying to anticipate the possible escape routes and to close them off is that it is easier to establish a belief about something that is neutral for the person than it is to challenge a conclusion that he has already come to, especially if that conclusion enables him to make sense of, and to reconcile, the apparent contradiction to his delusional belief.

3. Expose the logical inconsistency

When you have decided the time is right to expose the logical argument, you should consider how to do this in a way that will not be experienced by the other person as you triumphantly proving him wrong. The approach is the same as that used for exposing contradictory evidence (see pp. 159–164) and therefore will not be repeated here.

EXAMPLE OF USING LOGICAL REASONING TO MODIFY A DELUSIONAL BELIEF

A young man suddenly developed the unpleasant belief that there were little men in his head, based on the sensation of feet pattering from one side of his head to the other. This sensation seemed to be a mixture of touch and sound. He accepted that he had schizophrenia and knew from earlier therapy that this could produce some strange hallucinatory experiences, so it was not necessary to do any preparatory work to ensure that the alternative belief, namely that these sensations were caused by his illness, would be acceptable to him.

I asked myself why I did not believe as the man himself did and came up with a number of reasons including (a) that the man had a brain in his head and therefore could not have a cavern there as well, and (b) that the little men could not have got into his head without leaving a hole around the entry point.

I decided to develop these two lines of reasoning into watertight, logical arguments and then, if they were sufficient to modify his delusional belief, to support this modification by discussing my other reasons with him. Remember that the answers to the questions detailed below would have been obtained at different times before they were brought together into the two chains of logical reasoning.

How do you know the little men are in your head? How long have they been there?
I can hear them and feel them running from one ear to the other; they're in a large cavern, I can hear the echoes. They've been there a couple of days, since Sunday night.

How many of them are there?
About half a dozen, I think.

How big are they?
About one and a half inches high and half an inch wide.

How big is the cavern?
About seven inches by four inches.

How did they get into the cavern?
Through my ears; they can't have got in anywhere else because, as my friend pointed out, there are no scars on my face.

These questions produced the basic information required to indicate where the contradictions lay. It was important to establish the physical size of the little men and the cavern because it would have been unhelpful if, when faced with the argument that he must have a brain in his head and so there could be no room for the little men as well, the man had retreated to the position of a tiny cavern and tiny men, as these latter would have been harder to disprove than his original perception. It was agreed, therefore, that the men were $1\frac{1}{2}$ inches tall, and that the cavern must be at least 6 inches wide and 2 inches high for most of the distance across, in order to account for the pattering sound.

The contradictions to be used were based on the solid physical properties of the little men and the cavern in which they were running, so it would have been unhelpful if the man were to resolve the contradictions by modifying the delusion from physical to spiritual or ghostly men, as such entities might well be able to move through brain tissue. In order to prevent this modification from occurring it was established and agreed at an early stage that if he could hear and feel the men, this must mean that they were physical, solid objects of some sort.

The next set of questions was used to establish that the man could not have a cavern in his head as well as a normal, functioning brain. He had studied A level Human Biology and so knew about the brain and how it worked, and was able to answer the questions appropriately. Had he not done so, we would have had to establish the facts first, using a biology book and/or medical colleagues as the authority on these matters. We could not have proceeded with this line of reasoning unless and until the man had accepted the basic, biological facts about the brain being responsible for sight, hearing and speech.

Why do people have heads?
To hold their brains.

How big is the brain?
Almost the same size as your skull.

So normally the brain fills the person's head, with no gaps?
Yes.

What does the brain do?
It sees, hears and makes you talk.

So if someone can see, hear and talk normally does that mean their brain is normal?
Yes.

Can the brain ever get squashed up?
Yes, if there's a tumour.

Does a squashed-up brain work normally?
No.

Would it affect the way the person sees, hears and talks if their brain were squashed up?
Yes.

Can you see, hear and talk?
Yes.

So if you can see, hear and talk normally does that mean you have a normal brain?
Yes.

So if you have a normal brain, that's not squashed up, how can there be a big seven inch by four inch cavern in your head?
I suppose there can't be.

In establishing that the man had a perfectly normal brain we used functions that there could be no doubt about his being able to do. He had complained earlier that his thoughts felt a bit muddled so we were careful not to use thinking as an indication of normal brain physiology.

The next line of reasoning was used to add weight to the conclusion from the previous logical reasoning exercise and was set to establish that the men could not have entered his head through his ears without damaging his ears so badly that he would not be able to hear.

When I learnt biology I was taught that the passage in the ear led to an eardrum. Did you cover that in your course?
Yes.

What does the eardrum do?
It vibrates to sounds and this is turned into nerve signals that get sent to the brain.

So it can't do that if it is damaged at all?
No.

How do you know the little men didn't get in through your face?
Because it would have left a scar at least half an inch across, probably more, so I would have been able to see it.

I agree – I would have been able to see it, too. So if they had got in through your ears, they would have made a hole at least half an inch across in your eardrum, too?
Yes.

So you would not be able to hear through that ear with a hole that size?
No, that's right.

Can you hear with both ears at the moment?
Yes.

So you can't have a hole in either of your eardrums, and so the men couldn't have got in that way?
No, I suppose not.

And you know they can't have got in any other way because there are no scars on your head. And I guess there would have been quite a lot of blood around on your pillow on Monday morning if something as large as one and a half inches by half an inch had forced its way through your skin?
Yes, that's true.

So no little men can have got into your head? There can't be any little men in your head?
No.

So it sounds as if the **feelings** *you get of tiny pattering feet running across your head must be another example of your brain hallucinating, but this time through the sense of touch as well as sound. What do you think? It must be a horrible feeling, but I suppose at least it's reassuring to know that there aren't really creatures living in your head and that your brain is still perfectly OK.*

These two arguments were sufficiently robust that when they contradicted the delusional belief it was the delusional belief and not some element of the arguments that was changed.

Note: The series of questions reported above represents the course of the logical arguments pursued to expose the contradictions. In practice you would never fire a series of questions at someone in this way; the logical argument would be developed in a natural way during one or more discussions. Nor would you necessarily need to use all the questions in the series in order to develop the argument; depending on the strength of the person's delusional belief and their knowledge of the facts and arguments you are using, they may move readily through several steps in one jump.

You certainly do not want to bore or appear to patronize the other person by asking a lot of 'obvious' questions, but equally you must be careful not to assume that what seems obvious to you is obvious to them, not least because the delusional belief can have a powerful, distorting effect on the way the person perceives and understands things. For example, with the man above, it may seem silly to ask why people have heads and what the head contains, because within our own belief system it is perfectly obvious what is there, but for someone who believed he had a large cavern in his head it was not at all obvious that heads are for holding brains and therefore this had to be established. The stronger the delusional belief, the more meticulous you have to be to go step by step to make the argument watertight so that it cannot be disputed when it is set against the delusional belief.

REALITY TESTING

Reality tests are situations that are set up for the specific purpose of producing evidence that is directly relevant to the delusional belief and/or to the alternative, replacement belief. Providing they are set up properly, this evidence is clear and unambiguous and so can be very persuasive.

Usually the reality test that is used to disprove the delusional belief will, at the same time, support the desired alternative, but you should not make the assumption that this is so. If the reality test disproves the delusion but leaves open a range of possible alternative beliefs, then before you carry out the reality test you must ensure the desired alternative is the strongest one available so the belief change, when it occurs, will be in the direction intended.

The aims and details of a reality test are agreed by the therapist and patient/client working together, so it is not possible to engage in reality testing until the person is ready to explore and test out the parts of the delusional belief that are the subject of the test. Needless to say, it is not appropriate to set someone up to conduct a reality test under false pretences, for example by asking them to do something that would 'prove to other people that their belief was true'. Not only would such an approach be an unacceptable breach of the honesty, trust and respect that are integral to the therapeutic relationship but it would also almost certainly pose a dysfunctional challenge to the delusional belief before the person had been adequately prepared for it.

THE USE OF REALITY TESTS

There are four broad areas in which reality testing is used.

1. To test the evidence that supports the delusional belief or on which the delusional belief is based

These reality tests, if successful, do not directly disprove the delusional belief but weaken it by removing a piece of the supporting evidence. For example, for the belief 'I know I have special powers because I can predict the future', showing that the man cannot predict the future removes one of his reasons for believing he has special powers, but it does not prove that he has *no* special powers. Similarly, for the belief 'I have a large piece of metal in my leg that causes clocks to slow down when I am near them', showing that the clocks in the woman's residence keep normal time when she is near them removes a piece of evidence that was thought to support her belief, but it does not rule out the possibility that she has some metal in her leg.

The impact that successfully challenging a piece of supporting evidence has on the delusional belief itself depends on how important that piece of evidence is for the delusion. If, as in the first case just cited, the evidence is a major reason why the person believes their delusion to be correct, then disproving it will have a significant impact on the delusional belief and may even be sufficient to bring about a belief change. On the other hand, if the piece of evidence is just one among many, as in the second case cited, then the reality testing may not have any significant effect on the underlying delusion until many such pieces of evidence have been discredited.

Where the impact of the reality testing is potentially greater, you must be all the more careful that the person has been prepared for the disconfirming results and is otherwise ready for their belief to change. Conversely, reality testing of less significant evidence will have less of an impact and therefore can be conducted earlier on in therapy. However, in this latter case you should be careful not to make a big issue of the disconfirming results, because if you force the person to resolve the inconsistency between their delusional belief and the results of the reality test they may do so by distorting the interpretation of the reality test results.

Reality testing is essentially concerned with evidence produced in the here and now, but in some cases it may be possible to check out interpretations of events in the past. Although the identical situation can never be reproduced, it may be possible to set up a very similar situation to that experienced in the past so that a reality test can be run and the results can be used to at least cast doubt on the previous interpretation. For example, it was not possible to disprove that a shopkeeper had made derogatory remarks to a young woman the previous week, but we were able to reality test his reaction to her on subsequent occasions. As he was polite and pleasant to her on these later occasions we were able to suggest that this made her initial interpretation about her experience less likely and the alternative explanation, namely that it had been one of her voices again, correspondingly more likely.

2. To test an implication of the delusional belief, i.e. a prediction that, if disproved, would necessarily also disprove the belief on which it is based

For example, for the belief 'There are little men running around in my head', if the man tilted his head by 90° and found this made no difference to the sounds of the pattering feet, then this would disconfirm the prediction 'If there were little men in a cavern, they would fall to one side when my head was laid flat'.[5] Similarly, for the man who believed his sister wished him harm, if she responded warmly and helpfully to his request to be taken to buy some new clothes, then this would demonstrate that she cared for him, and therefore could not want to harm him.

Reality testing of implications is less powerful than directly testing the delusional belief itself because it involves more links in the chain of logical reasoning between the delusional belief and the reality test results, and so more stages where the line of argument can be weakened or broken down. For example, in the second case mentioned, if the sister takes him shopping this cannot be used as conclusive evidence against the man's delusional belief (a) if he can think of any other reasons why she might take him shopping other than to be kind to him (e.g. 'She can't resist going shopping' or 'She wanted to look good in front of the staff'), or (b) if he can think of any other reason why she might want to harm him other than feeling negative and aggressive towards him (e.g. 'She loves me but she's been threatened that her daughter will be harmed if she doesn't poison me').[6]

Some delusional beliefs cannot, by their very nature, be tested directly and so reality testing implications of the belief may be the only option available. Beliefs about supernatural beings and powers often fall into this latter category, as do delusional beliefs about future events, for example 'God wants me to stop eating and drinking'; 'I will go to hell after I die'; 'My neighbour invades my mind and puts in his thoughts'.

A particular type of implicational reality test is when the test is conducted on someone else, so the result has to be made relevant to the person themself via the logical reasoning 'If this is the result for "Y" then since you are both humans this would be the result for you too'. For example, for a man who believed a ghost could cut off his head, the therapist challenged the ghost to cut off her head instead. This sort of indirect reality test is usually done when the feared outcome is too dreadful for the person to be able to risk carrying it out on themself.

In some cases you may choose to reality test the implications of the belief even if that belief could be tested directly, either because it is a gentler form of challenge than a direct test or because the belief is so strongly held that you want these results to add further weight to the result of the direct test.

3. To directly test the delusional belief

For example, for the belief 'I can cause you to feel unwell by ill wishing you', if the results of a controlled experiment show that the person cannot affect the way other people feel by ill wishing them, then this constitutes proof that their belief is wrong. Similarly, for the belief 'I own a large house in the village of Stairways',

[5] In clinical practice, before setting the reality test in this case, you would want to ask, casually, if the man could still hear the feet pattering when he was in bed at night and if they sounded any different then. Firstly, this would check that tilting his head did not make a difference for some reason. Secondly, once the implications had been pointed out to him, his expectations might cause the results of the reality test to be biased; if this happened, it would be helpful to have his accounts of what had happened on other, similar occasions to counter this interpretation.

[6] This latter is an example of an escape route.

a search of the Land Registry will prove that they do not own any of the houses there, and for the belief 'I have solid little men running in a seven inch by four inch cavern in my head' an X-ray will prove this is not the case.

Where it is possible to directly test a delusional belief, as in the examples just given, then this is the most powerful use of reality testing. Since such a head-on challenge to the delusional belief is capable of bringing about a more or less immediate belief change you must be particularly careful not to conduct this type of reality test until the results will be beneficial.

Because of the power of a direct challenge to a delusional belief, this is often the final stage of a modification programme, introduced after all the preparatory work has been covered. Logical reasoning and evidence evaluation may be necessary to cast sufficient doubt on the delusional belief to make reality testing seem a reasonable and/or a safe thing to do, and then the direct reality test can provide the conclusive evidence to clinch the belief modification.

4. To directly test the alternative explanation or belief

For example, for the belief 'The pain in my stomach is due to indigestion, not the effects of poison', if the stomach pains after eating can be prevented by slowing down the person's rate of eating plus the use of indigestion tablets, then this would support the alternative belief that the pains were due to indigestion.

In some cases it may be better to target the reality test at the alternative belief rather than the delusional belief so that the results will actively strengthen the desired alternative belief. Furthermore, it is likely to be more pleasant for the person to conduct a test that proves them right than one that proves them wrong.

If the alternative belief is incompatible with the delusional belief, then this approach is as effective as a direct test of the delusional belief, and the same precautions about conducting it too soon apply. However, in some cases proving that the alternative explanation is possible, or applies, does not necessarily rule out the possibility that the delusional belief could be correct. If this is the case then testing the alternative belief could be useful as an early strategy that would not be sufficient in itself to eliminate the delusional belief but that would help to undermine it.

CHARACTERISTICS OF A GOOD REALITY TEST

It is important that reality tests are set up correctly in order to achieve the desired result. In particular, you must avoid inadvertently providing support for the delusional belief, or producing evidence that the person can interpret as positive support even though most people would not interpret it in this way. Reality tests should have the following characteristics:

1. The result of the test should be clear, precise and unambiguous

It is important that the reality test is set up so there can be no doubt or debate about what the results were. This means that the outcome must be clearly specified and measurable, and the test must take place within set time limits.

If you do not specify clearly what would count as 'positive' and 'negative' evidence, then there is a significant risk that the person will interpret something else that happens during the period of the reality test in line with the delusional belief and therefore regard this as positive evidence to support the delusion. This is certainly not what you want. Reality tests are set up to test out the delusional belief and to highlight the results obtained, and as such they will tend to magnify the significance of any positive supporting evidence, should it occur accidentally. We can use the example of the man who believed he could predict the future to illustrate this point. If the reality test he is set is to predict the outcome of the 2.30 p.m. race at Epsom, then there can be no doubt about whether or not his prediction was correct. If, however, you have not specified what the prediction of a future event is to relate to, but have left this rather vague, it is highly likely the man will interpret some other event as proof of his ability to predict the future; for example, he might have 'known' what type of biscuits were going to be brought into the group meeting that week.

Similarly, if you do not set a strict time limit to the reality test, then there is the risk that something will happen weeks later that the person will interpret as support for their belief, and at a time when you may not be around to discuss the interpretation they have made. For example, if a man believes there is a conspiracy to make him ill, then it is likely he will fall ill with at least a cold or flu at some time in the next year. If the reality test involves something happening within a time limit, we usually set the time period to be between one session and the next, though it can be much shorter, for example a few minutes within a single therapy session, depending on what is being tested.

2. The interpretation of the results should be unequivocal

You must ensure that you check with the other person how they will interpret the various possible outcomes of the reality test before putting it in motion. However convincing a test may be to you, there is no point in running it if the person themself would not accept or would be able to explain away the results. For example, a man in hospital believed his head was empty and that his brain had been removed. As he was going to have a full neurological examination we suggested the reality test of asking the neurologists for a copy of his head X-ray. We asked how he would interpret the X-ray if it showed a brain in place, like the example from a textbook that we were looking at. He thought for a while before replying that he would not believe it and that if the neurologist said that this was his X-ray, then he would know that the neurologists had switched them. So without any prospect of disproving his delusional belief, we did not attempt this particular reality test.

It is recommended that you and/or the other person makes a formal note of your agreed interpretations of the possible outcomes before running the reality test in order to clarify and strengthen them. Having a formal record also helps to prevent the person discounting these interpretations in favour of some other explanation when the reality test provides the expected contradictory evidence. Even so, should the person show any unwillingness to accept their pre-test interpretation of the results when they are obtained, be prepared to back off and wait until more work has been done before presenting the evidence again. If you attempt to force a conclusion when there is an apparent reluctance to accept the desired alternative belief, then there is a risk that the change made will be in the direction of another delusional belief. (See p. 196 for an example of this.)

Results that are open to different interpretations are not suitable for a reality test and so, wherever possible, the outcome of the test should be some publicly observable event or happening about which there can be no differences of opinion. For this reason, subjective experiences can only be used as outcomes if it is possible to make some objective measure of them. For example, it would be possible to set up an experiment to test the man's belief that he could make other people feel unwell by ill-wishing them. He would ill-wish the therapist for one hour in the week and the therapist would keep a record of how well or unwell she felt every hour to see if the hour she felt most unwell coincided with the person's ill-wishing her. By recording their experiences, the therapist and other person would convert their subjective feelings of being unwell into an objective and definite event that could not be reinterpreted later.

In actual practice the reality test for this particular man involved him and the therapist well-wishing rather than ill-wishing one another. The man was reluctant to ill-wish the therapist because he thought he would be successful and the therapist did not want the man to think she would ever wish him ill, even as part of an experiment aimed at helping him in the long run. As a general point, reality tests dealing with pleasant things are preferable to those that could potentially (for the other person at least) have an unpleasant outcome, because they are less stressful for the person concerned. However, because of the very nature of the unpleasant delusional beliefs being tested, it is usually the case that one cannot avoid at least some of the possible predicted outcomes being unpleasant ones. Indeed, this is why it is usually necessary to use logical reasoning and evidence evaluation to bring the person to the point of thinking that his delusional belief is quite possibly or even probably not true before he will be willing to reality test it.

3. The probability of a positive outcome due to chance should be very small

Since you are reality testing with a view to disproving the delusional beliefs you must avoid the risk of inadvertently 'proving' that belief with a positive outcome. Therefore, you should specify some outcome that is very unlikely to occur by chance; normally, we reckon that the probability of a positive outcome by chance should be at least less than 1 in a 100.

Do not assume the other person will interpret the results as you will, especially when you are dealing with probabilities rather than black and white certainties. For example, if you were conducting a telepathy experiment with four different shapes, you might be very satisfied that the patient/client guessed only 25% correctly, just what would be expected by chance, and consider that this result provided convincing proof that they had no telepathic powers. However, they might be able to ignore the items they got wrong but be impressed by how often they did get a correct answer and so take this as proof that they can do telepathy *sometimes.*

Be careful not to inadvertently risk a positive outcome occurring by chance by over-enthusiastically trying to reinforce the results of a test by repeating it. For example, if you are testing the person's telepathic powers by asking them to guess a number between 0 and 100, then it is within safe limits to do this once, i.e. the chance of their getting it correct by chance is low enough to risk. But if you were to repeat this a further nine times, then the chance of their getting one correct would then go up to 1 in 10 – too high to risk, as it is unlikely you would be able to explain the statistics of chance convincingly enough to persuade the other person that their guessing correctly on one occasion was not significant. Of course, it is perfectly safe to repeatedly test events that could not possibly happen, for example spontaneous combustion.

IF THE PERSON IS ANXIOUS ABOUT THE RESULTS OF A REALITY TEST

Although the person is unlikely to agree to a reality test of their delusional belief unless they recognize that there is at least a possibility the outcome will be negative, i.e. that it will disprove the delusion, a reality test would not be necessary if they were *sure* the delusion was untrue and that the reality testing would turn out well. Therefore, whenever the delusion is about some unpleasant or frightening matter, it is to be expected that the person will approach the reality test with some trepidation. There are three main ways in which you may be able to keep the anxiety to acceptable limits.

1. Although it is usual for the person to conduct the reality test themself, if the delusion is such that someone else (usually the therapist) could test it out, then this is likely to be much less anxiety-provoking. For example, if someone believed that alien forces would cause them to spontaneously combust if they said they did not believe the aliens existed, then you could express your disbelief loudly and firmly so that they could see what the aliens did to you, before risking the test themself. Although involving yourself rather than the person themself may provide a less conclusive test of the delusional belief, it may be sufficiently reassuring to allow the person to go ahead with the reality test on themself.

2. Another way of reducing the anxiety around a reality test is to test a watered-down version of it, or a non-anxiety-provoking equivalent. For example, for the belief that a ghost could cut off someone's head, you could challenge it to remove just the tip of a finger, or cut off a chunk of hair, or to cut a pencil in two. In another example, for someone who feared that a powerful entity could make them spontaneously combust, you could challenge it to make a sheet of paper burst into flame.

3. When the person is very anxious about the possible outcome of a reality test, then if it is possible to do so, the test should be carried out and completed during a single therapy session, so that you can give your support with the anxiety and also remind the person of all the logical arguments, etc. that have proved useful in casting doubt on the delusion. Depending on the nature of the

delusion, it may be possible to limit the test to a very short period, for example challenging the Devil to ignite a piece of paper in the next five seconds. When the outcome of a short reality test is seen to be negative, i.e. the feared outcome does not occur, then this may provide the person with the confidence to try over longer periods, including outside the therapy session.

THERAPIST PARTICIPATION IN THE REALITY TEST

If you are taking part in a reality test, you should always carry out your part in the test as agreed, however certain you are that the test will turn out in a certain way. For example, if you agree to well wish the other person for one hour during the week, then you should do so, and similarly, if you are supposed to be recording each hour how you feel, then you should do this genuinely. This is not just a matter of living up to the trust the other person has in you to do what you say you will do and not tell them lies, though these are, of course, very important considerations. Genuinely testing out a delusional belief is an important part of your acceptance that you could be wrong about it, and the other person could be right.

Sometimes the person elects to carry out the reality test on someone else, perhaps because you have been involved in helping to set it up. However tempting it may seem, you should not attempt to influence the results by 'warning' the other person of what will be happening. This is the same ethical point about integrity and respecting the genuinely collaborative approach of CBT as when you are directly involved in the test.

EXAMPLE OF REALITY TESTING THE BELIEF: 'PEOPLE CAN READ MY MIND'

The delusional belief 'People can read my mind' is a fairly common one in clinical practice. Having someone else read one's private thoughts would be an outrageous invasion of one's personal privacy, so it is not surprising that people find this belief a very unpleasant one. Added to that, some people are also worried or ashamed at the thought that other people might know exactly what they have been thinking. If this latter is the case, then it is appropriate to do some destigmatizing and normalizing work around the content of the average person's thoughts and automatic thoughts, before going on to reality test the accuracy of the delusion itself (see Chapter 6).

Since this belief is usually based on a strong feeling the person has that other people are reading their mind, the aim of reality testing is not only to provide convincing evidence that people cannot read their mind but also to provide them with a handy test they can use on subsequent occasions to confirm that people are unable to read their mind, should the strong feeling that this is happening occur again.

Before reality testing this particular delusional belief, we usually ask the following questions:

1. *Can you read other people's minds?* The answer to this is nearly always 'no'. (If it were 'yes', then you would have to devise a separate reality test to show that the person could not, in fact, do this.)

2. *Do you think that I (i.e. the therapist) can read your mind?* People usually express uncertainty, but regardless of the answer you can reassure them that you definitely cannot read their mind, while being sure to admit that of course you cannot speak for other people's ability to do so. None of the people I have reassured in this way has ever doubted what I have said and, apart from any reassurance this statement may give, it also serves the function of being a very gentle challenge to the implication that 'everyone' is capable of reading their mind.

3. *Can other people read one another's minds?* People often have to stop and think about this question, and usually the answer is 'no'. When this happens, it may be helpful to wonder aloud how the person's brain could come to be made so differently from everyone else's and, thinking along evolutionary lines, how strange it would be for everyone else's brains to suddenly have developed this power to read just one individual person's mind. Occasionally, the answer is 'yes', the person thinks that other people can read one another's minds. This can be countered easily by arguing that if people could read one another's minds, then they would not need to speak aloud to one another and certainly they would not spend such large amounts on telephone bills!

The reality tests for the belief 'People can read my mind'

The reality tests described below are just some that have been used with this particular delusional belief. Some provide more watertight evidence against the ability of people to read the person's mind than others, but as in all aspects of this work, it is what the person themself finds convincing that matters, not what you or anyone else would consider to constitute proof. As you move from level 1 to level 5, the tests become stronger in that the results are less easy to explain away.

If you are going to try any of these tests in your clinical work do not forget to discuss with the other person how they would interpret the different possible results. The general principle is that there is no point in running a reality test if the disconfirming results will be explained away, but on the other hand there is no point in conducting a complicated experiment if a simple one will suffice.

Level 1: Ask other people if they can read your mind

The reality test of asking other people directly about something applies to a wide range of situations and beliefs. It will be effective only if the person trusts the other people to tell the truth, but it is perhaps surprising how often people do accept the replies they get to this question, even where there is a paranoid flavour to their delusions. So in clinical practice, do not forget this very basic reality test; it is very simple and easy to use and can be effective.

The major practical caution with regard to this test is that the person should not question people who might give a positive response out of a misplaced sense of humour or for some other reason. In order to reduce this risk, you should discuss and agree who would be a reliable person to question before this is carried out. Another potential disadvantage of this test is that if overused it may become irritating to the people being questioned, and this in turn may lead to unsympathetic and even mischievous responses being given. If a reality test is to be used frequently, then it is better if it does not involve the active participation of other people.

When this level of test is used to check out mind reading, even if the person initially accepts the answers to their enquiries, if the strong feeling of mind reading persists, then they may come to doubt whether the people they asked were telling them the truth. If this happens, they would need to use one of the reality tests given at levels 4 or 5.

Level 2: Conduct a telepathy experiment

This would be set up with the person attempting to send telepathic messages to you or someone else who agrees to take part in this experiment. Of course, if you have already given your reassurance that you cannot read their mind, then you would have to involve someone else as the 'mind reader'. The test can be set up informally, with the two people together in a session, or more formally, with the sender and the receiver sitting in separate rooms. How you set it up will depend on what the other person feels is the most appropriate and impressive way of conducting the test.

The test stimuli should be something that is very unlikely to be guessed by chance, so four-digit numbers or unusual words are suitable – providing you get agreement that the guess must be *exactly* the same as the target in order to count; for example, for the number 4,791, the response 7,419 would be as wrong as 6,582. Do not use common, self-generated words as it is surprising how often words like 'apple', 'orange', 'cat', 'dog', etc. spring to people's minds, so there is too high a risk of getting a 'hit' by chance. It is also recommended that you do not use drawings for these experiments as it is all too easy to see features of the target drawing in the often rather vague efforts of the receiver.

In fact, telepathy experiments have no more power to disprove that the receiver can read the person's mind than simply asking the receiver if they can do so, because the former, like the latter, relies on the sender trusting that the other person will respond honestly and truthfully. Be that as it may, a few people do seem to find the formal set-up of a telepathy experiment more persuasive than simply asking the other person concerned, so if this is the case, then you should conduct the experiment.

Level 3: Think or send a request or instruction to another person, and monitor their response

Although the request would be for something that was unlikely to occur without the request being 'heard' through mind reading, the response itself does not necessarily have to be an unlikely one, because the most likely response to hearing nothing is to do nothing. For example, someone could test out a nurse's mind-reading ability by standing at the dinner trolley and 'thinking' their request for the jam tart pudding option, because even if there are only two options available, the most likely response of the nurse is to ask the person what they wanted rather than to give them one of the puddings without asking. The only potential problem with this kind of test is if the person is in a social situation where they would normally be asking for something, for example in a shop, in which case their apparent silence might come across as a bit odd, something that in general you would want to avoid. In order for this not to happen, you should discuss the request and the situation in which it is made to ensure that their silence will not be socially remarkable or embarrassing.

As far as interpreting the results of reality tests at this level is concerned, it is quite feasible to explain away the negative results as being due to the other person having successfully read the sender's mind but then not wanting or not being bothered to respond. If the person interprets it in this way, then a higher level test will be needed.

The advantage of this level 3 type of test over the telepathy type is that it does not require the receiver to know about the experiment in progress or to know anything about the delusional belief being tested.

Level 4: Send a message so important that anyone receiving it would respond, and monitor the response

Some people believe other people will not admit to being able to read their mind because for some reason they want to conceal this fact. The 'reason' for wanting to conceal this fact can be tackled using the CBT strategies described earlier in this chapter, but especially if they are unsure or quite vague about what reasons people might have for such a conspiracy, it may not be necessary to go through this lengthy procedure. If a reality test can provide conclusive proof that people cannot mind read, then the reason why people might be doing it, or concealing that they can do it, becomes irrelevant.

If what the patient/client is thinking about is sufficiently important to someone else, then it can be argued that if the person concerned could read their mind and knew what they were thinking, they *would* respond even though it would mean revealing they had got this information through mind reading. Below are some examples of messages of this type that people have found useful in clinical practice, not only for the initial reality testing of the delusional idea but also as an ongoing strategy to check out the feelings of mind reading whenever they occur. The most important criterion for these messages is that the person themself is confident they would provoke a response if they were 'read'.

1 (To a nurse) 'The hospital is on fire', ' "X" is about to abscond', 'You've left your car lights on.'
2 (To someone in the room) 'There's a wasp right behind you.'
3 (To someone about to sit down) 'There's a drawing pin on the chair, spike up.'

If one were being very precise, it could be argued that if other people could really read the person's mind, then they would also know the things she was thinking about were not really happening and so they would not need to respond to the messages they picked up from her mind. In practice I have never known anyone argue this way, but if this did happen, or if you thought there was a risk that the person might discover this logical flaw in the interpretation of the results some time after conducting the test, then you would need to use a level 5 test.

Level 5: Send a message that is true and so important that anyone receiving it would respond, and monitor the response.

1 'I have a £1 coin (or £10 note); anyone who asks me for it can have it.'
2 'I have a cigarette (or packet of cigarettes); anyone who comes to me and says "I like Christmas pudding" can have it.'

In order to make these tests watertight the person must agree that this is a genuine message and that they will carry out whatever they promise in the message, should their mind be read successfully. So in the examples given above they would have to have the money or the cigarettes they were offering to give away.

The big advantage of these tests is that they are simple and easy to do, and as the people being tested do not know they are involved, they can be repeated as often as necessary to counter the feelings of mind reading. The only thing you need to be careful about is that the person is not sending a message that might be responded to by chance. For example, if they are sitting in a room of cigarette-deprived smokers, it would not be advisable for them to send out a simple message 'If anyone asks me for a cigarette they can have it' because it is not unlikely that someone will ask for a cigarette anyway. In this case, you would add something very unusual that the receiver has to do or say (e.g. saying 'I like Christmas pudding' in the middle of summer) before they can claim their cigarette.

Sometimes the patient/client has a good reason for thinking that people are concealing their mind-reading abilities despite the advantages they would get from responding to the messages, for example the man who believed the doctors and nurses were pretending not to be able to read his mind because they wanted to make out he was ill so that he would have to stay in hospital. In these circumstances it would be easy to argue that such a reason would not apply to strangers, who could only stand to gain by responding to the message, and then conduct the reality test with strangers.

Level 4 reality tests have no advantages over level 5 tests except that they can be used when the person is not able to carry out the promises of the level 5 tests, for example if they have no money or cigarettes to give away. In practice, therefore, we now tend to go for one of these level 5 tests straight away in order to provide proof that other people cannot read the person's mind.

COMBINING THE CBT STRATEGIES INTO A COHESIVE TREATMENT PROGRAMME

The central CBT strategies of logical reasoning, evidence evaluation and reality testing can interact with one another at all levels and in all aspects of the treatment. Perhaps the easiest way of illustrating how this is done is by using the clinical cases of Jane and Stephen that have been described earlier.

Readers may wish to refer to Appendix 1, which gives a structure for the treatment approach used.

CASE STUDY JANE

(See also pp. 76, 95, 99, 136, 143 and 277.)

Belief: *I am an evil witch.*

Goal for belief modification: *I am not an evil witch, the thoughts and feelings I get/got are due to my schizophrenia.*

LESSENING THE DISTRESS CAUSED BY THE DELUSIONAL BELIEFS

The first step of treatment was to try to reduce the impact that the delusional belief had on Jane's life using some simple, practical coping strategies. These are reported on p. 277. (See Chapter 15.)

MODIFICATION OF THE UNDERLYING BELIEFS INCORPORATED INTO THE DELUSIONAL BELIEF (DEEP MEANING)

There was no significant deep meaning for this delusional belief. (See p. 136, Chapter 6.)

MODIFICATION OF THE UNDERLYING BELIEFS THAT ARE NECESSARY FOR THE DELUSIONAL BELIEF TO BE HELD (SURFACE MEANING)

The belief that witches have special powers and can do supernatural things was targeted for modification. (See p. 143, Chapter 6.)

LOGICAL REASONING AGAINST THE CORE DELUSIONAL BELIEF 'I AM AN EVIL WITCH'

In this case, the logical reasoning about Jane's belief that she was a witch was done at the same time as the evidence evaluation work.

The principal argument put forward was that an evil witch would enjoy making the bad things happen in Iraq, so the fact that she hated doing this, and wanted the war to stop, proved she could not be evil.

It was also argued that an evil witch would have the power to do good things as well as bad, but just choose not to do so. So it was argued that the fact that Jane could not do good things by supernatural means, for example make the weather nicer for people, indicated she did not have any special powers at all.

If Jane had believed all witches had cats as 'familiars', then it might have been possible to argue that she was not a witch because cats did not show a particular affinity for her (certainly none visited her flat or the hospital ward), but in practice this line was considered to be too flimsy to be worth pursuing. It also ran the risk that she might acquire a stray cat in the future, in which case linking 'having a cat' with 'being a witch' would be dysfunctional.

EVIDENCE EVALUATION

1. Evidence: *People can see I am a witch.*

The evidence on which this conclusion was based was:

(a) *When I pass people in the shopping centre they look away when I smile.*
From Jane's report of her experiences it sounded as if the non-smiling responses were appropriate to the situation, but in case there was some delusional misinterpretation as well (e.g. 'I can just sense they see me as evil') the therapist went to the shops with Jane to observe what happened there. This confirmed that people did break eye contact with Jane and did not smile, but in a perfectly appropriate way. This indicated that this part of the evidence fell into the category 'The evidence is true and accurately recalled, but has been misinterpreted' (see p. 149). In order to **eliminate this supporting evidence** a reinterpretation was suggested, namely that although people in hospital often exchange smiles when they pass, even if they do not know one another, it is normal *not* to smile at a stranger in a public place like a shopping centre; indeed, some people might even be a bit worried if strangers smiled at them, because it was so unusual. The therapist demonstrated how eye contact was normally broken in these circumstances. As a result of this discussion Jane stopped smiling at strangers and this ceased to be a worry for her when she went out.

If it had been necessary, the therapist would have conducted a **reality test** to test the alternative interpretation. Using himself as the subject, he would have smiled at strangers in unlikely places so that Jane could see that he, too, got no positive response. In doing such a reality test the therapist would have had to be careful not to get a different response from Jane, for example because he looked more 'respectable' for some reason, or smiled in more appropriate situations.

(b) *Some people stick out their tongues when they pass by.*
From my subsequent discussions about this case with other therapists I understand that in some parts of the country this behaviour would not necessarily be considered abnormal, but for the rather respectable town that Jane was visiting it certainly was. So it was not at all clear from her report what was going on. Therefore, the therapist

accompanied Jane to the shops and she told him whenever this happened. It was quickly apparent that what Jane was noticing was the tongue movements of people who were talking together as they passed by. This comes under the category of evidence 'The interpretation of an event is inaccurate or distorted' (see p. 150). This piece of **evidence was eliminated** by using an alternative interpretation based on what was really happening.

As a **reality test** for the alternative explanation, Jane was encouraged to watch the therapist whilst he was talking and to notice that she could see his tongue moving, too. It was also suggested she could watch her own mouth movements in a mirror as she talked.

Additional **evidence to support the alternative explanation** was the fact that people only seemed to stick out their tongues when they were with someone else and when they were talking to one another.

Two lines of **logical reasoning** were used against the evidence that people could see she was a witch. Firstly, it was argued that if people could see she was a witch, then they would be frightened of her and therefore would not risk offending her by sticking out their tongues. Secondly, it was argued that since she was unable to specify what it was in her appearance that people could recognize as indicating she was a witch, and since she could not say how her appearance had changed from the time when she had not been a witch, these things indicated that her fear that she looked 'different' in some way was based on a *feeling* and was not a fact. This led to some work on **feeling something to be true does not mean that it is true.**

When she checked in the mirror, Jane could not see any changes in her appearance, and the simple **reality test** of asking people that she trusted confirmed that they thought she looked just as she always did and in no way different from other human beings. It was not necessary to conduct any other reality tests to confirm this fact.

2. Evidence: *I can change the weather.*

Being able to change the weather was not in itself of any importance to Jane and did not carry any emotional overtones, so it was tackled before the issue of the Iraq war.

The evidence she had that she could change the weather was that on several occasions she had noticed the weather had changed just as she had expected it would. This falls into the category of evidence 'The interpretation is an exaggeration of the truth' (see p. 149). In order to undermine the supporting evidence, it was established that the 'new' weather had never been anything atypical for the time of year, and so the therapist suggested these changes *could* have occurred anyway, without her being involved. This would mean that she had *predicted* the change rather than *causing* it. The **alternative, normalizing explanation** for seeming to be able to change or predict the weather went along these lines: 'It is often possible to tell how the weather will change, for example because of the way the clouds are building up or dispersing. This is why we can often judge whether we need to take an umbrella or coat when we go out, and why farmers are good at judging what the weather will be like the next day. Some people are better at this than others, so you may be particularly sensitive to these natural cues. Perhaps on a couple of occasions you noticed that the weather had changed in the way that you thought it would. Believing you had special powers, it was not unreasonable for you to conclude that you could have been responsible for changing the weather so it turned out the way you thought it would. Having reached this conclusion, this would have supported your belief that you had special powers; this in turn would have supported your belief that you must be responsible for the bad things that were happening in the world, which in turn would have made you feel more fearful and guilty.'

The only times she had tried deliberately to change the weather for the better, she had failed to do so. This is an example of **contradictory evidence from the past** that is not recognized as such (see p. 157). She had interpreted this evidence as showing that she was unable to change the weather for the better, but the reinterpretation suggested was that since these constituted *all* the attempts she had made, then the results were consistent with her not being able to change the weather at all.

The therapist did not believe that Jane could change the weather because, amongst other things, very large forces (said to be equivalent to several atom bombs) are needed to produce the wind power to move the banks of cloud across the sky, either to bring rain to a clear sky or vice versa. So this formed the basis for the principal line of **logical reasoning** against this piece of evidence.

Having discussed how the different types of weather occur and the great forces needed, Jane was invited to conduct a **reality test** of producing a very small wind to knock over the therapist's cup, which she was unable to do. The full reality test was then conducted, Jane having agreed that if she was unable to change the weather in an experimental situation, then this would confirm she was not able to do so generally. She also agreed that this would suggest that on all previous occasions, when she thought she had changed the weather, it had just been good guesswork on her part. As the time of year was summer, the reality test used was for Jane to produce a snowstorm in the following four hours.[7] When no snow occurred, Jane accepted the result of the reality test and concluded that she could not change the weather after all.

3. Evidence: *I am responsible for events in the war in Iraq.*
The therapist then turned to tackle the evidence that Jane was responsible for world disasters, of which the war in Iraq was the most prominent, ongoing example. Having told Jane why he believed she could not be responsible, the therapist became more forceful and more challenging, asking her *how* she sent the messages to Iraq, *when* and *where* they went, and *what* they contained. The **logical reasoning** used was that

[7]If it had been wintertime, then the test would have been to produce sunshine and temperatures in the 80s. The less likely it is that the weather change will occur naturally, the longer the period you can safely set for the change to take place.

as she did not know these basic facts about the actions she thought she was doing, she could not be doing them. Related to this was the argument that as she did not know what atrocities had happened unless she saw them on TV or read about them in the newspaper, she could not have been responsible for them happening.

Other lines of logical reasoning included: How could she give instructions for the acts of violence when she did not know the places, geography or positions of military personnel? Why would military experts listen to her instructions, especially as she did not know their political aims? How could she give instructions to Arabs in the field when she does not speak Arabic? Jane was unable to answer these questions so she concluded her belief was based only on a very strong feeling of conviction that she had and not on any actual evidence. It had already been established that **a feeling is not valid evidence**, however strong that feeling might be, so it was suggested that since the only evidence she had for her involvement in the war was a feeling, this meant that she had no real evidence at all.

In practice Jane rejected her delusional belief at this point in the therapy, but if it had been necessary a **reality test** of her ability to influence events in Iraq would have been conducted. Since Jane would not deliberately cause bad things to happen, this would have taken the form of asking her to stop the war immediately, backed up by the **logical reasoning** that if she could influence events by causing them to happen, then she must also be able to cause them to stop.

REALITY TESTING THE CORE DELUSIONAL BELIEF

Having obtained from Jane what she thought an evil witch ought to be able to do, it would have been possible to reality test the core delusional belief about being a witch by putting these defining qualities and abilities to the test. For example, she believed she had the ability to cause wars, so a reality test that set her to cause a physical fight to occur between two of the nurses would have tested this ability. Similarly, setting her to cause a train crash at a set time and place would have tested her ability to cause disasters. In practice, direct reality testing of the delusional belief in this way was not necessary because the earlier CBT strategies of evidence re-evaluation and logical reasoning successfully modified the belief.

CASE STUDY STEPHEN

(See also pp. 78 and 97.)

Belief: *I get messages (which are always correct) from my spirit guide.*

Goal for belief modification: *I get messages from my spirit guide but it is possible for me to make a mistake in interpreting them because there is never perfect silence.*

This was a good example of those cases where it is very difficult to set the goal for the belief modification but where, once the appropriate goal has been set, then the actual therapy to achieve it is quick and easy.

Since the core delusional belief was beneficial for Stephen it would have been inappropriate to undermine it by modifying the associated **underlying beliefs.**

The aim of therapy was not to show that the messages were totally unreliable but rather that Stephen's interpretation of them *could* be unreliable, so it would only require evidence of the messages being wrong sometimes (theoretically, once would be enough), despite ideal conditions, to prove the point. Therefore, it was not necessary to **eliminate any supporting evidence** that Stephen already had of the messages being accurate.

The only instance of disconfirming evidence from the past, of which the therapist was aware, i.e. when a clear and definite message had turned out to be wrong, was when the spirit guide predicted who would win the Oxford and Cambridge boat race (Stephen had been a Cambridge undergraduate). Having assured everyone that Cambridge would win he had been clearly discomfited by the actual result, finally coming to the conclusion that perhaps the Cambridge crew had been celebrating prematurely the night before and this was the reason they had failed to fulfil their intended destiny. He was still so sensitive about this incident that the therapist considered it inadvisable to bring it up with him too soon.

It would be very easy with a reality test to prove the messages Stephen received were not accurate, so the only problem for therapy was how to introduce the notion of the test without Stephen experiencing this as a threat to his core belief about his spirit guide. A possible solution to this problem was suggested by Stephen's own report that he could make mistakes in interpreting the messages when there were other noises around. Since there are always some noises in the environment, even if very faint, perhaps the boundaries of what constituted 'uncertain' noise situations could be extended so that *all* situations were included as potentially uncertain.

First of all, the therapist confirmed with Stephen the fact that it was possible for him to make mistakes in his interpretations when it was generally a bit noisy. Secondly, she confirmed that there were no other ways that Stephen used to guarantee the messages were accurate other than the quietness of the room: this fact was discussed briefly in order to strengthen it. This was done in order to avoid the risk of his resorting to another reason for knowing the messages were accurate when the 'quietness' factor was shown to be unreliable.

Stephen also agreed that the exact cut-off point between 'quiet' and 'noisy' was vague. The therapist continued along the lines: 'So it sounds as if when it's noisy it is really difficult for you to know exactly what noises are part of the messages, whether or not two noises are supposed to go together to form a "no" or whether one is a "yes" and the other just a random noise in the environment. Is that right? I'm not surprised that sometimes you can misinterpret these noises. I appreciate that it gets easier the less noise there is around, but it seems to me that there must always be *some* noises occurring somewhere, so I would think that even when it seems pretty quiet to you there must be just a small possibility that perhaps a faint sound has occurred that you have missed, or that led you to misjudge the interval between sounds – what do you think? Have you ever noticed any occasions when it has sounded pretty quiet, so you thought you could be sure of the answer, but in fact there must have been some slight noises around because you made a mistake?'. Stephen agreed that perhaps he could never be absolutely sure that it was absolutely quiet when he was listening to the messages, and spontaneously recalled the incident of the boat race. It seems likely he was able to recall other incidents of errors from the past, as well as this one, because floating the suggestion of why these messages might always be susceptible to error was enough to bring about the belief modification required, namely that it was always *possible* his interpretation could be wrong even when the environmental conditions were apparently at their best. He was not asked about these other 'errors', however, because it was not necessary for the belief alteration to be effective, and the fact that he did not speak of them spontaneously suggested he was still sensitive about them.

If **reality testing** had been necessary, then it would have been suggested to Stephen he might try asking his spirit guide questions in order for him to check whether it was true that he could make mistakes even when it appeared to be very quiet. One wrong answer in apparently perfect conditions would be enough to achieve the goal of modification. In this particular case, it would not have mattered if the reality test appeared to confirm the delusional belief on many occasions, so long as there was one or more disconfirming results; this is very unusual for a reality test (see p. 181) and comes about because the belief being tested involves the notion of accuracy on *every* occasion. Indeed, since the aim of therapy was definitely not to challenge Stephen's functional belief in the messages as such, the reality testing would have been discontinued as soon as one, or at most two, incorrect interpretations had been made, because a series of incorrect interpretations would risk challenging the core belief itself, especially in someone who was sophisticated enough to appreciate the probabilities.

In practice Stephen gladly adapted his belief to include the possibility of error on his part, probably because this enabled him to account for previous incidents of incorrect interpretations that he had not been able to explain away for himself and that therefore had constituted a threat to his core belief about his spirit guide sending messages in this way. Be that as it may, once Stephen agreed it was possible for him to misinterpret the messages, then he also agreed it would be sensible to seek confirmation of these messages if they were important. For example, with respect to his medication, if he could not be sure he had interpreted his spirit guide correctly, then it made sense to consult the other experts available, namely the doctors, which is what he did.[8]

---

[8]Stephen agreed to continue with his medication. He was able to be discharged from hospital and he remained relatively well. Although he knew that he could not be certain about the replies, he continued to ask his spirit guide questions and to obtain spiritual support and guidance by this method.

CHECKING AND RECAPPING

As with all CBT, it is important to check the person's understanding of each piece of work that you do, so that you do not press on too quickly or in the wrong direction, or inadvertently present conflicting or confusing ideas and evidence. The art of skilful checking is to do it in such a way that the other person does not feel they are being examined on the work you have covered.

It is standard CBT practice for the therapist to recap frequently, both within and between sessions. Not only is this a powerful means of reminding the other person (and yourself) of what you have covered but it also reinforces it prior to the next therapeutic move. Recapping provides a summary of the relevant areas of work, allowing you to pull it together within a cohesive framework and giving you the opportunity to emphasize the key points. It is also one way of checking that your understanding of the implications and significance of what you have covered is the same as the other person's, a very important check to make.

Because of the fluctuations that can occur in the biological aspects of psychosis, with consequent fluctuations in delusional belief conviction and in insight, you should be particularly careful when recapping between sessions in case what was agreed in earlier sessions is rejected or regarded as too challenging for the present one. If you suspect that the other person's level of understanding has changed substantially between sessions, then it may be safer to ask them to remind you of the details of what you were talking about the last time this issue was discussed, rather than risking a recap that might be experienced by them as a direct challenge to their views and recollections.

Asking the other person to remind you of what you talked about may also be a useful strategy if you suspect that they have misunderstood a line of therapy that you had been trying to pursue. Paradoxically, if their understanding is quite different from your recapped version, then they may be more likely to signal agreement, not less, simply because they are too confused or are unable to see how to correct you.

A key feature of CBT practice is rephrasing what the other person tells you and then asking whether that rephrasing accurately reflects what they were trying to express. This is done not only to help you understand the other person's ideas and experiences but also to help them clarify these in their own mind. You should be aware that by rewording and clarifying what they are saying and getting their agreement to that rewording you may be subtly altering their perception and/or interpretation of events in the direction of that rewording. This being so, you must be careful of the changes you make and go slowly, and always check that you have understood properly. In your eagerness to reach a more rational phrasing, try not to move too rapidly in this direction as this may result in their feeling pressured to see things differently, or to their feeling misunderstood. If this does occur, you should be quick to apologize for having got it wrong and make another attempt. Remember that the least challenging reflection is that which uses the person's own words exactly; but although this is good for rapport, it will not further your understanding of what they meant by their words, and nor will it help to clarify or modify their thinking about the matter.

DANGER: MODIFYING A DELUSION IN AN UNWANTED DIRECTION

Despite careful planning and execution of your treatment, there may be occasions in your clinical practice when you inadvertently push the delusional belief in an unwanted direction.[9] The most likely reasons for this to happen are (a) that the replacement belief is not as acceptable and welcomed as you thought, (b) that the delusional belief has more benefits than you realized, (c) that the belief change is going ahead too quickly, and/or (d) that there is some additional factor(s) operating of which you are not aware. The immediate response to this situation is to back off, retreating if necessary to the original delusional belief (e.g. in case 1 below, retreating to the position 'I'm not sure whether the voices come from her ex-fiancé or not, but I'm certain they can't be from the Martians').

This is one occasion where you should not go away and think about the situation: you should immediately become more assertive and directive in order to close down the dysfunctional alternative. Since the person has only just come up with this new belief or explanation for events it is likely their conclusions will still be tentative, and so this is the time to move in swiftly to counter them. In this situation it is appropriate to disagree, stating (gently) that you do not think this alternative can be correct and giving all your reasons for thinking so. The following examples come from my own clinical practice.

CAUTIONARY TALES FROM CLINICAL PRACTICE

Case 1: This case demonstrates what can happen if you fail to appreciate that the other person's understanding about their illness may be quite different from your own.

A young man was distressed by threatening voices that he believed came from his girlfriend's ex-fiancé, so we undertook a reality test to prove that the voices, which seemed to come from buildings 50 or more yards away, could not be coming from a real person because real voices cannot travel that far. The first set of experiments produced the results I had expected and he seemed reassured and pleased about that. However, the evidence was not enough to change the delusional belief so we agreed to do some more tests next session. I noticed that although he was willing to participate in the second set of tests he seemed less keen than I was expecting, but I failed to appreciate the potential significance of this and carried out the tests anyway.

[9] Pushing someone into an alternative delusional explanation couched in terms of religious or supernatural powers can be particularly unwelcome. Not only are they capable of having profound effects on the person but, by their very nature, spirits and aliens may also be able to operate in ways that contradict rational argument and scientific experiment and as such are inherently difficult to challenge with cognitive-behavioural techniques.

They produced irrefutable proof that the voices he heard could not be coming from a real human being, and therefore could not represent real threats of harm from the ex-fiancé. In good CBT fashion, I asked him what he made of these results. He paused before suggesting that perhaps this meant the voices came from the Martians. This was not a helpful modification so I moved immediately to counter it, stating that I did not think this could be so (a) because we had tested how far we could hear voices and we certainly would not be able to hear voices from Mars, which is millions of miles away, (b) because no one else could hear the voices, which they would be able to do if they were just voices coming generally to earth from Mars, and (c) because Martians would speak a language of their own, not English.

The young man concerned had been in hospital for several years and I had been in several assessment meetings with him when his schizophrenic illness was discussed and noted that he used the term himself and appeared to be quite unconcerned. So I assumed he knew he had a mental illness and that this was perfectly acceptable to him: this was my mistake. It was only by discussing the possibility of mental illness as an explanation for the results of the reality test that I realized he was horrified at the thought his voices might come from within himself, because this would mean he was 'mad'. I immediately went into some normalizing and destigmatizing work around hearing voices and left the results of the reality tests until he brought them up again himself.

Case 2: This case illustrates the risk posed by not detecting fluctuations in psychosis and consequent fluctuations in insight.

I had been working with a woman for some weeks to identify ways that she might be able to distinguish between her delusional memories, which were very vivid and totally convincing (what we agreed to call her 'dream memories'), and real events. For example, on one occasion she was convinced she and I had been teaching in the same junior school the week before, and on another occasion that we had just come back from a trip to the local shops, even though I had never been outside the hospital with her. One of the ways that we found worked quite well was that when the memory included other people, she would ask them if they recalled the event as she did, with the agreement that if they did not recall it, then this would indicate it must be a 'dream memory' rather than something that had really happened.

On the occasion in question, the woman told me that the previous weekend she had been with her mother on a large boat crossing a street in Epsom. In this instance, I could be sure this was a delusional memory, but rational arguments about the geography of Epsom, which she knew well, were not persuasive for her and so I suggested we phone her mother. Her mother confirmed she had no recall of such an event, and after she put the phone down I asked her why this could be. I was dismayed when she thought for a bit and then concluded that the woman she spoke to on the phone must have been a 'double'. I had not appreciated that her psychosis had worsened to the point where she was no longer able to question her memories in the way that we had been doing in previous sessions.

This was certainly not a desirable shift in belief so I moved to close it down immediately by stating (a) that doubles did not and could not occur in real life, that the only double possible was an identical twin but she and all her family knew her mother was not one of twins, (b) that the woman who answered the phone had been at her mother's phone number and therefore must be her mother, (c) that the woman knew who I was, whereas a double would not, and (d) that the woman knew her and our plan of treatment, which her mother did but which a double would not have done. We discussed these points until she was reassured that she really had been talking to her real mother, and we agreed that perhaps her mother had just forgotten about the weekend trip for some reason. It was safer for her at this stage to have an erroneous memory about being on a boat in Epsom than for her to open up the possibility that people can have doubles. By its very nature, this latter would have been a very difficult belief to challenge. In its immediate presentation it could have had a significant affect on her relationship with her mother, and once the possibility of doubles had been established, then it could have been extended in the future to include other people as well. This would have been a very dysfunctional development because it would have provided an escape route to explain away many of the inconsistencies that I was already using, and planning to use, as challenges to the accuracy of her delusional memories, and also in other belief modification programmes.

9 ASSESSMENT, CASE FORMULATION AND GOAL SETTING FOR AUDITORY HALLUCINATIONS

ASSESSMENT

The assessment of voices is undertaken with the same gentle approach as that used for delusions. As with delusions, as far as possible you should frame your questions from within the person's own belief system, i.e. using their terminology and concepts rather than your own.

Basic information about the voice(s)

The initial assessment aims to identify and collect basic information about the principal voices. The information you will require about each different voice will include:

- What does the voice say (or what *sort* of thing does the voice say?)
  - What does that *mean* for the person?
  - Is the voice telling the truth?
- How distressing is the voice?
- Is it malevolent or benevolent?
- What does the voice sound like?
- Where and/or who does it come from?
  - (If appropriate) How does the person know the voice comes from a particular person or entity?
- How frequent is the voice?
- How does the person *feel* about the voice?
  - Does it have any power, or can it cause harm? What evidence does the person have for this?
- How does it affect the person's life?
- Does the voice command the person and, if so, how?
  - Is the voice difficult to resist?
  - What does, or could, happen if they resist?
- Does the person have any coping strategies for the voice, even if they are not recognized as such?
- What is the person's attitude to 'mental illness' or 'psychosis' as a possible explanation for the voice?

Obtaining the information

In the early stages of the therapeutic relationship people may be reluctant to tell you about their voices, especially what they say. It is important to reassure the person that you do not need to know the details, and with this reassurance they may be willing to tell you what sort of things the voices say and/or why they are distressing. For example, 'I understand that you'd rather not tell me what the voice says, and that's absolutely fine, there's no need at all to tell me. But I was wondering if it would be OK to just tell me what *sort* of thing it says, so that I could get a better picture of how it affects you? But only if you feel OK with that – and please don't tell me exactly what it says, unless you want to, it's entirely up to you'. It is often possible to start some useful work despite having only this general information and, knowing that you will not push them for more details than they are comfortable giving, people usually feel safe to start to talk about the exact content of their voices within a few sessions.

As we shall see in Chapter 11, in some cases the voices can reveal something about the person or their life history that they might not, in other circumstances, have wanted people to know or talk about. This being so, you should always approach the content of hallucinations and what they reveal as privileged information, to be treated with the greatest of respect.

CASE FORMULATION

As with delusional beliefs, the main purpose of case formulation for an auditory hallucination is to be able to understand why it takes the form it does and why it affects the person in the way it does, so that the relevant factors can be identified and targeted with appropriate lines of therapy.

The form taken by the voice

A very important aspect of the case formulation deals with the content of the voice and seeks to explain *why the voice says what it does*. A key question here is 'What do the voice's utterances *mean* for this particular person?', bearing in mind the possible deep meaning of what is said as well as the more obvious, literal meaning. This important aspect of the case formulation is discussed in detail in Chapter 11 (see pp. 215–216).

Another aspect of the case formulation is concerned with *why a thought has been heard as an external voice* and, if it applies, *why the voice is recognized as coming from a particular person*. There is essentially only one physiological explanation for the phenomenon of voices per se, though this explanation can be couched in different ways. However, there can be different reasons why this physiological response occurs (see Chapters 2, p. 33, and 12, p. 234).

Why the voice affects the person in the way that it does

What the voice says and *the beliefs associated with what it says* are important determinants of how the voice will affect the person hearing it. This part of the case formulation is closely related to the case formulation for the content of the voice (see Chapter 11).

As well as what the voice says, it is important to consider *what the person believes about the voice* because these beliefs can have significant effects on how the person feels and responds to their voice. For example, the voice may cause distress because of delusional beliefs about who or where it comes from, about its power and authority or about its malign intent towards the hearer (see Chapters 12–14 for more details).

The occurrence of the voice may be distressing because of the *implications of 'hearing voices'* (see p. 228), or the sheer *irritant effect* of not being able to get away from the noise of the voice (see p. 211), so these factors may also be relevant when case formulating for why the voice is dysfunctional and distressing.

What is maintaining the voice?

The model described in Figure 1.2 (p. 2) and the ABC model (p. 17) may be helpful when constructing this part of the case formulation, which is particularly concerned with identifying the factors maintaining or exacerbating the voice. Some examples of maintenance cycles are:

- What the voice says causes anxiety, which increases arousal, which in turn increases the voices.
- The experience of hearing the voice triggers the negative thought 'I'm out of control, it will take over my mind', which in turn triggers feelings of fear, which leads to increased arousal and increased cannabis use to try to reduce the arousal, which increases the voices.
- A paranoid voice warns that the man opposite is sucking out the hearer's soul, so the hearer tries to protect himself by stabbing the man, which leads to arrest, which leads to increased arousal and confirmation that people are against him, which leads to more paranoid voices.

As with delusional beliefs, it is usual for case formulations for the form of the voice and the beliefs about the voice to expand as new relevant factors emerge during therapy, but the preliminary formulation(s) is sufficient for goal setting purposes when you are satisfied you have identified the major factors involved, i.e. when the formulation provides an adequate explanation for what it sets out to explain. (See case examples of Sanjay and Richard, below.)

GOAL SETTING

The goal(s) for an auditory hallucination may involve one or more of the following:

- Reduce the frequency/loudness of the voice.
- Modify the belief(s) associated with the content of the voice.
- Modify the belief(s) about the origin of the voice.
- Modify the belief(s) about the power and authority of the voice.
- Modify the responses to the voice's commands.

These different types of goal are discussed in detail in Chapters 10–14, but as a general principle, beliefs about the voice are treated like any other delusional belief. Total and partial modification goals may be set and considered, and their relative merits compared; and, as with any other belief, when a total goal is set, then a functional replacement belief must be specified and, if necessary, prepared in order to ensure it is acceptable and functional for the person concerned.

Where there is more than one voice these should be considered separately because the different voices may require different goals. For example, the goal for one voice may be to modify the dysfunctional beliefs that underlie what it says, whilst the goal for another voice may be to take away its power and authority.

Before starting any modification work it is important to consider the possible impact that the modification of beliefs about one voice may have on beliefs about another, and/or the effects that modifications of one aspect of the voice may have on another aspect of that same voice. For example, working to bring about the understanding that the bad voices were internally generated memories and not messages from a dead father would almost inevitably weaken a belief that the encouraging voices came from a dead mother. Similarly, working to show that a voice had no power and was ignorant would have significant implications for a belief that it came from an archangel.

As with the non-psychotic beliefs underlying a delusional belief, goals set for the beliefs underlying the content of the voice should be set so that they are consistent with the person's socio-cultural-religious background (see pp. 83–86).

CASE STUDY SANJAY[1]

(See also pp. 214 and 225.)

CASE HISTORY

Hostel staff where he lived had noticed that Sanjay, a man in his late 60s, sometimes became upset by his voices. He had heard voices for as long as he could remember and recognized that they were part of his 'illness'. They were sometimes male and sometimes female; he did not recognize them as anyone he knew. They talked about what he was doing; sometimes they were critical but often they were just banal. When asked for examples, he described a recent occasion when a voice had called him 'clumsy' and 'a messy old man' when he had spilt some tea, and his example of a banal comment was 'Oh look, he's hurrying downstairs because he's worried that he'll miss dinner'. Sometimes he could not hear what the voices were saying but he found this irritating as well because they would mutter on and on and he could not get away from them. There was nothing at all that he liked about the voices and wished they would go away.

CASE FORMULATIONS AND GOALS OF TREATMENT

1. Sanjay wanted to get rid of the voices, not only because the critical ones upset him but also because the mere presence of the other voices irritated him.

[1]The course of therapy for Sanjay is followed through at appropriate points in Chapters 9-14.

Goal 1: *Block the voices or at least reduce their loudness and/or intensity.*

2. The criticisms made by the voices tended to centre around untidiness and messiness, and implied (a) that he had an underlying belief '*It is important to be clean and tidy*', and (b) that he perceived himself as falling below the required standards in these areas of functioning.

The most functional goal of modification for this underlying belief depended on whether Sanjay was, in fact, being unusually clumsy and messy. If he was not being messy and untidy, i.e. if he was misinterpreting situations and being over critical of his own behaviour, then the existing underlying belief about the importance of cleanliness and tidiness could be left intact, and the modification would have been around him changing his evaluation of his behaviour. In these circumstances the goal would have been: '(It is important to be clean and tidy): I *am* clean and tidy, to a good, acceptable standard.'

In fact, Sanjay had become clumsier than one would expect for a man of his age because he had developed a slight tremor, and because the negative symptoms of his illness meant that looking after his room and personal hygiene had become increasingly difficult for him. Furthermore, he was nearing 70 years of age and therefore these features were likely to get worse over the coming years. For this reason, the modification chosen targeted the underlying belief about the importance of not being messy and untidy.

Goal 2: *'It doesn't matter when I am messy or untidy; some people are and some people aren't – lots of people prefer to live like that. Being messy or untidy doesn't affect the value of a person, and other people don't look down on me if I am sometimes messy and untidy.'*

3. Sanjay did not know what his voices were or where they came from, and did not recognize that they were his own thoughts. His rather vague belief that they were 'part of his illness' was functional, and in this particular case it was considered that understanding the critical voices to be his own thoughts might actually have been unhelpful since it would have made it harder for him to distance himself from what they said. Therefore, no attempt was made to change or develop his belief about the voices' origin.

Goal 3: *Leave the belief about the nature/origin of the voices intact.*

4. The voices were not perceived to have any power or authority and they never gave commands, so case formulation and goal setting for these aspects did not apply.

CASE STUDY RICHARD[2]

(See also pp. 214, 226, 246, 262 and 278.)

CASE HISTORY

Richard was a man in his early 20s. In his late teens he joined a religious sect that believed every member had a duty to pray regularly, using a set form of words, in order for the world to be saved. Eighteen months after joining, Richard left the sect and was admitted to hospital within days with an acute psychotic episode.[3]

He described his current problems along these lines: 'Sometimes I have to get out of bed in the middle of the night, even when it's cold and I'm tired, because a voice tells me that I have to say the prayer I learnt whilst with the religious sect. It's particularly frightening when it's dark in my room. I have to kneel by my bed and repeat the prayer over and over again for two hours. I have tried ignoring the voice but it tells me I must pray in order to save the world, and I am frightened something awful will happen to me if I don't do what it tells me to do. I've no idea where the voice comes from. Every night when I go to bed I pray that I will sleep through the night until morning, and sometimes that works. I feel much better the next day when I have had a good night of uninterrupted sleep. I feel a bit safer in this ward, but I'm only in hospital because I had a row with my parents and I would like to go home soon.'

Richard was religiously minded, and at the time of his referral he was discussing joining the Church of England with the hospital chaplain.

CASE FORMULATIONS AND GOALS OF THERAPY

1. Richard wanted the voice to go away and would pray not to hear it. Obeying the voice was made more distressing by the physical discomfort this involved.

Goal 1A: *Block the voice, or at least reduce its loudness and/or intensity.*

Goal 1B: *Reduce the distress caused as a result of hearing the voice.*

2. The content of the voice suggested that Richard was still concerned about leaving the sect and feared that not praying in the way they did was tantamount to defying and displeasing God. In the daytime he no longer believed this to be true: he was never troubled by a voice or even a thought that he ought to pray at other times during the day when the sect would have been praying together. But when he was in his room in the dark, at night, the greater sense of insecurity allowed the feelings of guilt and fear surrounding this issue to be reactivated, i.e. the beliefs instilled by the sect were still there, overlaid by his new religious beliefs, and these earlier beliefs could still be triggered by appropriate cues and circumstances. Having been

[2]The course of the therapy for Richard is followed through at appropriate points in Chapters 9–15. [3]There is no suggestion that the sect was implicated in the development of his illness; indeed, it seemed likely that the very structured regime actually enabled him to survive outside hospital for longer than he otherwise would have done.

reactivated, these old beliefs then enhanced the impact that the voice was able to make on him, and a self-maintaining cycle was established. Therefore, the second goal was to further weaken the non-psychotic but dysfunctional belief underlying the content of his voice. If successful, this would serve the dual purpose of (a) breaking the maintenance cycle, so that even if the voice should occur at night it would not lead to feelings of guilt or fear, or be able to compel his behaviour, and (b) ensuring that he would not have any lingering fears about leaving the sect that might re-emerge at some time in the future.

In the statement of the goal, the sect was described as being benign rather than malign in intent. Apart from the fact that this was almost certainly fairer to the sect concerned, this description was more functional for Richard because it helped to remove some of his fear of the sect members and of their beliefs.

Goal 2: *'Members of the sect genuinely believe what they say is correct, but they are mistaken. God does not require me to say this prayer repeatedly, and he does not require me to be a member of this sect.'*

3. Richard had no definite theory as to where the voice came from, but he assumed it must be some sort of powerful spiritual force. The therapist was careful when questioning Richard not to force him to come to some more specific conclusions about the origin of the voice because she wanted to avoid the risk of Richard interpreting it as coming from God. For religious people, God is the ultimate source of power and wisdom and therefore any form of 'challenge' would be completely inappropriate.

Although Richard's explanation for the origin of the voice was vague and imprecise, he was sure it had power and that it was able to cause him harm or kill him. The voice would lose its power completely if Richard were to come to an understanding that it was no more than a thought coming from within himself, reflecting a superstitious fear, and so his belief about the origin of the voice was targeted for modification. This was a total modification and so a replacement belief had to be identified. The fact that he gave a non-illness reason for his admission to hospital, despite the fact that staff members would have talked to him about his psychosis and the need to take medication, strongly suggested he had some dysfunctional beliefs about mental illness and therefore that any replacement belief couched in these terms would not be acceptable to him and would need to be 'prepared'. Fortunately, the common occurrence of voices in the general population means that it is not always necessary to explain their occurrence in terms of mental illness, and so a non-illness replacement belief was used for Richard whilst attempts were made to prepare him for the notion of mental illness.

Goal 3A: *'The voice is not from some external entity: it is a vivid thought produced by my brain that I hear out loud because it makes me feel so frightened and stressed.'*

Goal 3B (Possible extension/development of goal 3A, for the future): *'The voice does not come from an external source: hearing my thoughts out loud is a feature of my (psychotic) illness.'*

4. The main reason the voice was able to cause Richard such distress was that he feared what would happen if he failed to do as it instructed him. Removing his fear of the voice would not only mean that he would no longer have to obey its instructions but would also enable him to challenge it, and to use coping strategies against it, without fear of retribution and without significant increases in arousal. There were two stages to reducing Richard's fear of the voice, namely changing his belief about the voice's possible displeasure and ill intent towards him, and then showing that the voice could not inflict harm.

Goal 4A: *'The voice does not want to harm me.'*

Goal 4B: *'The voice is not able to harm me.'*

5. The fear of what the voice might do to him if he disobeyed was the only reason for Richard getting up to pray during the night, so it was predicted that if this fear could be removed, then it should be relatively easy for Richard to stop this behaviour.

Goal 5: *To be able to ignore the voice and go back to sleep.*

It was anticipated that some interim steps might be needed for this goal, wherein Richard would use a distraction task and/or an anxiety-reducing task whilst he ignored the voice's commands. Depending on what turned out to be effective in this respect the interim goals might include: '*Ignore the voice and go and talk to nursing staff*' or '*Ignore the voice and listen to my Walkman®*', etc.

CHECKING THAT THE GOALS WERE ACCEPTABLE AND FUNCTIONAL

During the assessment Richard was very definite about his preferences for his current religious beliefs and his wish that the night-time voice would go away for good, so little was needed in the way of checking out the goals for acceptability. We could imagine no advantages for Richard in these beliefs except, just possibly, a sense of importance because the voice was talking to him. However, Richard did not think this implied he was special for any reason other than that he had left the sect.

ORDER OF TACKLING THE GOALS

The first step of the therapy was to see if any practical strategies could be used to help reduce the distress of the situation (see p. 278).

Goals 1A and B (reducing the voice and the distress it caused), 2 ('The sect is wrong'), and 4A ('The voice does not want to harm me') could be pursued immediately. The goal setting exercise had highlighted the fact that modification of his belief about the nature/origin of his voice would not be acceptable and functional until the replacement belief had been adequately prepared, but goals 1A and B, 2, and 4A did not impact on this belief and so could be pursued safely. Work on these goals was carried out in tandem, so that it was usual to pursue some aspect of each of the lines of treatment in every session.

Showing the voice was not able to harm him or make things happen in the physical world would not challenge Richard's belief that it came from some external, spiritual source, and as such it was considered safe to move on to goal 4B ('The voice cannot harm me') at an early stage. This work was carried out alongside that on the four goals above.

Before being able to move to goal 3A ('The voice is my own thoughts') it would be necessary to prepare the replacement belief. The preparation work would involve giving information about how people's brains work; this is not unpleasant or stigmatizing, so it was anticipated this would be relatively easy and quick to do. The potential problem with goal 3A was the possibility that Richard would move on immediately to goal 3B, before the replacement for that modification had been prepared, i.e. that he would move from 'The voices are my own thoughts' to 'They are hallucinations, so people were right when they said I had a mental illness'. Therefore, the destigmatizing work around the diagnosis of psychosis was started early on, whilst the other 'safe' goals were being pursued. It was anticipated this work would also lay the foundations for actively pursuing goal 3B in the future should it become apparent this would have some benefits.

Note that it was not necessary in this case to move towards acceptance of mental illness in order for Richard to have a rationale for taking medication. Under the conceptualization of his experiences given by goal 3A ('I hear my thoughts out loud because they are so frightening'), the medication would be useful in helping to control the recurring fragments of memory and old beliefs that surfaced so strongly from time to time that they sounded like real voices.[4]

---

[4]This latter is just as accurate a conceptualization of Richard's experiences as the one in terms of psychosis and biochemical abnormalities, but it applies at the cognitive, subjective level rather than the biological, objective level.

10 PRACTICAL INTERVENTIONS FOR VOICES

WALKMAN® AND EARPLUG

In addition to the more general coping strategies described in Chapter 15, there are some specific interventions aimed directly at blocking or reducing the intensity of the voices. Two of these, the Walkman and the earplug, are particularly helpful strategies. They are effective in a large number of cases, they require very little effort to use, they do not prevent the person from getting on with other aspects of their life, and they can be used for long periods at a time.

The Walkman can be suggested as early as the first session, because if a Walkman stops the voices, this implies nothing about their nature or origin since a Walkman might reasonably be expected to block any sound coming from an external source. The earplug is more problematic in this respect, though in practice most people do not seem to question why a single earplug should stop external voices and are just glad that it does. However, as with all CBT interventions, if you have any doubts about the implications of stopping the voices by this method, then you should check with the person themself how they would interpret this possible outcome before suggesting they use it.

You should also be sensitive to how the person responds to your suggestion of trying something that might stop their voices, especially if there is any sign of reluctance, because if they are not keen to accept the suggestion, then this may indicate some ambivalence with respect to the voices and possible undetected benefits. For example, I was asked to see a woman who became very agitated and angry when she heard her voice. She did not want to talk to me about it or, indeed, about anything else, so I offered her a Walkman. She did not seem keen to take this but I left it anyway, with the suggestion that if the voice got really nasty and upsetting for her, then she might like to give it a go. When I approached her some days later, she tried to kick me. The Walkman had been effective, but this had caused her to doubt the origin of her voice which, though it made derogatory and critical comments, was her only contact with her mother.

The Walkman and earplug are usually introduced along the lines 'Some people find this seems to block voices a bit like yours' or 'You might like to try this out just to see if it helps at all'. The advantage of offering these practical suggestions early on is that, if they work, they provide the person not only with immediate respite from the voices but also, possibly for the first time, the realization that they have a certain amount of control over them.[1] It is usually best to try just one

[1]Occasionally, the practical strategies are found to be effective but the voices, then command the person to stop using them. If this happens, it is probably less stressful for the person to discontinue their use until cognitive work can be done to disempower the voices and their threats (see Chapter 13).

of the practical coping strategies at a time so you can determine which are the more effective.

The personal cassette/CD player player (Walkman)

Most people gain some immediate respite from their voices by using a cassette player with headphones, though when the voices are very troublesome the volume may have to be turned up very loud. As well as being the most effective this is also the most popular way of controlling the voices.

Although there are good theoretical reasons to suppose that listening to taped speech would be more effective than music in combating the voices, the large majority of people prefer to listen to music. The type of music does not seem to matter, though there is some evidence that aggressive pop music (e.g. heavy metal) can provoke agitated behaviour and actually increase the voices. Whilst we do not attempt to stop people listening to music of this type if this is their choice, we do warn them of the potential risks and help them to carefully monitor the effects on their voices. Very occasionally, people have reported hearing messages from the words of vocal music, in which case a switch to non-vocal music is usually successful.

The cassette player probably has its beneficial effect on auditory hallucinations in two complementary ways. Firstly, auditory hallucinations are known to be adversely affected by stress, so if listening to the music is pleasurable and relaxing, then this may indirectly result in a reduction in the voices. Secondly, the cassette player diverts attention or awareness away from the voices; this is likely to occur at two levels. People report that the louder the music, the more effective it is at blocking the voices, suggesting that some of the attention-switching effect occurs at a level that is under neurological rather than conscious control: the music literally 'drowns out' the voices. This is why it can be effective even when the person is paying no attention to it. However, the more meaningful and attention-demanding the input, the greater the effect on the voices seems to be, suggesting that there may also be some attention-switching effect that occurs at a higher level of information processing and control.

The earplug

A number of people with auditory hallucinations benefit from putting an earplug in one ear. At best, the earplug stops the voices altogether, though for some people it works by distorting or reducing the volume of the voices or even by changing the nature of what they say.[2]

Wax earplugs (Boots 'Mufflers®', cut in half for greater comfort, cost less than £2 for a box of 10) are easy to obtain and cheap to replace if lost or dirty.[3] You should demonstrate how to warm and mould the wax in your fingers before

[2]It is not immediately obvious why this latter effect should occur, but it may be mediated by a reduction in anxiety, which is a result of the reduced intensity of the voice.

[3]Black people may prefer darker coloured earplugs because they are less conspicuous. Some industrial and camping equipment suppliers have alternative colours to the standard pink.

inserting it into an ear, and normalize their use by explaining that they are commonly used for pop concerts, when using loud machinery, or to help sleep in planes or other noisy situations. Sponge-foam earplugs are more expensive but some people find them more comfortable to use, so they should be considered for longer term use where people find this strategy useful. Cotton wool earplugs appear not to be as effective or comfortable as wax or foam.

You should encourage the person to experiment with the earplug in their left and right ear as some people do report marked ear preferences. Wearing earplugs in both ears at the same time is not normally recommended because of the potential interference the resulting 'deafness' might have with everyday functioning. However, some people try two earplugs for themselves and find the effects so beneficial that they continue to use them this way.

The most likely explanation for the effectiveness of the earplug seems to be that the distortion in sound that it produces causes the brain to pay particular attention to the sounds coming from external sources and hence diverts attention away from the internally produced sounds/voices: this diversion of attention occurs at a neurological level outside our conscious control. If this explanation is correct, and the effect of the earplug depends on the brain's response to the novelty of the sound distortion, then this would suggest that the earplug should not be used for long periods as this may result in habituation to the effect. Over the years we have found in a few cases that this does happen, though only after many months of continual usage, but for this reason we do suggest to people that they use the earplug only when the voices are bothering them. Nevertheless, occasionally people are so troubled by their voices that they choose to keep an earplug in all day and night.

Although earplugs can be very effective in interrupting the voices (indeed, they are effective in the majority of cases), some people are unwilling to use them, whilst others find them too uncomfortable to use regularly. Occasionally people are worried about what might happen to the earplug if they put it into their ear; if this is the case then it may be helpful to show them a diagram of the ear and discuss its workings so they can see that the earplug cannot get 'lost'. With respect to the discomfort of the earplug, it is recommended you try wearing an earplug for a couple of hours yourself, as this may help you understand why people may refuse to use this method even though it stops the unwanted voices. Apart from anything else, without experiencing the discomfort it is easy to conclude that the voices 'cannot be that bad' if the person will not use such a simple method of stopping them.

Long-term effects of the earplug and Walkman

For most people, the effect of the earplug or Walkman on the auditory hallucinations is limited to when the strategy is being used and for a short period immediately after use, but for a few there appears to be a longer-term beneficial effect as well, with a gradual reduction in the occurrence of the voices when the strategies are used over several weeks. In a handful of cases, chronic voices have stopped altogether for many months. These longer-term effects are thought to be mediated by a reduction in anxiety and arousal levels, which is brought about not only by the treatments themselves but also by the sense of control over the hallucinations these strategies give. Put another way, knowing you can stop the voices if they become very bothersome reduces your fear of getting them, and reducing your fear of getting them reduces their occurrence: a beneficial cycle has been established.

Walkman and earplug as the main treatment strategies

Some people are not bothered by what their voices say, perhaps because the content is insignificant or because the voices are so indistinct they cannot quite catch what they are saying, yet they find the unwanted interruptions intensely irritating, especially if they continue for long periods unabated. In these cases, where the primary cause of distress is the irritating presence of the voices, then an earplug or Walkman, if effective, may be all that is required in the way of treatment. For example, one woman was plagued by a babble of meaningless words that continued throughout her waking hours. This made her agitated and irritable towards others, causing arguments and even occasional physical assaults. Using an earplug stopped the voices, thereby breaking the negative cycle of voices leading to stress, leading to more voices, leading to more stress, etc.

A few people want to get rid of their unpleasant voices but keep their pleasant ones. It is likely to be very difficult, if not impossible, to modify beliefs about the power and origin of the unpleasant voices without modifying the beliefs about the pleasant ones in the same direction, and in these circumstances the selective use of the earplug and Walkman to target and block just the unwanted voices may be the most effective CBT strategy you can offer.

These simple strategies, which require little contact to set up or administer, may also be the only (and, therefore, the most useful) CBT strategy you can use with people who do not want to engage in any sort of interpersonal relationship.

OTHER STRATEGIES

The strategies detailed below are more difficult to put into practice and are usually less effective than the Walkman and earplug, so they are not the first choice for stopping voices. Furthermore, some of them imply that the voices are internally generated and therefore should not be introduced until the person accepts this explanation for their voices. However, it is useful for someone to have more than one method of stopping their voices because their chosen method may not always be available to them, or it may be inappropriate in certain situations (e.g. using a Walkman in the cinema).

Pointing, 'look and name'

The verbal areas of the brain responsible for producing voices are essentially the same as those used for spoken speech, so if these areas are being used for some other verbal task, then there is less capacity left to create the voices. A simple task of this sort is naming objects, so one way of temporarily stopping the voices is to point to things around the room, naming each one out loud and moving rapidly from object to object to maximize the involvement of the verbal brain areas. If this is found to be effective, then the person should also practise just looking at the objects and naming them silently to themself, so that the strategy can be used in social and public situations.

Despite the sound theory behind it, this strategy does not work for everyone. It requires a lot of focused attention and so can only be used for short periods, and it cannot be used if the person is trying to focus on something else. However, it can be useful in some situations, for example in public places such as waiting in a supermarket queue, where the anxiety has caused a temporary increase in the voices and where other strategies are not appropriate or available.

Subvocal speech or singing under one's breath

Talking out loud can be an effective way of blocking auditory hallucinations but it may not be socially acceptable for the person to suddenly start talking to themself, for example if they are walking along a shopping street or sitting alone in a railway station. In order to avoid social embarrassment, they may be able to use subvocal speech, i.e. talking quietly to themself so that no one else can hear. The theory is that providing there are minor movements in the vocal cords, then this will be sufficient to prevent the vocal cord movements that accompany at least some auditory hallucinations. Some people do report beneficial effects from subvocal speech but one of the major practical obstacles is that many people find it difficult to understand the concept of subvocal talking and are unable to put it into action.

Singing under one's breath is easier to understand and to do, and as such may be preferable to subvocal speech, even though there are theoretical reasons for supposing it would be less effective. Another major practical difficulty is that keeping up a flow of subvocal speech requires concentration and effort, so it is only suitable for use over short periods. Repeating sequences of numbers (e.g. 1–10) may be less attention-demanding but quickly becomes tedious; subvocal singing may be less effective but it is easier to keep up over longer periods.

Despite the limitations of subvocal speech and singing, this may be a useful practical strategy if it is important to stop the voices and there are no other means to hand, for example if the person is in a public place when the voices start and they have no earplugs or Walkman with them.

Concentrating/focusing on the voices

In some of the early clinical work with hallucinations, people were asked to complete homework assignments recording details about their voices, and it was found that in some cases focusing on the voices in this way actually seemed to reduce the frequency of their occurrence. This reduction may occur, in part at least, because adopting a scientific or objective attitude towards their voices helps people distance themselves from them and from the power that they have. This effect may be exploited for therapeutic purposes by setting a homework task requiring details of the voices to be recorded on a formal chart, as and when they occur, for discussion at the next therapy session. A secondary gain from this exercise is that the additional information about the voices that it provides may suggest other coping strategies; for example, the man who discovered that his voices occurred most frequently in the television room decided to avoid this room until his voices got better.

Focusing is not a commonly used coping strategy, not least because most people with active psychosis are unable to complete this type of formal homework assignment. Furthermore, you should check that the person does not become more agitated or distressed by concentrating on the voices. This is particularly likely to occur if the content of the voices is very unpleasant, especially if one of the present coping strategies is avoidance. If you test this by asking the person to focus on their voices during a therapy session, you should bear in mind that the distress the voices causes is likely to be quite a bit higher outside the safety of the session, when the person is on their own and without your calming influence and support.

Restricting the time spent listening to the voices

This is a variant of a CBT strategy used for worrying. The person attempts to limit the intrusiveness of their voices in their everyday lives by setting aside a set period in each day when they will listen or respond to them. Having set aside this time, they are better able to ignore or to refuse to listen to the voices at other times.

In practice this strategy seems to be used by only a very small minority of people who, typically, have a long history of hearing voices and a good understanding about the nature of these experiences; so the most appropriate time to consider suggesting this strategy to someone would be in long-term management.

Switching the voices on and off

A few people are able to bring on their voices within the therapy session. It may not have occurred to them to try this before, so asking them to imagine the voices talking may help to bring them on. Once the voices have been voluntarily produced in this way the person tries to turn them off again, either by fading them away or by terminating them suddenly. Having practised switching off the voices that have been produced voluntarily, some people are able to transfer this learnt ability to switch off the voices to when they occur involuntarily. This technique is not suitable for people who do not have insight into the origin of their voices, and so should not be used either before insight has been achieved or in cases where full insight is not the desired goal of therapy. During my own clinical practice I have not encountered people who were able to produce their voices voluntarily in this way, but there are reliable reports in the research literature that this technique can work so it may be worth a try.

Although voluntarily producing the voices has irrefutable implications about their origin, the same is not true for dismissing voices that have occurred involuntarily, and so this latter can be used whilst there are still delusional ideas about the voices. Some people do report that they can sometimes get rid of their voices by telling them to go away, though the relief is usually short-lived. Commanding the voices to stop seems to be more effective if shouted out loud, but because of the social difficulties this may cause it is worth practising to see if the person can gradually reduce the volume until they can stop the voices by just saying the command word quietly to themself. This may be particularly important as some people find that swearing at the voices in a disrespectful way (e.g. 'F *** off!') is more effective than telling them politely to stop. There is, however, a caution with this particular strategy. If interacting with the voices in an aggressive way increases arousal levels, then it may actually increase their persistence, so it is useful to monitor both the immediate and the longer-term effects.

CASE STUDY SANJAY

(See also pp. 202 and 225.)

Goal 1: *Block the voices or at least reduce their loudness and/or intensity.*

As a first treatment strategy Sanjay was offered wax earplugs, which he used appropriately, in one ear. The plan was to offer him a Walkman later so that he would have a choice of options available for stopping the voices when they were irritating him. In practice the earplugs were so successful that he did not want to try the Walkman.

CASE STUDY RICHARD

(See also pp. 204, 226, 246, 262 and 278.)

Goal 1A: *Block the voice or at least reduce its loudness and/or intensity.*

In the early stages of therapy, Richard was too frightened of the voice to use the earplug or Walkman to block it once it had started talking. However, both of these were very effective strategies once the voice had been sufficiently disempowered for them to be safe to use (see p. 263).

(It has been suggested to me that Richard could have tried going to sleep with an earplug already in place, as this might have prevented the voice occurring as he woke up. This is certainly a good idea, but as we did not think of it at the time it is not possible to say if Richard would have agreed to it, or whether it would have been effective.)

Goal 1B: *Reduce the distress caused as a result of hearing the voice.*

(See p. 278 for the practical coping strategies to help to achieve this goal.)

11 Modifying the beliefs that influence and underlie the content of the voices

Introduction

Different people can hear a voice that is saying the same thing but for completely different reasons. For example, there are many possible reasons why a woman might hear a voice accusing her of being a murderer, including (a) she has actually committed murder, (b) someone has accused her of being capable of murder, (c) she has a delusional memory of committing murder, (d) she believes she is responsible for the flood that killed hundreds of people, (e) she has had an argument with someone at work and wants them dead, (f) she has had an abortion, (g) she has 'murdered' someone's reputation by telling lies about them, (h) she has been frightened by a film in which people screamed 'murderer' at the heroine, etc. It is easy to see from this example why it is necessary to identify *why* the voice is saying what it does in the individual case, in order to set appropriate goals and to plan appropriate lines of treatment.

Case formulation for the content of a voice

'Surface' and 'deep' meanings of what the voice says

When considering the meaning of the content of the voice, it is important to bear in mind that it may contain a deep or symbolic meaning as well as the more obvious, surface one. For example, in the case above, the line of treatment for the woman who feels guilty about an abortion will be quite different from that of the woman whose voice is based on a memory of someone accusing her of murder. The surface meaning of the content of the voice is obvious, but the therapist may need to speculate about the possible underlying deep meanings and then check these out with the person concerned to see which, if any, apply. This aspect of the work is essentially the same as that involved in identifying deep as opposed to surface meanings of delusional beliefs (see p. 133) and so will not be repeated here.

It is inevitable that in some cases you will not be able to identify the factors that underlie what the voice is saying and in these circumstances you should proceed with some caution, keeping alert for any indication of any beliefs, memories or experiences that might be involved. For example, a man was troubled by a voice accusing him of being evil but we could find no reason for him to believe this. Having worked to strengthen his functional belief that he was not evil, he then asked his voice directly if it had any evidence to prove what it said.[1] His voice replied that he was evil because he smoked too much. Perhaps it is not surprising that we had not elicited this explanation because we would not have been alert to the possibility that smoking could be viewed in this light. Interestingly, the belief seems to have developed as the result of an antismoking campaign and confusion about the meaning of the word 'bad'. The man had taken on board the message 'Smoking is bad' and his subsequent line of unconscious reasoning seems to have gone 'Smoking is bad, therefore if I smoke I am bad: "bad" means "evil", so if I smoke I am evil'. Having uncovered this confusion we were able to draw a clear distinction between 'bad' meaning physically harmful and 'bad' meaning morally evil, as result of which the voices became less frequent and then disappeared altogether.

Why the voices say what they say

As we saw in Chapter 2, voices are automatic thoughts that are heard out loud and so voices, like thoughts, may be influenced by any of the different factors in the CBT model. Some of the more common reasons for the voices saying what they do are given below.

- They reflect an underlying worry, fear or concern.
  For example: 'You're fat.'
  'He's going to hit you.'
- They reflect something that the person has read about, heard or seen that frightened them, or that seemed significant or important for some other reason.
  For example: 'I will make you spontaneously combust.'
  'You are responsible for the earthquake.'
  'The spy satellites will vaporize you if you don't obey.'
- They reflect the person's belief about something; this belief may or may not be delusional.
  For example: 'They want you to be sent to hospital again.'
  'You are a disgusting pervert.'
  'Dr Smith is trying to poison you.'
- They are an accurate memory of something heard in the past.
  For example: 'Whore, prostitute.'
  'I hate you.'
- They are a distorted memory from the past, or something that was imagined or anticipated in the past.
  For example: 'I'm ashamed of you.' (This was implied but never said.)
  'Don't go near him, he's got fleas.' (He had had fleas, but this was not the reason that people avoided him.)

[1]Directly questioning a voice in order to get information should only be done with great caution, and as a last resort, as you must be able to deal with whatever emerges. The material produced by the voice might contain information or memories that the person has suppressed from conscious awareness and for this reason this strategy should always be undertaken within a formal therapy session.

- They are automatic thoughts, made important by being heard aloud or because they occurred at the same time as psychotic feelings of great significance.
  For example: 'The paper cups are the majestic answer.'
  'Close the curtains.'
  'Look at the number plates.'

These explanations are not mutually exclusive. For example, a voice accusing a man of being a paedophile might be based on recent TV news programmes about antipaedophile vigilante groups, plus the memory of having been accused of being a pervert by a neighbour, plus fears that he might be a secret paedophile because he enjoyed reading *Lolita*.

In theory, each voice and each different utterance of each voice should be considered separately for case formulation because different factors might be involved. In practice, although a voice may say different things on different occasions it is often the case that these different utterances can be grouped together into one or more 'theme(s)', for example 'The Mafia are out to get me' or 'I'm inferior to other people', in which case it is appropriate to case-formulate for each theme rather than for each individual expression of it. Where the content of the different voices is obviously different (e.g. when one voice is critical and another is supportive), then separate case formulations and goal setting are essential. Accurate case formulation will enable you to set the goals and target the treatment appropriately and effectively.

Sharing the case formulation

Understanding *why* the voice is saying what it does may help to reduce the impact it has on the person. For example, if I understand that I hear my father's voice telling me I am a disappointment to him because this is what I feared and imagined he might have thought when I dropped out of university, then this will give me a sound reason for why the voice says what it does, other than this being what my father really thinks about me. As another example, if I hear a voice warning me I have an alien growing inside me that will burst out of my stomach soon, then this may seem a less frightening prospect if I am aware that this idea has come from watching one of the fictional *Alien* films a few months ago.

Sharing the full case formulation for the content of the voice is usually only appropriate when people understand that the voice is their own thoughts, coming from within their own brain. However, even when there is a delusional explanation for the voice, it is often possible to make use of the case formulation as a way of explaining why what the voice says is so upsetting. For example, 'It's not surprising you feel really frightened when the voice threatens you with spontaneous combustion, because you read that really scary magazine article about people suddenly bursting into flames'. This would be developed during therapy into something along the lines of 'Fortunately, we know that magazine goes in for sensationalist and inaccurate reporting, so we can't believe a word it says, and the reassuring thing is that modern science has explained why spontaneous combustion is completely impossible'.

Guilt and shame associated with the content of the voices

If the guilt or shame is associated with the understanding that the voices are 'my thoughts', then work to normalize and destigmatize the automatic thoughts is carried out as described in Chapter 6 (pp. 120–123).

If the guilt or shame relates to the beliefs, memories and/or experiences that are directly referred to by the voices or that underlie what they are saying, then the approach would be to identify why this belief, memory, etc. causes feelings of guilt or shame in this person, and then apply CBT accordingly. For example, a voice is referring to the time when the hearer stole a charity collection box when it says 'They wouldn't want to know you if they knew what you'd done'. Therapy in this case would focus on (a) reappraising the event, including developing a compassionate understanding of why it had happened, and (b) re-evaluating other people's likely responses to an incident like this from someone's past.

MODIFYING THE BELIEFS ASSOCIATED WITH THE CONTENT OF THE VOICE

If the voice is based on an underlying belief of fear, then this is treated in the same way as the non-psychotic beliefs that underlie a delusional belief (see Chapter 7). So, for example, if the voice reflected an underlying worry about being fat or a fear of spontaneous combustion, then a major part of the CBT would be to address these issues. Similarly, *if the hallucination is voicing a delusional belief*, then this delusional belief would be considered for modification in the same way as any other delusional belief (see Chapter 8).

If the voice is based on a memory, then it is helpful to establish whether this memory is accurate or not. If it is not accurate, or if the voice is distorting what happened, then showing that the voice has got it wrong will remove one of the sources of distress. For example, if the accusation 'I'm ashamed of you' was never made and did not reflect the accuser's true feelings, then establishing that this was a false memory would minimize the impact the voice could make. If the memory is accurate, then the treatment approach would be to determine why the memory is upsetting, and to apply CBT to the issues uncovered.

If the voice is based on inaccurate knowledge, for example the voice that said the spy satellites could vaporize the hearer, then the approach is to challenge and correct the inaccuracies.

If the voice is an otherwise insignificant automatic thought that has been given inappropriate significance because it has been heard out loud or has been associated with a significant psychotic experience, then the approach is to explain how this could occur, for example explaining to someone how their brain could attach the feeling of significance to an ordinary thought like 'close the curtains'. Using 'the brain' to explain the feeling of significance may impact on the person's belief about the voice's origin and so it may not be appropriate to use this particular line of work until the person is ready to recognize the voice as coming from within themself.

Work on the content of the voice may or may not impact on the belief about its nature and origin, depending on whether or not the content is associated with the perceived source of the voice, and how it is associated. As a practical guideline, if you are not ready to start modifying the belief about the nature of the voice, then you should be careful to consider for each piece of work that you do on the content whether or not this will threaten the belief about the voice's origin.

The content of the voice is untrue/inaccurate

The truth and accuracy (or otherwise) of what the voice says is an important factor in determining the lines of treatment taken and, crucially, the order in which they are tackled.

As a general guide, if the voice is not telling the truth, then a major part of your treatment will be disproving what the voice says, and you will be able to start on this work early on in the treatment. The major exception to this is when proving the voice gets things wrong would have wider, dysfunctional implications at this stage of the therapy. This is most likely to occur in connection with beliefs about the origin of the voice. For example, proving the voice gets things wrong would have significant implications for a belief that the voice came from God, and so this line of work should only be pursued once the person is ready to have their belief about the voice coming from God modified.

In some cases, there is little or no significant deep meaning to what the voice says and it is the surface meaning that is the important one as far as causing distress is concerned. If this is the case, then proving the voice is wrong may be the only treatment necessary in order to reduce the person's distress. For example, a woman was distressed by a voice that said it could turn her into a pillar of salt, which was based on a church sermon that she had heard: she was completely reassured when it was proved that it could not do so.

In other cases, what the voice is saying may be untrue at a surface level but its deep meaning may indicate a dysfunctional underlying belief, or it may be based on a memory that is causing distress. In these circumstances, even though the voice is not literally true, hearing it say what it does will not only cause immediate distress but will also tend to reinforce the associated underlying beliefs.

Starting treatment in such cases by proving what the voice says is untrue at the literal level is likely to be helpful, but work on the underlying beliefs may, in the long run, be as or even more important for the person's well-being than what the voice is actually saying. For example, for the woman who had had an abortion many years ago and was now being accused by her voices of being a murderer, proving that she did not meet the criteria for 'murderer', and therefore that the voice was wrong to make this accusation, might help to limit the immediate distress caused by the voice when it spoke but it would leave intact her grief and guilt about the abortion. Working on the underlying dysfunctional beliefs is likely to take quite a bit longer than disproving the literal meaning of the voice. This aspect of the work is usually undertaken at the same time or after the work on the surface meaning.

The voice makes mistakes. The voice is 'ignorant' or 'tells lies'

The content of inaccurate voices can be subjected to evidence evaluation and logical reasoning in the same way that delusions are (see Chapter 8). Therefore, as a first step, you need to find out if the person has any evidence to suggest the voice could be telling the truth so that you can 'eliminate' this supporting evidence by re-evaluating it with alternative interpretations. Evidence to contradict what the voice says can be built up from anything that the person has noticed in the past that seemed to be inconsistent, plus evidence collected during the course of therapy and from reality testing. When you have collected all the evidence and arguments against what the voice is saying, the most persuasive pieces can be summarized on a card for the person to carry with them, to help them challenge the voice when it 'speaks' outside the therapy session.

If the voice says a number of different things that are untrue, then each one is approached in the same way, with different summary cards being developed for each different topic. These different strands of work can be carried out concurrently. Proving that 'The voice can be wrong' on one topic can help to undermine what the voice says on the other subjects as well, especially if the person had up until now accepted whatever the voice said unquestioningly. For this reason it may be helpful in the early stages of therapy to work on at least one of the voice's sayings that is easy to disprove.

Even if the person does not believe what the voice says, it is still good practice to build up the evidence against it as this will help to strengthen the person's opposing, functional belief(s).

EXAMPLE OF USING EVIDENCE TO DISPROVE WHAT THE VOICE SAYS

A woman was accused by her voice of being mentally retarded. Since this was clearly not true, we were able to set about disproving the accusation straight away. This was achieved easily with a combination of logical reasoning and evidence evaluation. The card summarizing this work is given below.

I am not mentally retarded because:

1 I can read and write.
2 I can have a normal conversation with another person.
3 I've got an O level in French and sat for eight other O levels (therefore, I must have been brighter than those pupils who didn't sit for exams – and this was a normal school for non-retarded children).
4 I have good personal hygiene – I can look after myself.
5 I can cook, shop, etc.
6 If the nurses tell me I'm not retarded, then I'm not. They have been working with me so that I can get a true understanding of my condition and have not told me lies about anything else.

Note that the evidence included was couched in the woman's own words and represented the items that *she* found the most convincing. Item 3 on this list was not produced spontaneously by her, but because it was possible that at some time in the future she would encounter people with learning disabilities who could read and write, have a normal conversation, had good personal hygiene, etc., the more solid piece of evidence about her academic achievements at school was elicited from her for inclusion. (*Note*: With respect to item 6, we do encourage people to rely on their own reasoning abilities rather than asking other people for their opinions, but in this case the woman wanted to include this as a piece of hard evidence and so it was included.)

EXAMPLE OF WORKING WITH BELIEFS UNDERLYING WHAT THE VOICE SAYS

Successfully disproving what the woman's voice said, as described above, had some positive effect on its frequency but it still occurred from time to time. We felt it was likely the voice reflected some underlying fear that she might be retarded, even though she was unable to come up with any reason or evidence to base this on. So whilst she was using arguments and evidence to successfully counter the voice whenever it said she was mentally retarded, we were constantly alert in our sessions to pick up on any comment or hint as to what might underlie the fear, because whilst that fear was still present we predicted that the voice would continue to recur from time to time.

After several weeks we picked up the missing links: she believed that 'Too much sex makes you demented' and also believed that she had been promiscuous in the past. Having elicited these two underlying beliefs we were able to modify them using the standard CBT techniques of logical reasoning and evidence gathering. We discussed the old-fashioned belief about overindulgence in sex and dementia, and agreed that it came from the time when syphilis was a cause of dementia. She was confident she did not have syphilis and so did not need to fear dementia from this cause. We also used the arguments that married people, who have sex regularly, do not die earlier with dementia than single people or nuns, and that there were not large numbers of ex-prostitutes in the elderly dementia wards of our hospital (fortunately she did not require proof of this; she knew some of the patients and knew that they had been in hospital for very many years, so their opportunities for sex would have been very limited and certainly less than the national average).

The woman herself was not promiscuous and had not been promiscuous in the past, but this was her underlying fear. We explored this issue and she was able to readjust her evaluation of herself. As it turned out, her sexual activity was probably below the average for her age, so she was able to use this in another line of reasoning to counter the fear, which went 'Even if it were true that too much sex makes you demented (which I know it's not because of all the reasons and evidence we found that proved it wasn't true), I have not had more sexual contacts than other women of my age, so even in days gone by that old saying would not have applied to me'. (*Note*: If there had been a history of frequent promiscuous sexual contacts, then we could not have 'disproved' this particular belief about herself. In this case, we would have had to rely on the arguments and evidence about sex and early dementia or subnormality not being related in order to break the dysfunctional chain of thinking.)

This case is a good example of how work with hallucinations and delusions may set off a chain of CBT work that encompasses areas unrelated to the psychosis as such. In this case, the content of the voice and its associated deep meaning for her suggested that the woman might be concerned about her sexual behaviour, now or in the past, and this led to CBT work with her dysfunctional underlying beliefs about sex and sexual relationships.

The content of the voice is true/accurate

If the voice is telling the truth, either at the surface and/or deep meaning levels, then the most important part of the work will be with the beliefs or fears that are revealed by the voice. As a general guide, this work with the underlying beliefs should be done before tackling the voice itself, though you can offer an earplug or Walkman as a temporary way of stopping it. For example, in the case of the man whose voice accused him of being fat, it was not possible to challenge the voice on the accuracy of what it was saying because he was significantly overweight. Therefore, the only way to reduce the distress caused by hearing the voice was to attempt to modify his beliefs about fatness being a matter for scorn and derision.[2] Note that we did not discuss dieting with him because this would have implied that we agreed with his voice and that we, too, thought that his fatness was undesirable and shameful and that it would be better if he were thinner. From his past history we could be fairly certain that dieting would not work, so it was certainly not worth risking inadvertently supporting his dysfunctional beliefs about fatness when there was only a very low chance he would be able to reduce his weight by dieting.

In our experience, once the person is no longer bothered by what their voice is saying, because the underlying belief has been modified, then the voice stops saying this particular thing, or only says it very rarely indeed. For example, in the

[2] I have been asked how it is possible to modify this belief when it *is* undesirable or shameful to be overweight (!). The first step is to recognize that this is a widely held belief or opinion and not a fact that cannot be disputed. Indeed, classic art suggests that in the past 'fatness' was seen by society as being desirable and beautiful, as it is in some non-Western cultures. The second step is to ask 'Are there any people in this position (i.e. overweight) who do *not* have negative beliefs about it?'. Even if they are few in number, the fact that *some* people do not share these negative views indicates that it is *possible* to replace the negative attitudes or beliefs with more positive ones.

case mentioned above, if the man were no longer worried about his weight, then he would no longer be distressed by the voice's comments, and so one of the maintaining cycles would have been broken.

A person's voice can say different things for different reasons. Each 'theme' and its associated underlying dysfunctional beliefs are worked on separately. These different lines of work can be carried on concurrently, priority being given to whichever of the voice's sayings the person themself most wants to work on.

EXAMPLE OF WORKING WITH VOICES WHOSE CONTENT COULD BE TRUE

A woman was distressed by persistent voices calling her 'whore' and 'prostitute'. This had been occurring for many years and it had become the practice to reassure her that what the voices were saying was not true ('Of course you're not a prostitute!'). The beneficial effects of this reassurance were short-lived and she would seek reassurance again, wearing down the patience of the staff in the process. The problem was that, unknown to the staff caring for her, there had been a time in the past when she had attempted prostitution, only on a couple of occasions but, nevertheless, often enough to provide some support for what the voices were saying. This being so, simple reassurance was not appropriate and could not be successful in the long term. Furthermore, implicit in the reassurance given by the staff was confirmation that they believed reassurance was appropriate, i.e. that of course it was insulting to be accused of prostitution because being a prostitute was, indeed, shameful.

Since the voices' accusations were related to a true incident and reflected her feelings of shame at what had happened, it was decided to tackle her belief that 'Prostitution is wrong and dirty and so anyone engaging in an act of prostitution should feel guilty and ashamed'. Firstly, we looked at what was meant by the term 'wrong' and came up with the definition that morally wrong meant doing something deliberately to hurt or offend against someone else. We then looked to see who had been hurt by her actions and concluded that she was the only one who had suffered in any way, by her feelings of guilt and regret. Hence we concluded that her acts of prostitution had not been morally wrong and therefore that she should not feel guilty about them.

In a wider context, we were aware that if we successfully modified this woman's belief about prostitution being morally wrong, then this would remove what might be an important factor in controlling her present sexual behaviour, so at the same time that we looked at the moral issues around prostitution we also looked at the practical side. We went through the health risks associated with prostitution (we also took the opportunity of doing some safe-sex education) and considered other disadvantages of the lifestyle, for example the risk of being a victim of violence and the fact that some people in society, whether rightly or wrongly, do disapprove of prostitution and prostitutes. We also included in the list of disadvantages the fact that her past history indicated she would be very worried afterwards, for weeks if not months and years, that people would find out about it.

Having looked at the advantages and disadvantages of prostitution for her, the woman decided the disadvantages were much too high a price to pay for the few packets of cigarettes that prostitution would bring her. We noted that most women come to similar conclusions, though for a few people the advantages seem to outweigh the disadvantages and so they choose to become prostitutes. The final conclusion from this exercise was 'Prostitution is not morally wrong; if that's what other women want to do that's OK, but it wouldn't suit me because I would worry so much about the risks that it just wouldn't be worth the money I'd get'.

She still blamed herself for what she had done when she was younger and all the subsequent upset it had caused her, so we also looked at the context of her brief move into prostitution so that she could better understand why it had happened. We considered why it had seemed like a reasonable option at that time, understanding and knowing what she did then, and why she felt differently now. This enabled her to view her young self less critically and with more compassionate understanding, as well as appreciating her present, greater maturity.

Viewing the acts of prostitution in the past as potentially unwise (though fortunately no physical harm had come to her), rather than morally wrong or shameful, took the sting out of the voices' accusations and this may have been an important factor in their reduction. We also involved the care staff in the treatment so that instead of 'reassuring' her on the rare occasions when the voices did recur with this particular accusation, the staff would adopt a more neutral attitude of 'I don't know whether what the voices are saying is true or not, but it wouldn't matter to us one way or the other. We like and respect you just as you are'.

The truth/accuracy of the voice is uncertain

Whenever you set about disproving a voice that offends or upsets the person, then you are implicitly agreeing with them that it is appropriate for them to be offended or upset by it (see the case example above). Therefore, if you are in any doubt about its accuracy it is safer to treat the content *as if* it were true and to attempt modification of the associated beliefs *before* tackling what the voice actually says. For example, a young man was accused by a voice of being a 'gay queer'. He vehemently denied he was homosexual, but in view of his strong negative beliefs about the subject it would have been very difficult for him to acknowledge any inclinations that way. So even though there was no evidence to suggest he was homosexual, we considered it safer to attempt to modify his underlying beliefs about homosexuality being disgusting rather than seeking to show that what the voice said about him was untrue. If he were exclusively heterosexual, then gathering supportive evidence would have been a quick and easy way to counter the voice and reduce the distress it was able to cause. However, there was a significant risk that taking this approach would imply our tacit acceptance or even approval of his negative views of homosexuality, so if it had turned out that he did have unacknowledged homosexual tendencies, then this would have compromised our position to carry out what would, in these circumstances, have been the most effective element of the treatment, namely to modify his beliefs about homosexuality.

CASE STUDY Sanjay

(See also pp. 202 and 214.)

Goal 2: *To modify the underlying belief about being messy or untidy in order to end up believing 'It doesn't matter when I am messy or untidy; some people are and some people aren't – lots of people prefer to live like that. Being messy or untidy doesn't affect the value of a person, and people don't look down on me if I am like that'.*

This was an example of a voice whose content was essentially true, so treatment focused on modifying the underlying beliefs about the importance of messiness and untidiness.

We started off by finding examples of people who like to live in an untidy room or house and choose to live that way. This established that tidiness and cleanliness are not universally held ideals.

We then challenged the presumption that 'Tidiness and cleanliness are best' by taking a neutral stance and looking at the advantages and disadvantages of being neat, clean and tidy. The main advantage that emerged for him was the approval of other people, whilst the main disadvantage was the time and effort it took to achieve. We suggested that people's different levels of tidiness and cleanliness had nothing to do with any sort of moral value but merely reflected how they rated the relative importance of these two factors. Whilst doing this work, we noted with approval those people who were able to spend their time on what they wanted to do rather than worrying about what other people thought of them.

We also explored where the belief had come from, and found that it had been learnt from his mother. We suggested his mother had chosen to keep a clean and tidy house because for her the end result was more enjoyable than spending her time doing other things, but that he did not have to view it the same way or make the same choice.

In order to address the issue of feeling shame when he was clumsy or messy, we looked at how he viewed other people when they spilt their tea, etc. In fact, he was not critical of other people and so we were able to use this as evidence that other people would not be critical when these things happened to him. We noted that he, like other people, tended to be more critical of himself than he was of other people, and so an additional strategy was to remind himself of this fact whenever he found himself being self-critical. (*Note:* If Sanjay *had* been hypercritical of others, then the approach would have been to establish that other people were not as sensitive to or critical of these behaviours as he was, and thereby to argue that his reactions were not a good guide as to how other people regarded his clumsy behaviour.)

We also undertook some general self-esteem work, which included looking at the characteristics he found important in friends and acquaintances and noting that tidiness etc. was not included as a factor that affected their value and worth.

We did *not* suggest his clumsiness was due to illness, medication or old age because 'excusing' the behaviour would have implied it did matter, even though people did not blame him for it.

CASE STUDY RICHARD

(See pp. 204, 214, 246, 262 and 278.)

Goal 2: *'Members of the sect genuinely believe what they say is correct but they are mistaken. God does not require me to say this prayer repeatedly and he does not require me to be a member of this sect.'*

On direct questioning, Richard admitted he still had occasional feelings of fear about having left the sect, though he reported that this did not worry him as much now as it had done in the past. He was rather vague about the sect's exact teaching on the duty of members to stay within the sect, so one potential approach would have been to consult with sect leaders. If, perchance, Richard had misunderstood the sect's attitude to people leaving their ranks, then the leaders' correction of this misunderstanding would have been very powerful in undermining his fears. However, the therapist decided not to use this approach because, from what the clinical team knew of the sect, it seemed probable the leaders would confirm that it was a sin to leave them and this would only have served to fuel Richard's fearful beliefs. (*Note*: CBT is a collaborative approach so it would not have been appropriate for the therapist to approach the sect leaders without informing and involving Richard.)

The therapist used the line of argument that other religious sects exist that believe just as adamantly as the sect Richard left that theirs is the only correct way for personal and world salvation. Not all the sects can be correct; indeed most, if not all, must be wrong. Therefore, adamant belief that they are correct is certainly no guarantee of correctness. Even if one were generous in estimating the size of this particular religious sect at 25,000 people, given that the world's population is over 5,000 million this would mean that fewer than 1 in 200,000 people believe as the sect does, i.e. the vast majority of people in the world believe the sect in question has *not* got it right. It was also argued that all the many millions of religious people in the world, including Christians, Muslims, Jews, Hindus, etc., would certainly support chanting the prayer if they thought this was what God really wanted, but they and their spiritual leaders were certain it was not.

In a separate line of approach, the therapist argued that the voice did not seem to be bothered whether Richard chanted the prayer or not. As evidence for this, she noted that the voice did not always wake Richard up at night to say the prayer. In the early stages of therapy Richard believed the voice had the power to wake him whenever it wanted to, so clearly the fact that he sometimes slept through meant that the voice did not want to wake him on these occasions.

A little later in therapy, the therapist also stated that because he had never heard the voice in the daytime this must indicate that it did not want Richard to say the prayer then, even though the rest of the sect would be saying it at that time. This positive interpretation of why he had not heard the voice in the daytime was presented as a statement by the therapist rather than taking what would have been the more usual approach of asking Richard for his opinion and discussing the implications with him. This was done in order to avoid the risk that when this 'omission' was brought to Richard's attention, he might worry about not saying the prayer during the daytime and therefore start to listen out for the voice, and to hear it for this reason. The therapist reinforced the argument that the voice was not really bothered whether Richard chanted the prayers or not by offering to chant them at night on his behalf, if the voice instructed her to do so. It did not.

It was fortunate that Richard was pursuing Church of England membership when these hallucinations were at their height because this meant he had available to him a replacement set of religious beliefs that were incompatible with the religious beliefs of the sect. The therapist suggested that Richard was not alone in deciding the sect was not the appropriate form of religion for them, and Richard confirmed that other people had left during his stay. The hospital chaplain discussed and strengthened the alternative position and beliefs of the Church of England. In particular, the chaplain was firm in noting that it disagreed with the sect's teachings about the need to say these particular prayers and was very definite that the sect had 'got it wrong' and had no special status and authority with respect to God. As a recognized authority on spiritual matters, the reassurance of the hospital chaplain on these issues was more powerful than that of the therapist.

12 MODIFYING THE BELIEF ABOUT THE NATURE/ORIGIN OF THE VOICES

INTRODUCTION

The impact of what the voice says and its ability to cause distress depends not only on what it says but also on where or who the voice is perceived to come from. For example, if a man's voice says 'You are going to burn in hell', this will be more frightening if he believes it comes from God than if he believes it comes from an unpleasant neighbour, because only God can actually carry out this threat. Similarly, if a woman hears the words 'You're a waste of space – I wish you'd never been born', it is likely they will be more distressing if delivered in her mother's voice than if they are from some unrecognized or unimportant source. Therefore, modifying the person's belief about the nature/origin of their voice(s) can be a very important step in reducing its ability to cause distress. The approach to modifying delusional ideas about the origin of a voice is the same as that used for other delusional beliefs.

Delusional ideas about the source of the voice are often supported by the content of that voice and vice versa, so when this is the case these two lines of therapy are intertwined and normally proceed together. For example, in the case of God's voice predicting the future death of the hearer, proving the voice cannot accurately predict the future would not only show that it cannot be believed when it predicts the woman's death in three years' time but also that it could not be God talking: alternatively, proving the voice was not from God would immediately take away its authority to predict her future death.

THE IMPLICATION OF 'HEARING VOICES'

Although delusional beliefs about the nature/origin of the voice usually exacerbate the distress it causes, in some cases it is *not* having a delusional belief for its occurrence that causes the distress, i.e. when people are disturbed by the implications of hearing voices. For example, one woman was concerned primarily about her voices because she knew that hearing voices could be a sign of schizophrenia, and she was horrified by this notion because she believed that if she had schizophrenia then this meant that she might suddenly go berserk and kill someone. Treatment in such cases is aimed at modifying the underlying dysfunctional beliefs about voices and schizophrenia/psychosis, using the strategies described for promoting insight in a helpful way (see Chapter 6, pp. 108–119 and this chapter, pp. 233–234).

GOAL SETTING FOR THE BELIEF ABOUT THE NATURE/ORIGIN OF THE VOICE

Modification of the belief about the nature/origin of the voice may be total or partial, and the specified goal should include not only what the person will stop believing about the nature/origin of their voice but also, in the case of a total modification, what new belief will replace it. As with any other delusional belief, although you will probably not be able to discuss the goal with the person themself in the terms in which you have written it down, you must check out indirectly, using words that do not conflict with their way of conceptualizing their experience, how they would feel if they came to believe the goal were true. For a belief about the nature/origin of a voice this means checking out both parts of the goal, namely how they would feel (a) if the voice did not come from who it appeared to come from, and (b) if the replacement belief about the origin of the voice were true instead. Work to modify the belief should not be started until the replacement belief is acceptable and preferred to the delusional one.

You should be careful to think also about the possible wider implications of a change in belief about the source of the voice as you will need to take these into account when weighing up the advantages and disadvantages of the modification. For example, some voices may be unpleasant in what they say but, nevertheless, the person does not want to lose the relationship with the source of the voice or the sense of purpose or self-esteem this relationship provides. This is most likely to occur when the source of the voice is important for religious reasons or when it is a valued friend or family member. In these circumstances you should not go for a belief modification about the voice's origin unless there are compelling reasons for doing so. For example, the voice of God might be welcomed, but if it were suggesting that the person kill themself or others, then this consideration would almost certainly outweigh the former when you were goal setting.

We have already noted that if there are both wanted and unwanted voices coming from different identified sources, then it will probably be impossible to change the belief about the origin of the unwanted ones without also bringing about a change in belief about the wanted ones. In these circumstances, the relative benefits of modifying all or none have to be weighed up and checked out informally with the person themself. For example, a man disliked hearing his neighbours criticizing him but was comforted by hearing his mother speaking words of encouragement when he was sad and lonely. When asked the 'hypothetical' question of whether he would rather hear both voices or neither, he said he would not want to lose his mother's voice. Therefore, modification about the origin of the neighbours' voices was not attempted for fear this would destroy the ability of his mother's voice to provide comfort.

TOTAL MODIFICATION OF A BELIEF ABOUT THE NATURE/ORIGIN OF THE VOICE

The total modification for a belief about the nature/origin of a voice takes the form:

The voice does not come from...	(negation of the delusional belief)
+	+
The voice comes from...	(the replacement belief)
or: *The voice is...*	

REPLACEMENT BELIEFS FOR THE ORIGIN OF THE VOICE

The replacement belief that is used to explain the nature/origin of the voice should be the one that makes best sense to the person concerned. The three broad types of explanation most commonly used, with common variations, are given below.

- 'Inner-speech loop' model (described on pp. 30–33)
  - vivid thoughts
  - superior auditory imagery
- Vivid memory
  - trauma memory
  - 'broken record' (for repetitive voices)
- My illness/psychosis
  - part of my brain being overactive
  - part of my brain dreaming whilst I am awake.

Although any one of these explanations can be sufficient for the replacement belief, in some cases a fuller explanation may be obtained by combining more than one. For example, 'My brain is mishearing the information coming from my inner-speech loop, because this is an effect of my psychosis' or 'The vivid memory keeps coming back because part of my brain goes into a dream-type state, so I hear it aloud as if I were in a dream' or 'I hear the memory out loud because the memory makes me very agitated, and when that happens a part of my brain makes the mistake of thinking it has come from outside and so hears it as real sound'. Or, if you were progressing slowly towards recognition of illness, you might start with the notion of an overactive brain and then move on later to the idea that this overactivity is caused by an illness.

Not all explanations will be relevant to any one person. For example, you can only use the notion of superior auditory imagery if the person is indeed able to remember or imagine voices very clearly. Similarly, the vivid- and trauma-memory alternatives can only be used if memory is an appropriate explanation for what the voice is saying.

The 'broken record' explanation can be used for all repetitive voices, including those where the content is not based on an actual remembered event. In these latter cases it is the memory of the voice itself, speaking out loud, that constitutes the memory that is being repeated.

The biological explanations apply to all cases but may be unacceptable or dysfunctional for the person, especially in their strongest forms of 'schizophrenia' and 'psychosis', and so this level of explanation is the one most likely to require preparation before it can be used.

PREPARING FOR THE NEGATION OF THE DELUSIONAL BELIEF

If there are some positive aspects to the belief about the voice's origin, for example in terms of self-esteem or reassurance, then you should try wherever possible to provide alternative sources of these positives before you modify the belief itself. For example, a woman believed she was only respected by other people because they knew that an archangel spoke to her, so evidence was collected to show her that people liked and respected her for herself. In practice this work also helped to prepare the way for the modification itself, because by her enquiries she discovered that other people liked and respected her despite not knowing or not believing that she was in communication with the archangel.

In some cases, a helpful delusional belief about the nature of the voice may be lost as a result of effective medication and improved psychosis. In other cases, an unwanted modification of a belief about positive voices may be the price that has to be paid for the benefits obtained from a related modification of negative voices. When a helpful belief about the voice is lost in this way you should try to 'reframe' the voice in as positive a way as possible. For example, if the voice's comfort and advice had added value because it was thought to come from an angel, then the reframing might take the following lines: 'The fact that it is your own brain producing this helpful and insightful voice shows there is a really strong, caring and understanding bit of you, your "inner wisdom". The fact that this inner wisdom and support comes from within yourself rather than from an angel is better really, because it means you will always have it with you. It has been very helpful to you in the past and you can use it to help you again in the future, anytime you need it.' Or as another example, if the loving words spoken by the voice were treasured because they were thought to come from the hearer's mother, then the reframing might take the lines: 'The voice is not actually your mother talking but it does come from your deep knowledge and close relationship with her and that is why it says just the sort of things she would say to you if she were here. Lots of people like to think about what their mother would say to them, so they would think you are lucky to be able to hear it so vividly, in her voice.'

PREPARING THE REPLACEMENT BELIEF

1. Replacement beliefs in terms of 'my own thoughts, heard out loud'

The inner-speech loop model (see pp. 30–33) can be used to explain why a thought is heard out loud and why it sounds like a particular person. It can also explain why the thought is not recognized as one's own.

Essential preparation for this replacement belief is to check out and ensure that the person is comfortable with the notion that the content of the voice is his or her own thoughts. If you are not sure about its acceptability, when discussing what the voice says you may find it helpful to casually ask 'Do you ever get thoughts like this?' as the response may give a good indication of how the person would feel about such a possibility. Even where there is some recognition that the content of the voice is very similar to some of their own thinking, it is still important to spend time giving information about automatic thoughts and normalizing/destigmatizing them. This work is described in Chapter 6 (pp. 120–124) and so will not be repeated here.

The issues of guilt and/or shame at what the voices say can be particularly important. When the person themself considers the content of their voice to be undesirable or shameful ('I would *never* have thoughts like that!'), then gentle but thorough preparation work is essential before any attempt is made to bring about a modification that results in the person concluding that the voice comes from within themself and is their own thoughts.

Having understood how the brain produces auditory hallucinations, the person may well go on to ask why this is happening to them, so you should also have this next step prepared. The fact that voices are heard by many people in the general population may be sufficient reason ('You just happen to be one of those people whose brain is able to do this'), especially if the voice hearing can be linked to times of increased arousal ('. . . and most people are more likely to hear voices if they are upset or agitated about something/have not been sleeping or eating properly/have been taking street drugs, etc.').

If it applies, the ability to image sounds very clearly and vividly may be a positive way of explaining why thoughts are heard as voices. People differ greatly in the clarity of their auditory imagery and so you would need to check out the viability of this alternative by asking the person to remember or to imagine someone talking and then asking how clear and 'real' this sounds to them.

However carefully you prepare the ground for a non-illness replacement belief, there is always the risk that once the person no longer believes the voice comes from a real external source, then they will make the connection with illness/psychosis for themself. After all, it is highly likely that friends, family and members of the mental health profession have all been arguing for this particular alternative explanation. Therefore, as far as you can, you should also prepare for this possibility (see 3, below).

2. Replacement beliefs based on 'memory'

If they apply, the memory alternatives are very easy to use because they are so 'normal' that they do not need preparation work to make them acceptable, and they are much less likely to trigger a jump to an unwanted 'mental illness' explanation.

People may ask why their memory is so vivid that it sounds real. It is generally well known these days that trauma events can cause people to 'relive' their experiences in vivid flashbacks, so this analogy may be helpful in explaining and destigmatizing the 'realness' of the sound of the voice.

The 'broken record' explanation for repetitive voices can be prepared by giving examples of recurring thoughts from everyday life in order to normalize this experience. For example, if one is anxious or excited about something, then thoughts about it will keep intruding, or if you hear something repeated often, then it springs readily to mind. If it helps, you can include a neurological explanation, with a diagram showing how nerve cells tend to grow towards one another when they are repeatedly activated together. For example, your explanation might go along the lines: 'Because you've heard the voice say this so often, these few cells in your brain have got linked together in a small loop so now they just keep repeating it round and round, without any real sense of meaning – rather like a song goes round and round in your head when you hear it too often.' This sort of explanation, and the term 'broken record', can be helpful in reducing the significance and importance of the content that is being repeated.

3. Replacement beliefs in terms of 'brain function' and 'illness'

The preparation work when 'brain function' or 'illness' explanations are used as a replacement belief for the origin of the hallucination follows the same lines as when they are the replacement for a delusional belief and therefore this section should be read as an addendum to Chapter 6, pp. 108–115.

(a) As with delusions, insight about auditory hallucinations is developed within a *normalizing framework*, which in this case means regarding the hearing of voices in psychosis as an extreme form of what is an essentially normal phenomenon, a phenomenon which is of no importance in itself and that only matters if it bothers or upsets the hearer.

(b) As with the sharing of 'odd ideas' (see pp. 109–110), *sharing any experiences of hearing voices* that you may have had will help to demonstrate that the actual hearing of voices as such is not weird and nothing to be ashamed or frightened of. Whether you are doing this work as part of a group discussion or during an individual session, it may be helpful to know of some other people's experiences to back up your own, particularly if your own are not very impressive. The examples of hearing voices given below are those reported by people on our CBT courses who have agreed that they may be shared more widely.

- A mother, in an empty house, heard 'Mummy' being called.
- Someone walking in the country on a windy day twice heard his name being called from behind.
- A student working one evening heard 'Go out and enjoy yourself.'
- The same student about to leave his room heard 'Go back and finish your work.'
- A therapist often heard her own thoughts spoken aloud.
- A woman heard her recently deceased husband talking to her.

(c) Although most non-psychotic people hear only isolated words, some people do hear phrases and sentences and even continuous speech, much as people with psychosis can do, though they have no other signs or symptoms of a psychotic illness. This phenomenon can be disturbing when it first occurs but most 'hearers', as they are sometimes called, learn to recognize and accept their voices for what they are. Studies to investigate the prevalence of voices in non-psychotic people have come up with different results, but some suggest the incidence could be above 70%: in one study, around 15% of the people reported they often heard their thoughts being spoken out loud. In a large gathering of psychologists, a show of hands indicated that between 70% and 80% had heard voices at some time in their lives. Whether psychologists are particularly prone to voices or whether they are just more willing to admit to it I do not know, but these figures clearly show that *hearing voices is really quite common* and as such quite normal. It can be very helpful to share these prevalence figures; certainly most people with hallucinations find it both surprising and reassuring that the incidence of voices in the general public is so high.

When sharing your own experiences of voices you should make clear that you are not suggesting your voices are the same as the psychotic person's voices, or that they are as disturbing or as distressing. Your aim at this stage is just to demonstrate that it is possible for the brain to mishear things and that there is nothing stigmatizing about that. If the person is not ready to understand their voices in terms of coming from within themself, then you should be careful to avoid implying that their hallucinations are the same sort of voices as those that you are talking about.

(d) The factors that increase the likelihood of non-psychotic people hearing voices are the same as those that increase vulnerability to delusional ideas (see pp. 110–111). A useful fact is that most people, if deprived of sleep for only 48 hours, will begin to hallucinate, demonstrating that it is really quite easy to push the brain into this state.

Voices are more likely to occur in noisy surroundings, especially where there is a loud and monotonous background noise with no foreground noise clearly discernible above it, for example sitting under a hair dryer, mowing a lawn or in a noisy party. The person you are working with may have found that their hallucinatory voices are more frequent in some situations than others and be able to recognize some of these factors as being relevant for them.

(e) In order to destigmatize voice hearing, it may be helpful to know that the following famous people heard voices: Moses, Socrates, William Blake, Joan of Arc, Carl Jung and Ghandi.[1]

MODIFYING THE BELIEF ABOUT THE ORIGIN OF THE VOICE

As with any other delusional belief modification, the CBT treatment programme for a delusional belief about the origin of a voice is tailor-made for the individual

[1]These names appear on several web sites.

person and their voice(s), but some commonly occurring strategies are described below.

RE-EVALUATE THE SUPPORTING EVIDENCE

The ways in which the supporting evidence is re-evaluated depends on the type of evidence that the person has. This usually falls into one or more of the following four general categories.

1. 'The voice *sounds* as if it comes from an external source'

Usually our sense of hearing is reliable and entirely persuasive and so it is not surprising this should be a major reason for believing the voice really does come from an outside source. The evidence that the voice *sounds* as if it comes from an external source is re-evaluated by establishing that our senses *can* be unreliable, so just because the voice *sounds* as if it is a real voice this does not mean that it *does* come from an external source.

Establishing that our perceptions can be wrong involves using the appropriate strategies from the 'being convinced that something is so does not mean that it is so' line of work described in Chapter 6 (pp. 101–103), with the following adaptations for hallucinations.

(a) When working with hallucinations it is particularly helpful to include *misinterpretations of everyday events* that involve the five senses; for example, 'I bend down to pick up a piece of mud on the carpet but discover it is an ink stain'; 'I walk along and the moon seems to follow me wherever I go'; 'I can hear the sound of the sea when I put a seashell to my ear', etc.

(b) Since hallucinations are themselves *misperceptions at a physiological level*, this aspect of the insight work is particularly pertinent for voices. The following examples may be useful for normalizing and destigmatizing these sensory misperceptions.

Visual illusions

In our version of this exercise we show the person a number of visual illusions, each of which is printed on a coloured card (see Figure 12.1 for examples).[2] In each case we ask them what they see and then invite them to discover their 'mistake' by using a shape or measure cut from a piece of differently coloured card. For example, in the first illusion shown in Figure 12.1 a piece of card the same shape and size as the two (identical) shapes on the illusion card is provided for the person to lay over the shapes in the illusion: this clearly demonstrates that the shapes are, in fact, the same size, even though the top one looks bigger than the lower one. When the other person responds to the illusion, it is important you agree that the figure looks bigger to you, too. You should do this before you give them the piece of card to check their response so that when they find they

[2]Readers wanting to construct their own set of visual illusions will find examples and explanations for the illusory effects in most introductory psychology textbooks.

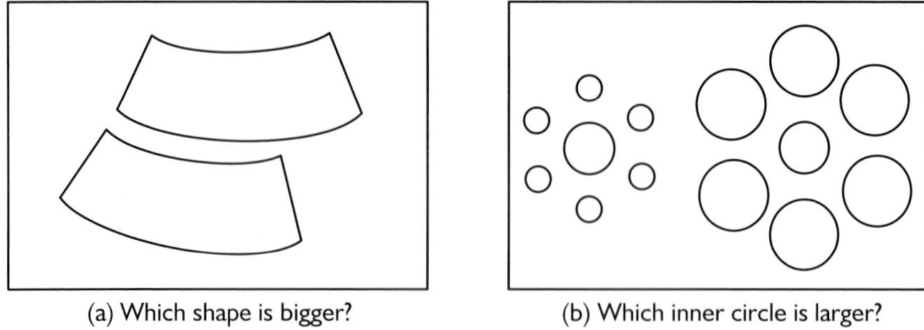

(a) Which shape is bigger?

(b) Which inner circle is larger?

Figure 12.1 Examples of visual illusions used to show that the brain can mislead.

are mistaken, then it is clear that you have been mistaken too. Your aim is not to make them feel foolish for making an error but rather to be curious about why this occurs.

Having noted how interesting it is that our brains can misinterpret what they see in this way, we usually offer some sort of explanation for each of the illusions used, in order to make the point that there are perfectly good reasons why, on occasions, the brain can misinterpret what it sees and hears. The explanations we give for the two illusions illustrated are as follows.

In illusion (a), the lining up of the left-hand edges of the two figures suggests that the double figure is actually stretching backwards into the picture: this perspective suggests that the top figure is further away than the lower one. The two figures are actually the same size, so the images they make in the eye are the same size. But the image that an object makes in our eye gets smaller the further away the object gets, so if two objects at different distances make the same sized image in the eye, then the object that looks further away must be bigger.

In illusion (b), when the centre circle is surrounded by smaller circles the contrast in size makes the centre circle seem bigger, whilst when it is surrounded by larger circles the contrast in size makes the centre circle seem smaller.

Pressing one's eyeball

Pressing one's eyeball from the side will produce immediate distortions in the way objects are perceived. This effect is stronger if you keep the other eye shut. As the eyeball is pressed, objects can be seen to 'move'. This effect occurs because pushing the eyeball distorts the lens in front of the eye so that the image of the object on the back of the eye moves, misleading the brain into thinking the object itself must have moved.

Stick in water

If an object, such as a stick, is half immersed in a glass of water it looks as if it bends at the surface of the water. This is because the light waves are bent as they leave the water, so it appears as if the bit of stick under the water is also bent.

The light waves bend as they leave the water because water and air have different densities.

Listening to stereophonic music through headphones
Stereophonic music coming through two stationary earpieces can sound as if it is coming from a moving source outside the head; special effects tapes of moving trains, etc. can be particularly effective in producing this sensation. With some tapes, the music can actually sound as if it is coming from inside one's head and is moving from one ear to another through the head. These effects are produced because the brain assumes the sound is coming to the two ears from a single source and therefore it combines these to 'hear' where that single source must be.

Phantom limb
This is a very useful example for showing how the brain can misinterpret where something is coming from, because the brain assumes that if a particular nerve is active, then this must mean that a particular area of the body has been stimulated. For example, a patient who has had a lower leg amputated might feel pain in his right toe even though the foot no longer exists. This is because the nerve that would have ended up in the right toe has been activated at the point where it was cut off at the knee. As far as the brain knows, this nerve still ends in the right toe and therefore it 'feels' the pain as located in the right toe.

The phenomenon of referred pain is very similar to that of phantom limb and can be used in the same way.

Use of the dream analogy
Whilst we are dreaming, we are not aware of anything abnormal about what we are hearing in those dreams. We are convinced it is real sound, even though we realize on waking that it was not.

Persistence of the physiologically based misperceptions
Some people feel that they ought to be able to control their voices once they know they come from within themselves. The examples of misperceptions described above also continue to occur even though we know exactly what is happening, so they can be used to demonstrate that the higher, rational parts of our brain are not able to override the misperceptions of the more automatic parts. Similarly, voices come from the more automatic parts of our brain and this is another reason why we are not able to override them.

2. The voice is the voice of 'X'

If the voice is recognized as someone, then it is possible to re-evaluate this 'evidence' purely by establishing that our senses are not always reliable and can be misleading, as described in 1 above. In particular, we can hear voices that we recognize in dreams but these voices come from our own brains.

A more detailed and perhaps more persuasive alternative explanation for the evidence 'The voice sounds exactly like "X"' makes use of the extended inner-speech loop model that accounts for why a voice can be recognized as coming from a particular person (see p. 32).

If it applies, the other most viable alternative explanation for the voice sounding like someone known to the person is in terms of memory.

3. The voice says it is 'X'

If the evidence for the voice coming from 'X' is that the voice itself has claimed this to be the case, then this piece of evidence would be re-evaluated by establishing that 'Claiming something to be true is no guarantee of its truth' (see p. 256 for strategies). It is very easy to establish this fact through logical reasoning, and there are plenty of examples from politics and elsewhere to reinforce it.

4. The voice is assumed to be that of 'X'

If the voice is assumed to come from 'X' because of the sort of things it says, rather than because it sounds like or claims to be 'X', then the first step is to note that this is only an assumption the person has made and therefore that it could be wrong. You would then proceed as with a voice of unrecognized origin.

COLLECT EVIDENCE THAT THE VOICE DOES NOT COME FROM AN EXTERNAL SOURCE, OR FROM 'X'

Possible inconsistencies

One or more of the following questions may elicit inconsistencies with the voice coming from a real, external source.

1. Does the voice sound *exactly like* a real voice (e.g. the therapist's)?

It is quite often the case that although the voice sounds as if it is coming from outside it does not sound *exactly* like a real person's voice, though the hearer may not be able to put into words what the difference is. If it applies, this can be used as evidence that the voice does not come from a real, external source.

2. Can you tell *the gender* of the voice?
3. Can you tell what *direction* the voice is coming from?
4. Could you hear someone from *that far away*?
5. Does the voice change in *volume and/or clarity as you move around*?

Normally we can identify the gender and direction of someone who is talking to us, so if we are unable to do either of these, then this suggests the voice is not a real one. If the voice appears to be coming from a further distance than words would normally travel, then this, too, can be used as evidence it is not coming from that source. Similarly, it is normal for the volume and clarity of what we hear to change as we move with respect to the source, for example by walking away or moving into another room and shutting the door, so if the voice does not change in these circumstances, then this is also evidence against it coming from a real external source.

6. Do *other people* hear the voice?

The large majority of people who hear voices, if asked, will say that other people do not seem to hear their voices, and yet they do not seem to have recognized that this is a powerful piece of evidence against the voice coming from an external source. (This is an example of the way a strongly held belief can ignore contradictory evidence.)

If someone believes their voice comes from a real person, then this is very obviously inconsistent with their observation that other people cannot hear it. You should not jump in to expose this inconsistency too soon, in case this causes their belief about other people not hearing the voice to be modified rather than their belief about the voice coming from a real person. It would be unhelpful if the person concluded: 'You are right, if the voice is coming from "X" they *must* be able to hear it, too – I wonder why they are pretending they can't.' To err on the safe side you should be content in the early stages to agree that the voice is 'somehow' different from ordinary voices and to confirm that other people seem to be unable to hear it.

Before exposing this particular inconsistency it may be helpful to establish that the voices of 'real' people can be heard by everyone in the same area. For example, you might discuss how we cannot voluntarily shut off our hearing so that if we are in a room with a loud TV set we cannot avoid hearing it, and everyone else in the room would hear it, too. You can back up the person's own experience of hearing everything that is going on in their vicinity by explaining to them why this is so, in terms of sound waves coming from the mouth and expanding out to cover all areas of the room. Having established that if a real person is talking, then other people in the hearer's vicinity *must* also be able to hear what he says, this can then be used as an argument against the voice coming from a real person.

Having clarified and agreed that other people do not hear the voice, then this piece of evidence can be 'exposed', when the time is appropriate, as part of the treatment plan; i.e. the person's attention is drawn to this fact so that they cannot avoid it, and its implications and significance with respect to the origin of the voice are discussed.

In some cases, people have already recognized the potential contradictory nature of the fact that other people deny hearing their voice and so they have gone down the escape route of concluding that other people do hear the voice but will not admit to it for some reason. In these circumstances, the first step is to establish that other people do not hear the voice. If the person trusts you, then a good starting point is to reassure them that *you* cannot hear the voice, though at this early stage you should be careful to admit that you can only speak for yourself and not for anyone else. Alternatively, the person may be able to use one or more trusted others to ask them whether they hear the voice when the hearer hears it. This will establish that *some* people cannot hear the voice. Even if it is only some other people who cannot hear the voice, this is good evidence against it coming from an external source.

You might also use logical reasoning to question why other people would want to deny hearing this particular voice and, if it is widespread, how such an extensive conspiracy could be organized, and by whom.

If other people are not trusted (which is perhaps surprisingly rare), then you might be able to use the reactions of strangers to indicate whether other people can hear the voice or not. For example, you might be able to argue that people standing in a supermarket queue would not just carry on regardless if there was a loud, threatening or obscene voice. Therefore, if they do not react when they hear the voice, then this would indicate that other people cannot hear it.[3]

LOGICAL REASONING

Possible lines of logical reasoning

One or more of the following lines of logical reasoning may apply.

1. Could the voice be stopped by an earplug or Walkman, etc. if it really came from 'X'?
Most people who are able to obtain some relief from their voice by using a practical coping strategy do not go on to consider what this implies about the origin of their voice (which is why it is usually safe to use these practical methods from the earliest stages of therapy). However, at the appropriate point in therapy you can expose this contradictory evidence by putting forward the argument that these strategies would not stop a real voice. This can be backed up by reality testing to show that the person can hear you talking even when they are using the thing that blocks their voice.[4]

2. Does medication stop or reduce the voice?
If the person recognizes that medication helps to reduce the voice, for whatever reason, then this is incompatible with it coming from an external source since medication makes no difference whatsoever to being able to hear ordinary people talking. Some people use alcohol or drugs to help to alleviate their voices: where this is the case the same line of logical reasoning can be used as with medication.

3. Does the voice say the sort of thing that 'X' would say?
If it does not say the sort of thing that the identified source of the voice would say, then you can argue this makes it unlikely it is coming from that source. For example, a woman heard a fellow resident using very coarse, explicit sexual terms in her accusation of promiscuity. In everyday life the elderly resident was pleasant to the woman and never swore or spoke about sexual matters, so this was used as evidence to strongly suggest these words were not coming from the resident. In another example, the Archangel Gabriel was heard being critical and making threats which, it was argued, was not compatible with coming from a supremely good and caring being.

[3]If you were a truly dedicated therapist you could confirm this logical argument with a reality test, by standing in a queue of lots of people and shouting out what the voice says so that the other person could see the reaction that this produced. [4]The only time this may not work is if the coping strategy is listening to very loud music through headphones.

4. Has the voice been disempowered?
If you have been successful in taking away the perceived power of the voice (see the next chapter), then this becomes evidence against it coming from a powerful entity. For example, showing that the voice cannot wake the therapist at night indicates not only that it has little power but also, by implication, that it cannot be a powerful voodoo force.

5. Other logical inconsistencies
There may be other logical inconsistencies about the voice or what it says that you can exploit to suggest that it does not come from the source it is believed to come from. For example, a man heard President Bush talking to him during the daytime, but if the voice really came from the President, then one would expect him to make contact during *his* working day, not when he would have been in bed and fast asleep.

Since some of the logical inconsistencies you can use will be idiosyncratic to the individual case, you have to use your own logical reasoning to detect them. As with other delusional beliefs, a useful question to ask yourself is: 'Suppose this voice really did come from "X", what might I expect it to say or sound like? Or how might it react? And are there any inconsistencies between my expectations and how the voice actually presents?'

Where the voice is not believed to be transmitted by sound waves

Some people do not consider that their voice comes via normal sound waves even though it is thought to come from a real person, whilst a voice from an alien or spirit force nearly always comes via radio waves or some sort of telepathic communication. In these cases, reality testing to prove the voice is not a real one would be inappropriate and irrelevant.

The voice is thought to be transmitted via radio waves
You may find the following lines of argument useful if the person is attributing their voice to radio waves.

The human brain is not made in a way that enables it to send or receive radio signals, because if it were:

- we could talk to one another without speaking out loud
- we wouldn't spend so much money on telephone calls
- we could pick up TV and radio programmes in our heads without requiring TV and radio sets – and we would not need to buy an expensive TV licence
- other people would be able to pick up and hear the voice as well
- like radio waves, the voice reception would be affected by being indoors or outdoors, and by hills, metal barriers, etc.
- if the voice only occurred at a specific frequency, then we would have to have tuning devices in our heads, and possibly tuning knobs that we could see and use
- if we had tuning devices in our heads, we would have control over the voices and be able to switch them 'on' and 'off'

- radio and TV waves have to come from, and be received by, things that are made up from metals but our brains are made of squashy, non-metallic material[5]

The voice is thought to be transmitted via telepathy
Where the means of communication is believed to be some type of direct, telepathic link it is very much harder to challenge it. None of the following lines of logical reasoning are strong ones and at best will instil doubt.

It might be effective to ask the person and/or their voice how the communication works, and then either (a) note that there is no apparent explanation, or (b) challenge and test the explanation given. It might be helpful to challenge the voice to use its telepathy to communicate with you or other people, and show that it cannot do that.

If the voices come from a number of different people, then you might attempt to argue this would imply that all human beings could engage in telepathy, in which case you would then set about disproving that this is the case. You might be able to argue that if other people could use telepathy they would not need to speak out loud or use telephones, and if everyone had the skill of telepathy, then the person themself would have grown up knowing about it. Alternatively, if it is only one person who seems to have the power to project their thoughts via telepathy, then you might be able to argue against the feasibility of just one person being born with such an advanced ability when normally new abilities like this would take thousands of years and generations to develop.

If the person can hear what direction the voice is coming from, then it may be possible to use this as evidence against the voice being transmitted by telepathy since telepathy is direct communication from one mind to another and therefore would not be expected to be heard as coming from a particular direction. Depending on the person's understanding of telepathy, it might also be possible to argue that the very fact the voice is heard as real sound is not consistent with mind-to-mind communication. Furthermore, if the earplugs and a Walkman are effective then this, too, would be inconsistent with telepathic communication.

Modifying the belief about the nature of the voice in an unhelpful direction

I am always aware that using logical reasoning and other modification strategies to prove the voice cannot be a physical sound might force the person to explain their experience in terms of radio waves or some more esoteric means of communication. This would be an undesirable belief change because this type of explanation is potentially much harder to disprove than the sound wave one. In practice I have found these unplanned alternatives do not arise providing you do not confront the person too soon, before you have adequately prepared them for the alternative belief about their voice coming from within. Nevertheless, as we

[5] I am not quite sure why this is so; fortunately I have never been asked to explain it, but no doubt a physics or electronics book would have the answer.

saw in Chapter 8, it is always possible to misjudge these situations, so if such an undesirable belief change were to occur, then you should close it down immediately by stating firmly and unequivocally that you do not believe this alternative is possible, giving as many reasons as possible to support your conclusion.

REALITY TESTING

Reality testing in connection with the origin of the voice is commonly used for one or more of the following purposes.

1. To establish and test the facts used in the logical reasoning and evidence evaluation

The following are examples of reality tests used to establish the 'facts' on which commonly used lines of logical reasoning are based. When conducting this type of reality test it is recommended the therapist takes part in them as well. Discovering the facts alongside the other person will put you in a better position to discuss the results and their implications.

(a) To establish that the person *can* locate the direction of a real voice a test situation is set up in which three or four people surround the person, who wears an eye-shield or puts their hands over their eyes. The other people take it in turns to speak; the person in the middle points to the person speaking and then checks whether they have done so correctly.

(b) To establish the distance limit of normal hearing, a test situation is set up in which the person listens to someone talking continuously as they move away, move into another room, go behind a tree, etc. The person notes how the volume of what they hear changes according to the distance and the other factors. They note the distance and situation when they can no longer distinguish what is being said, and when they can no longer hear the sound at all.

(c) A similar situation to (b), but with the person themself doing the moving, is used to establish how sounds change in volume and clarity as the person changes their position. This establishes that the voice *ought* to change in volume and clarity as the person walks away or moves from one room to another.

2. Ask the voice to do something it ought to be able to do

Examples of this sort of reality test are:

(a) Ask the voice of the Devil to set light to a flimsy piece of paper. This should be very easy for the Devil to do.
(b) Promise the voice of a greedy relative £100 if he or she sends the person a picture postcard of a gorilla in the next three days.
(c) Ask the voice of the head of MI5 to write to confirm that the person should travel to Russia as soon as they are discharged.

3. Ask the voice a question that it ought to be able to answer

If you are using this type of reality test, then you *must* make sure the person themself does not know the answer to the question and is not able to guess it.

Therefore, having agreed a likely question, you should check with the person 'If you had to guess, what would your guess be?'. Examples of this type of reality test are asking the Archangel Gabriel the names of the other cherubim and seraphim, and asking the voice of a dead accountant father an obscure technical question on accountancy.

Both types of reality test outlined in 1 and 2 above can only be used if the person believes the voice can hear you and/or them and also that the voice would respond to the challenge or question if it could. The logical reasoning used in these situations is described in the next chapter (p. 256).

EXAMPLE OF MODIFYING A BELIEF ABOUT THE ORIGIN OF A VOICE USING 'MEMORY' AS THE REPLACEMENT BELIEF

CASE HISTORY

David was a young man who was admitted to hospital during his second year at university. After receiving nearly two years of treatment he was able to move out of hospital but was not well enough to hold down a job. His family, who lived about 10 miles away, had broken off all contact with him because they claimed he was just lazy and had chosen to opt out of a difficult college course. When referred for treatment he described his problem in this way:

'I left university two years ago because I tried to work too hard and I had to be admitted to hospital with mental exhaustion. I live on my own now, which I like, but I wish my father would stop going on at me about being a failure. I can hear him when I'm sitting quietly or trying to get to sleep.

GOAL SETTING

1. Probably the most important goal of therapy for David concerned his underlying, non-psychotic belief about being a failure. The end goal for this modification was for David to end up believing '*Academic and occupational success are no measure of a person's worth. Working is only important if you enjoy it or if the money it provides enables you to buy greater comforts and pleasures in life. Work has no deeper, hidden value and is not a thing of worth in itself. Everyone is a unique person, of unique value and worth, and that includes me. Some of the things about myself that I particularly like are...*' The line of treatment to achieve this goal is not reported here.

2. David was under the care of a mental health team, who spoke to him about his mental illness and need to take medication. Moreover, he had been unable to return to his studies or to get a job because of the effects of his illness and this was likely to continue for some time in the future. Therefore, another goal was to modify David's dysfunctional beliefs about mental illness and psychosis in order (a) to prepare him for this level of understanding about his situation and, (b) to protect him from the

prejudiced beliefs of his family. The line of treatment to achieve this goal is not reported here.

3. It seemed probable the voice would have less power to wound David if he did not think it was actually his father talking. However, in setting the goal in terms of what David would end up believing, it was apparent there was a problem around the replacement belief. The way David described his past history as 'mental exhaustion' rung immediate alarm bells that warned that explanations in terms of mental illness and psychosis would not be acceptable as things stood at that time. This caution was reinforced by the fact that his family, too, had apparently refused to admit that he had a psychiatric illness, despite his hospitalization, preferring to reject him as a dropout instead. To be effective, the replacement belief would have to be in terms of the voice coming from within himself rather than from his father, but we wanted to avoid the notion of mental illness. David's antipathy to this term indicated that preparing for an 'illness/psychosis' replacement belief was likely be a lengthy process. Since David's recollection was that the voice was saying essentially the same things now as his father had actually said to him in the past, the memory option provided a valid and acceptable alternative explanation for the voice.

Goal: *'The voice does not come from my father. It is a fragment of memory that keeps recurring very vividly because it made me very upset when my father said those things.'*

PREPARING THE REPLACEMENT BELIEF

The therapist asked David again about how he had felt at the time when his father accused him of being a failure. She noted that he was already upset and agitated when this happened because he had had to leave university and go into hospital, and she suggested this must have been a very distressing time for him. He agreed that it was. Information was given about how clear and sharp memories of this type of situation can be, and this was discussed. The therapist then suggested to David that perhaps his voice might be of this type, and he was happy to consider this.

MODIFYING THE BELIEF ABOUT THE VOICE'S ORIGIN

Once David had an acceptable replacement belief, the actual modification of his belief about the origin of the voice was easy. The therapist quizzed David about how someone talking 10 miles away could be heard in his room at night, and he agreed this was not really possible. This point was reinforced by discussing the normal limits of sound or speech travel. Another argument used was that David often heard the voice late at night when his father would be expected to be asleep. At this stage he concluded the voice could not be a real one and must be a vividly recurring memory.

Understanding his voice to be a fragment of memory helped to protect David from the implication that his father was still being actively critical and unpleasant to him whenever he heard the voice.

CASE STUDY RICHARD

(See also pp. 204, 214, 226, 262 and 278.)

Goal 3A: *'The voice is not from some external entity: it is a vivid thought produced by my brain that I hear out loud because it makes me feel so frightened and stressed.'*

Goal 3B – for later: *'The voice does not come from an external source: it is a feature of my psychotic illness.'*

Shortly after the assessment and goal setting sessions, another member of the clinical team, not involved in the CBT programme, had sat down with Richard to talk about his diagnosis of psychosis and medication. As a result of this, although he was still certain that the voice he heard in the night was a genuine one, the link between internally produced 'voices' and psychosis was now too close to be able to achieve Goal 3A without also bringing about Goal 3B, so the two goals were combined.

PREPARING THE GOAL

When Richard told his therapist about his talk with the psychiatrist, she adopted a 'detached but interested' approach and asked what he understood by the term 'psychosis' and how he had felt about this suggestion. This led naturally to a discussion about psychosis in general, which enabled the therapist to correct some misinformation and to start to provide some more positive information.

When 'hearing voices' came up during one of these discussions the therapist took the opportunity to tell Richard that hearing voices was very common anyway, occurring in some form in probably about 60 to 70% of the general population. She then went on to explain how the brain produces voices and the factors that can increase this happening.

MODIFYING THE BELIEF

It would have been too distressing, and therefore dysfunctional, to attempt to challenge the origins of the voice whilst Richard still feared its authority and power to harm him, so some work to disempower the voice was carried out first (see p. 263).

When the work to establish that God did not require Richard to chant the prayers was well under way (see p. 227), the therapist returned to preparing the replacement belief for the voice's origin. She mentioned that the voices that people hear often express what they are concerned about, and explained why this is so. She then observed that Richard's voice also reflected something that worried him and floated the idea that perhaps the voice he heard in the night was something like that.

When Richard accepted the floated idea by agreeing this was possible, she pointed out that if the voice was a reflection of his own worries, then this would account for why it had been unable to harm or contact her when it had been challenged to do so, why the voice had never in fact done any harm to Richard, and why it was unable even to wake him up on the nights he slept through. It would also account for why the voice was saying something most religious people did not agree with, namely that it is necessary or required to chant a prayer repetitively.

At this stage, the work to disempower the voice (see p. 263) went hand in hand with the work to modify the belief about its origin. By now, the work on his beliefs about the sect were well advanced and Richard was fairly confident the voice was not too bothered whether he chanted the prayer or not and that it had no ill intent towards him. Furthermore, the disempowerment work had instilled sufficient doubt about the power of the voice for him to be able to use an earplug or Walkman when he woke up, and the effectiveness of these simple ways of controlling the voice provided more persuasive evidence against the voice coming from a powerful or real external source.

Moreover, after distracting and grounding himself by going to talk to the night nurses when he awoke, he started to go back to bed and sleep without chanting the prayers: when nothing adverse happened to him this provided yet more supporting evidence about the power and origin of the voice.

PARTIAL MODIFICATIONS OF A BELIEF ABOUT THE NATURE/ORIGIN OF THE VOICE

A partial modification of the belief about the origin of a voice takes the form:

The voice comes from 'X' but …

Usually this 'but' involves some unwanted or dysfunctional feature of the voice. For example, 'It is the voice of my father *but* he makes mistakes so it is not a good idea to put large sums of money on the horses he recommends' or 'The voice comes from my neighbour *but* it is not able to put thoughts into my mind or make me act against my will'.

The other main type of 'but' concerns how other people view the voice. For example, 'My voice comes from God *but* other people cannot hear it and so they do not believe it comes from God; therefore, I cannot expect other people to follow my instructions without question'.

Partial modifications of delusional beliefs about the nature/origin of a voice are treated in the same way as partial modifications of other delusional beliefs. This is described in Chapter 8, pp. 88–95.

13 MODIFYING THE BELIEF ABOUT THE POWER AND AUTHORITY OF THE VOICES

DISEMPOWERING THE VOICE

The first aim of disempowering the voice is to take away its power over the person who hears it, to show that it is weak and ineffectual and cannot actually *do* anything, other than sound like a voice and perhaps be irritating for that reason. A related aim is to take away the voice's authority by showing that it is ignorant, gets things wrong and/or tells lies. The third aim is to empower the person by showing that they are actually *more* powerful and *more* knowledgeable than the voice.

If the power of the voice comes from its perceived origin (e.g. the Devil), then work to disempower the voice will be closely interwoven with the work to modify the belief about its origin. It is often necessary to make some progress on disempowering the voice before the person feels safe to challenge its origin. However, where power and origin are closely interlinked the replacement belief about the voice's origin must be prepared before the disempowering work reaches the stage of threatening this belief. For example, showing that the voice has no power and is ignorant of the sort of things the Devil ought to know will not only disempower it but will also undermine the belief it comes from the Devil.

The approach to modifying a belief about the power and authority of a voice is essentially the same as that used with any other delusional belief and the same basic modification strategies described in Chapter 8 apply. The present chapter details how these strategies might be adapted and used for the purpose of disempowering the voice.

CHANGING THE BELIEF ABOUT THE VOICE'S MALIGN INTENT

Where the voice is feared, it is likely to be helpful, as a first step, to attempt to move the person's perception of it from being malign to being benign. Whether or not this is possible will depend on factors such as the perceived source of the voice (for example, it would not be possible to argue that an evil spirit could be benign), whether it has spoken aggressively or threateningly to the person, and in what terms, and whether it is believed to have caused actual harm in the past. Some people assume the voice means them harm or could do them harm if provoked, even though no threat has been made, because they feel frightened when they hear it.

Where it is possible to change the belief about a malign intent this will not only be a benefit in its own right but may also help to reduce the actual occurrence of the voice via a reduction in arousal levels. Viewing the voice as essentially benign will also mean the person will be less fearful and more willing to discuss it and to put it to the test in reality testing.

RE-EVALUATE THE EVIDENCE SUPPORTING THE VOICE'S POWER AND/ OR AUTHORITY

An important aspect of this part of the assessment is to ascertain what evidence the person has that their voice is powerful and/or authoritative. Whatever this evidence is, it has to be weakened by re-evaluation, whilst evidence against the voice's power and knowledge is collected and built up.

In some cases people may be so frightened of the voice, or so frightened of what will happen to them if they talk about it, that they are unwilling to give you any details. If this is so, then it is better to work as best you can with the notion of 'something awful' being threatened than to risk raising the person's anxiety levels even higher by persistent questioning. Once the therapy has started to be effective, then it is likely that they will feel safe enough to risk telling you more.

The voice has power to cause harm

Very often the power of the voice is assumed or feared because of the threats it has made to harm the person or someone close to them. In some cases the person may be unsure of what that harm could be but has a general feeling of the voice's power and its malevolent intent. It is harder to establish that the voice cannot harm someone mentally than physically and even harder to establish that it cannot harm someone spiritually. Therefore when, as part of your assessment, you are trying to obtain details about a 'vague' harm, you should avoid pushing the person towards coming to a conclusion that it must be some mental or spiritual harm they risk. To help prevent this happening, wherever appropriate you should accept and agree that the harm threatened is physical.

1. *If the voice is believed to have caused harm in the past*, then each incident of this happening must be explored with a view to re-evaluating it. The first step is to establish that the incident (or incidents like it) *could* have happened without any involvement of the voice but without questioning the voice's involvement in this particular incident at this stage.

It is your role as the therapist to consider what other possible explanations there could be for what happened and to explore these options by asking more questions. When you have determined the most likely alternative explanation(s), you would float the suggestion that this *might* be how the incident actually happened, with the implication that the voice was not involved and had not influenced the outcome. At this stage you would probably not be suggesting *all* incidents involving the voice had another explanation, only that the particular one(s) under consideration could have. As the number of re-evaluated incidents builds up you will reach the point where you can suggest that perhaps all the incidents from the past are of this type and therefore that the voice never has been able to cause harm.

Two examples of re-evaluating incidents of harm thought to be caused by a voice are: (a) A woman thought her voice was carrying out its threat to harm her when she kept tripping over in her flat. When her community psychiatric nurse visited it was apparent she was tripping because she wore very old slippers. A new pair of slippers not only prevented her hurting herself but also demonstrated that the voice was not really able to trip her up. (b) In a similar case, a woman feared her voice because she believed it had pushed her downstairs on a couple of occasions. An ABC analysis showed that when her voice was very persistent she drank large amounts of gin to try to quieten it and it was on these occasions that she fell downstairs. This alternative explanation was discussed and she was given earplugs and a Walkman to help block the voice. These were effective and so she no longer needed to resort to alcohol and the voice lost its power to push her over.

2. *If the voice has threatened specific harm in the past but failed to carry it out* (e.g. 'Your car will crash'), then the person is likely to have interpreted this as indicating that the voice changed its mind, or decided to be merciful on this occasion. If you are in the early stages of therapy and seeking to change the person's belief about the malevolence of the voice, then your reinterpretation of this would be along the lines: 'If the voice is able to harm you, then this is certainly in keeping with the voice not *wanting* to harm you – perhaps it is just trying to frighten or impress you for some reason.'

Later on, a stronger reinterpretation of this failure to carry out a threat would be 'The voice makes threats that frighten you but it is incapable of carrying them out'. For this stronger reinterpretation you would use logical reasoning to argue that threatening something and being able to carry it out are two totally different things (described in 'Logical reasoning', below) and then, when the person felt ready, move on to a reality test to prove the voice's powerlessness (described in 'Reality testing', below).

If one of the goals of therapy is for the person to understand their voice as coming from within their own brain, then it may be appropriate during the disempowering work to float the notion 'The voice seems to know exactly what you fear', moving on to 'The voice seems to have insider knowledge about your fears'. Asking the person whether they ever get fearful thoughts about the same sorts of things as the voice predicts or threatens is another way of helping to prepare for this replacement belief.

3. *If the voice has threatened harm without specifying what this will be*, the approach is to reinterpret this as indicating that it does not specify the harm because it *cannot* do so, and that it cannot do so (a) because it does not know what bad things are going to happen in the normal course of events, and (b) because it cannot, itself, actually cause anything bad to happen. It may be helpful to discuss how bad things happen to all of us from time to time, as part of our everyday lives, to make the point that it is not clever for the voice to predict that 'something bad' will happen, as something bad or harmful is likely to affect every one of us in the next few weeks.

Be careful to distinguish when the voice has claimed responsibility for a specific harmful event *after* it has happened. Everyone can do this, so it is not clever; indeed, the voice can be dismissed disrespectfully as trying to impress in this immature way because it is actually powerless to cause anything to happen.

4. *If the voice is that of the real person and it is the person that is feared rather than the voice as such*, then the most effective way of disempowering the voice is to modify the delusional belief about where it is coming from (see Chapter 12).

This modification may take some time to achieve or may not be possible to achieve, so it is worth considering whether you could reduce the distress (a) by showing that the person whose voice it is would not be able to carry out the threat in practice (if this is true), and (b) by arguing that the person would not attempt to carry out the threat because the penalties he or she would have to pay would far outweigh the gains. This latter argument can be strengthened by pointing out that since the person hearing the threats has told other people (including you) about them, the perpetrator would be identified immediately should he or she attempt to carry them out and so would not get away with it.

You may also be able to use the argument 'The source of the voice *cannot* cause harm' for voices that come from non-human sources. In these cases the logical arguments and reality tests used to substantiate your argument will depend on the perceived source of the voice. For example, if the voice was feared because it came from a ghost, it might be possible to argue successfully that ghosts cannot interact with material objects and, therefore, that the ghost making the threats could not hurt the person concerned.

5. *Sometimes the voice is feared because it comes from a powerful entity that could cause harm, even though it has never actually threatened harm.* The absence of threat is a very positive feature so you should try to strengthen it by interpreting it as 'clear evidence the voice has only good intention towards you'. Note that the usual approach of floating a suggestion and asking for the other person's opinion implies your suggestion might not be true, and allows for other interpretations to be possible, which would be unhelpful in this particular situation. Therefore, this is one of those occasions when you should be much more definite and present the interpretation as something that seems, to you, to be obviously true.

6. *Occasionally, it is the voice itself that is feared rather than the entity or person from which the voice comes* (for example 'The voice says it can cut off my head' and 'I am sure the voice could stop my heart if it wanted to'). This is most likely to occur when the person experiences the voice as powerful and invasive but has no clear theory about where or who it comes from. As far as possible you should try to firm up the person's conclusion that it is only the voice itself that seems to have the power and that nothing else is involved. This is done in order to reduce the risk of a move towards 'It is the source of the voice that can harm me' as you start to use logical reasoning to challenge the ability of the voice to cause physical harm.

The principal lines of logical reasoning used in these circumstances are (a) that *feeling* that something is so (in this case that the voice is 'powerful') does not mean that it is so (see pp. 155–156), (b) (if a threat has been made) that making a threat does not mean it can be carried out (see p. 256), and (c) that voices are not made of solid matter and so cannot interact with or damage physical objects or bodies.[1]

With respect to this last line of reasoning, the fact that real voices in general, and the person's voices in particular, are not solid can be demonstrated by the fact that they cannot be seen or touched and they go through walls and other solid things. In contrast, solid objects, including the person's own body, are made of atoms and molecules that are tightly bound together so that only another object that is also made of atoms and molecules could force its way in between and separate them, for example a knife cutting through an apple. Since the voice is not made of solid atoms and molecules there is no way it could cut or otherwise physically affect a solid object like the person's body. Indeed, this is why the voice, if challenged in a reality test, cannot so much as cut a piece of paper or pick up a pencil.

The voice has power and/or authority because of what it says and does

As with the power of the voice to cause harm, anything else that the voice has done or said in the past that has been interpreted as indicating it has power or authority should be disputed and re-evaluated so that it no longer supports this interpretation.

EXAMPLE OF DISEMPOWERING A VOICE BY RE-EVALUATING THE EVIDENCE AND REALITY TESTING

A woman believed her voice had power because it could tell when her phone was going to ring and, often, who would be ringing. Two lines were taken and explored in order to decide the most likely alternative explanation for this 'evidence'. Firstly, discussion confirmed the therapist's initial speculation that most of her phone calls came from 'regulars' who tended to call at the same time of day; for example, her father phoned every evening at 6 p.m., and when her sister called she usually did so in the early afternoon. She accepted that for these calls it was not surprising her voice could predict who it would be.

Secondly, the bias towards noticing confirming and ignoring disconfirming evidence was discussed and on the basis of this the therapist suggested to the woman that perhaps it was possible that sometimes in the past the voice had failed to predict the phone ringing, or guessed wrongly who it would be, but that if this had happened then it would be 'normal' for her to have forgotten these occasions. She also suggested that if the voice predicted the phone would ring and it did so several hours later, then she might understandably have taken this as confirmation of the voice's foreknowledge – but since she usually had several phone calls a day it was more likely

[1]Although I have not yet encountered it in clinical practice, I am aware of the possibility that the person may know about high-frequency sounds being used to break up material objects. If this were to happen, then the argument used would be that the voice cannot be this type of high-frequency sound because if it were then the person would not be able to hear it.

than not that the phone would ring within that time span and so it could not be counted as a 'prediction'. These suggestions were accepted and the woman concluded that probably some, at least, of the voice's predictions could have been based on informed guesswork.

In order to investigate the accuracy of the predictions the woman agreed to keep a detailed diary noting every time the voice predicted a call and who it predicted would be calling, and noting the time and caller for all her telephone calls. An important aspect of this reality test was to get the woman's agreement that, for the reasons given above, regular callers did not provide a valid test of the voice and, therefore, that its ability to predict phone calls could only be judged from its ability to predict unexpected and irregular callers. In order to ensure she got some of this latter type of caller it was agreed that the therapist would ring at some time(s) during the next couple of weeks. The therapist rang only a couple of times, to avoid the risk of chance 'hits'. She rang outside office hours, having surmised correctly that the woman would expect her to make the calls from her office, and chose times when the woman did not usually get phone calls, like early Saturday morning. The evidence provided by the reality test was overwhelming and conclusive.

In some cases, the authority of the voice comes from the fact that *it seems to know all about the person who hears it*. The alternative explanation for this evidence is that the voice knows about the person because it comes from their own brain. This re-evaluation requires the belief about the voice's origin to be modified (see Chapter 12).

If the voice *claims to be able to do powerful things*, for example broadcast the person's thoughts or influence the psychiatrist's decisions, then each of these claims would be challenged separately using evidence evaluation, logical reasoning and reality testing. Having shown that the voice cannot do these powerful things, its false claims can be added to the list of evidence that the voice tells lies (see below), or makes boastful claims because it wants to impress the person, or whatever other functional description of the claims you are using in order to reduce the credibility and hence the power of the voice.

If *what the voice says is untrue or inaccurate*, then the CBT work done on the content of the voice to show that it is untrue will also have the benefit of taking away some of the power of the voice and also some of its authority and control. Even if the content is essentially true, modifying the associated beliefs underlying it, so that it is less able to cause distress, may help to reduce the voice's perceived power (see Chapter 11).

The voice has power and/or authority because of what/whom it comes from

The strategies used to disempower a voice can be used for voices that are believed to come from a powerful source *providing* the person feels it is safe to test the voice's power and knowledge in this way. As noted earlier in this chapter, if it has been possible to argue that the voice is essentially benign towards the hearer, then he or she will be less fearful and more willing to put the voice to the test.

When the power and/or authority of the voice is based on who or what it comes from, then the most effective way of disempowering it is to modify the belief about its nature or origin (see Chapter 12), but such a significant modification may take quite a time to prepare and achieve. Disempowerment is generally quicker and easier to achieve than a change of belief about the source of the voice because 'power' is only one aspect of that source. For example, it would be possible to show that a spirit voice had no power but this would not necessarily be enough to prove the voice did not come from a spirit.

Whether or not it is possible to disempower a voice without modifying the belief about its source depends on whether or not 'being powerful' is an essential characteristic of the source. For example, power is not a necessary quality of ghosts so in this case it should be possible to disempower the voice before the belief about its origin is changed, i.e. for the person to believe 'The voice is a ghost, but it cannot harm me'. In contrast, if the voice was that of a violent drug dealer, then it would not be possible to disempower the voice without also changing the belief about its origin because the partial modification 'The threats are coming from the drug dealer, but he has no power to harm me' would not be tenable in this case.

The power and/or authority of the voice is known intuitively

Sometimes voices are accompanied by feelings of great significance or mystical power that are not directly related to what it says or who it seems to come from but that, nevertheless, imbue the voice itself with a sense of power and authority. The first step in re-evaluating this type of evidence is to establish that *feeling* something to be significant or powerful does not necessarily mean that it is so, based on the 'Believing or perceiving something to be so does not mean that it is so' lines of work (see Chapters 6 and 12). The second step is to provide an alternative explanation for the feeling, for example 'The brain activity [psychosis] that triggers your voices also triggers the area of your brain that recognizes the significance (or mystical quality) of things, so you get the *feeling* that something significant (or mystical) is happening even though it is not: not surprisingly, this feeling has become linked to the voices because they occur at the same time'.

EVIDENCE AGAINST THE VOICE'S POWER AND/OR AUTHORITY

Build up evidence that the voice has no knowledge or authority, that it is ignorant or tells lies

Showing that the voice can get things wrong, even if it is only for some of the time or on some occasions, can be an effective way of reducing its authority and importance. Furthermore, if the voice can get it wrong, then the person need not believe it when it threatens or says unpleasant things. The fact that it makes mistakes can be used at either the reasoning level ('The voice has said things in the past that turned out not to be true, so what it is saying now may well be untrue, too') or as a direct confrontation to the voice ('You're always making mistakes, so why should I believe you now?').

Inaccurate voices can be labelled as 'ignorant' or 'liars' depending on which view is more helpful for the particular person. The advantages of 'ignorant' are (a) it does not imply the voice has any malign intent, and (b) it suggests less knowledge and less importance than deliberate lying. If the voice is ignorant, then its opinion of the person, the information it gives and/or the threats it makes are not valid and not worth listening to.

For this line of work it is helpful to get as many examples of the voice 'getting it wrong' as possible. The person may be able to recall incidents in the past where this has happened but often such evidence, if it exists, has been forgotten and so it is collected during the course of therapy. Where work is ongoing to disprove the accuracy of the voice's content, each time the person concludes that the voice is not accurate about what it says this can be included in the list of evidence about it making mistakes. In addition to the evidence obtained from this more formal work with the content of the voice, it may be possible to catch the voice getting it wrong in some of its more trivial utterances, too, so you should keep alert for reports of this kind. Once the person has realized their voice can make mistakes, then they may be able to formally record instances when they arise. For example, one woman noticed that her voice wrongly predicted which nurse would be on duty in the afternoon, and that she would be called in to see her psychiatrist.

Of course, on some occasions the voice may tell the truth, but fortunately it is not necessary for the voice to always, or even usually, get it wrong to be able to undermine its reliability, knowledge and authority. It is sufficient if the person concludes that the voice makes mistakes and so what it says cannot be trusted and is not worth attending to.

EXAMPLE OF BUILDING UP EVIDENCE THAT THE VOICE GETS THINGS WRONG

(See p. 220 for an example of the more detailed work done on one of these incidents.)

The example given below is of a card built up during the course of treatment to show that a woman's voices lied about many things.[2] Underneath each incident is just one of the key pieces of evidence that was used to show that they had lied.

[2] If I were working with this woman now, for the reasons given above I would encourage her to label her voices 'ignorant' rather than 'liars'.

The voices are liars – in the past they have said:

1 That N. R. is Hitler. (Hitler would be over 90 years old if he were alive today.)
2 The nurses wanted to keep me on the locked ward so they would get extra pay. (Nurses' pay is fixed however many patients they have.)
3 I am mentally retarded. (I can read, cook, look after myself, etc.)
4 I was the only person alive in the universe and that everyone else was a ghost. (I can *see* everyone else around me, alive.)

Build up evidence that the voice has no power

When this evidence is obtained from reality testing and naturally occurring incidents, it should be collected together and summarized on cards so that the person has a ready reminder for when they are on their own with the voice.

Although incidents from the past when the voice did not carry out its threat may initially be attributed to the voice 'not wanting' to do so, as the person's conviction about the voice's power lessens, then these earlier incidents can be re-evaluated and added to the list of 'things the voice cannot do'.

LOGICAL REASONING

Logical reasoning is an integral part of the evidence evaluation and reality testing work. Some of the common lines of reasoning that are used for the power or authority of a voice can be summarized as follows.

1. Claiming to have power/authority does not mean that the voice has got power/authority

An important line of work is to draw a clear distinction between what the voice says and what it can actually do. This distinction may seem rather obvious but in fact even many non-psychotic people exhibit this sort of magical thinking, for example when we feel slightly uneasy about putting our fears into words in case this should make it more likely to happen.

In addition to your logical reasoning and collecting evidence of occasions when people have said they will do things and then not been able to do them, it may be helpful to actually demonstrate that *saying is not the same as doing*. One way of doing this is for you and the other person to 'claim' that you are able to do things and then go on to reality test if you can really make them happen.

If you are demonstrating that saying is not the same as doing, it is worth noting *why* you cannot do what you claim to be able to because this may be helpful for later, when you are looking for specific reasons why the voice could not do as it claims. Reasons include (a) because you do not have the ability, or (b) the power to make it happen, for example claiming 'I can play a Beethoven sonata' or 'If I ring Buckingham Palace, the Queen will be keen to talk to me', and (c) because what you claim is contrary to the laws of nature, for example claiming 'I can turn your hair green in the next five minutes' or 'I can make you float up to the ceiling' or 'I can blow that tree down'.

2. The voice is only a voice and therefore cannot *do* anything

This line of logical reasoning applies only to those people who believe it is the voice itself that has the power, rather than the source of the voice. It follows the same approach as that used for showing that a voice or sound has no power to cause harm, as described earlier in this chapter, namely that a voice or sound cannot interact with the physical world (see p. 252). The particular explanation given should be adapted to the particular power that the voice is deemed to have, for example explaining why a voice could not push someone off their bike or add poison to a plate of food. Where it applies, the opportunity can be taken to point out that the person themself could do what their voice is claiming to be able to do but cannot, and therefore that the person is more powerful than the voice.

3. If earplugs/Walkman/medication or other coping strategies work, then the voice cannot be powerful

Practical coping strategies are usually used from the earliest stages of therapy so it is a matter of clinical judgement when it is appropriate to use their effectiveness as a challenge to the voice's power. You should be careful not to use it too soon if there is a risk that exposing the challenge would lead the person to become too frightened to use these ways of stopping their voice.

The line of logical reasoning used is essentially the same as that described in Chapter 12 (p. 240) in relation to the origin of the voice. For the purpose of disempowering the voice, the argument is that a 'powerful' voice would not be stopped or reduced by something as simple as an earplug, Walkman, medication, etc. This line of logical reasoning is particularly beneficial because it is easy to extend it to show that the hearer is more powerful than their voice. For example, it is easy to demonstrate that the person can make themself heard when someone else is wearing an earplug or Walkman, or when someone is taking medicine, etc. – but the voice cannot overcome even these very minor barriers to make itself heard.

4. If the voice gets things wrong, it cannot be knowledgeable/ authoritative or, by implication, powerful

If the voice has been shown to be ignorant and to make mistakes (see above), then it may be appropriate to argue that it cannot be authoritative and, therefore, that it cannot be important or powerful.

Asking the voice questions it cannot answer (see 'Reality testing', below) will provide more evidence of its ignorance. Although the person themself will not know the answers either (if they did, you would not be able to use those particular questions to test the voice), you can argue that other human beings do know the answers and therefore that the voice is not as knowledgeable as these other human beings. Furthermore, you can point out to the person that they *could* have known the answers, just by reading a book or watching a TV programme on the subject, so potentially they, too, are more knowledgeable than the voice.

5. If the voice cannot meet the challenges put to it in reality testing (see below), then it cannot be powerful and/or knowledgeable

When the voice first fails to meet a 'challenge' that is put to it, it is not uncommon for the person to conclude that this was because the voice did not want to do what it was challenged to do, for some reason. Therefore, it is important to be able to argue why the voice *would* respond if it could.

Using logical reasoning to support the results of the reality test
The general line of reasoning taken is 'It is in the voice's best interest to prove to you that it has got power to do these things (or to do the things it says it can) – otherwise I, you and other people will think it is just a bag of wind. It seems to like to try to assert control over you and frighten you so it would want to prove to you that it really *does* have some power – otherwise it is inevitable that you will start to doubt it and then you won't listen to what it says any more or do what it tells you to do.' Providing the person is happy for you to take this approach, you might strengthen this argument by being rude and belittling to the voice and then reasoning that it would not tolerate such a deliberate insult from you if it was able to do anything about it.

REALITY TESTING THE POWER AND KNOWLEDGE OF THE VOICE

Reality testing the knowledge and power of the voice can expose its lack of knowledge and authority and can provide impressive evidence of its inability to do what it threatens or, indeed, to do anything at all.

Unfortunately, but entirely to be expected, when people believe their voice to be powerful, they are not willing to risk putting it to the test. Fortunately, they have an ally, the therapist, who, having a different set of beliefs, should have no qualms about challenging the voice and its power. The big advantage of reality testing the voice on yourself, apart from the obvious one of causing much less distress to the person who hears it, is that you can do this test early on in therapy whilst the person themself still firmly believes the voice to be telling the truth.[3] Needless to say, if challenging or reality testing a particular voice would make you feel too uncomfortable or too vulnerable, then of course you should not do so. This is very unlikely to happen but could occur if, for example, the voice is believed to come from some evil force that is compatible with your own religious or cultural upbringing or beliefs. If this should occur, then you might wish to

[3]When you start to challenge voices to harm you, you may experience some slight apprehension due to superstitious thinking. This feeling of unease should disappear as you collect evidence from your own practice to confirm that other people's voices really cannot harm you in any way. But this is another good reason for clearly describing exactly what you are challenging the voice to do to you, namely to avoid the risk that *you* will misinterpret subsequent bad luck in a superstitious way.

examine your own underlying beliefs, using CBT principles, to discover why you feel this way about something that, in other circumstances, you are so sure is a symptom of an illness!

In the early days, you *must* take full responsibility for the outcome of any challenges you make to the voice. As the person becomes more confident, then they may start to challenge the voice on their own behalf.

1. Challenging the voice to do to you what it is doing to the person who hears it

Examples of this from my own clinical practice are challenging the voice:

- to speak to me
- to wake me up at night
- to threaten me
- to tell me to do things
- to put thoughts into my mind
- to make my telephone ring.

2. Challenging the voice to do to you what it has threatened to do to the person who hears it, or what it is feared that it *could* do

Examples of this from my own clinical practice are challenging the voice:

- to cut off my head. (Milder versions of this would be to challenge the voice to cut off a little finger or hand, or to cut a piece of meat that has been brought into the session, or to cut a piece of paper.)
- to make me spontaneously combust. (A milder version of this would be to make a sheet of paper burst into flames.)
- to break my television set
- to harm me by causing me to have a car accident within the next week that was so severe I would be in hospital for at least a month.

Before making the challenge you should explain why you are confident that the voice cannot carry out what you are going to challenge it to do. This is done not only to reduce the person's concern on your behalf but also as an opportunity to start to build up the logical reasoning against the voice's power.

As with reality testing of any other delusional belief (see Chapter 8, pp. 179–182) the reality tests of the voice's power should be set precisely, including time limits for the voice to respond.

Note that the milder versions of the challenges are not only less stressful for the person but also show the voice to be even feebler. Why fear a voice that threatens to make you spontaneously combust when it cannot even set light to a teeny-weeny piece of paper?

Using logical reasoning to support the results of the reality test

When the results of the test are known, the person may reason that although the voice is unable to do these things to you this does not mean it is unable to do these things to them. Although this is a logically valid conclusion to draw, nevertheless the results clearly limit the voice's power ('Its power must be very limited indeed if it can only affect you'). Furthermore, you can argue that the other person's body is made up of the same physical stuff as your own, so if the voice cannot affect your body, then the logical conclusion is that it cannot affect the other person's body either. The logical reasoning to argue against the interpretation of the voice *not wanting* to respond when you challenge it is detailed in section 5, on p. 258.

3. Challenging the voice to do something it ought to be able to do because of who or what it comes from

Examples of this are:

- challenging the voice of an archangel to speak out loud to the hospital chaplain, before this time tomorrow
- challenging the voice of a ghost to make an appearance so that everyone can see it, now
- promising the voice of a neighbour £100 if she comes in to collect it within three days.

4. Challenging the voice to answer questions it ought to be able to answer

Examples of this are:

- asking the voice of the Archangel Gabriel how many Christians there are in China
- asking the voice of a distant uncle for the name of his sister-in-law.

As already described (see Chapter 12, p. 243), the questions used should be selected to ensure not only that the person does not know the answer but also that if they were to guess the answer their guess would be wide of the mark.

The most common response to this type of direct questioning is for the voice to say nothing, which you can interpret as evidence that it is unable to accept the challenge. (See p. 258 for how to counter the interpretation that the voice did not want to accept the challenge.)

When the person themself feels confident to question their voice in this way, then the inability of voice to answer them back is very empowering for the person. In some cases it can render the voice mute for periods of an hour or more, which firmly hands the control back to the person who has challenged it. Even if the voice should attempt a response, then the fact that it gets it wrong is also disempowering, and the incident would be added to the list of the voice's 'foolish mistakes'.

5. Challenges that show the voice to have less power or knowledge than the person who hears it

Many of the challenges used in 1 to 3 above involve actions that the person themself could do easily. Therefore, when the voice does not respond, it not only shows the voice to be powerless but also specifically indicates that the voice is not as strong and powerful as the person themself. For example, using the examples given above, the person themself would have no difficulty in waking you up at night, or cutting up a piece of meat, or breaking your TV set, etc., but the voice is unable to do these things. Similarly, if a 'powerful' voice is unable to lift up a single sheet of paper during the session, or write its instructions with the pencil and paper provided, then this shows it is clearly of vastly inferior strength to the person themself, who can lift hundreds of the sheets, and write pages of words, without any difficulty at all.

GENTLY MOCKING THE VOICE

If, through any of the approaches described above, the voice can be shown to be weak, ineffectual, ignorant, wrong or frightened of the challenges, then this will help to overcome the person's feelings of awe and powerlessness in its presence and give the person a sense of control or even superiority over it. As this work progresses, it is likely to be helpful if you start to treat the voice with the lack of respect that it deserves, as this will tend to further diminish its aura of importance and superiority.[4] Examples of this are: 'I am definitely unimpressed by what it has shown me so far, which is nothing'; 'It just burbles away making idle threats'; 'It seems to me that it's like a bag of wind, all air and no substance'. As with more direct challenges to the voice's power or authority, in the early stages you should phrase these remarks as clearly indicating that they are *your* opinions, and not involving the other person.

As gentle mockery is a form of challenge to the voice's power you should introduce these remarks gradually, checking that the person is comfortable with mild levels of disdain before moving on to greater levels of disrespect. When the person themself is ready to do so, then it can be very empowering if they can express their lack of respect for the voice in their own words, too; for example, 'It gets confused and frightened when I challenge it'; 'It can't answer any of the questions I ask it'; 'When I argue with the voice, it never wins because it can't think about the issues or argue about them as well as I can'.

Whilst encouraging the person to feel superior to their voice you must be careful that neither you nor they mock it in any way that could be interpreted subsequently as mocking the person themself, if and when they reach the understanding that the voice comes from within themself and not from some external source. When this insight is achieved, one way of retaining the person's sense of superiority over their voice and the confidence and self-esteem that this may bring, whilst not demeaning the person for being the source of the voice, is to describe the voice in terms of a 'lower level' of brain functioning, which we all

[4]The therapy described in this book is concerned with beliefs and voices that are not wanted by the person who has them and so this affects the attitude that the therapist adopts towards them. It would clearly be inappropriate to mock a voice that the hearer considered to be a valued friend.

have, rather like automatic thoughts and dreams, and contrasting it with the higher-level rational thinking of the person themself.

CASE STUDY RICHARD

(See also pp. 204, 214, 226, 246 and 278.)

Goal 4A: *'The voice does not want to harm me.'*

The therapist started on this line of work by noting that the voice had never actually threatened to harm Richard. She also pointed out that, even though they had got some things wrong, the sect was benign and wanted good for the world, and so any voice associated with the sect and its teachings would also be benign and want what was good for Richard. Furthermore, she noted specifically that the sect, and therefore any voice associated with it, did not advocate harming people to achieve these ends; indeed, causing harm to someone would have been against their beliefs and teachings.

Using the work being developed on the beliefs underlying this voice, the therapist pointed out that the vast majority of people living in the world, including very religious people, do not consider it necessary to repeat these particular prayers for two hours each night in order for the world to be saved, but the voice does not bother to instruct any of *them* to chant the prayers, so why should the voice be bothered with Richard in particular? She followed this line of argument with a reality test, by saying that if the voice considered it necessary for someone to say these prayers, then she would offer to say them instead of Richard for the next few nights, providing the voice woke her up and asked her to do so. When this did not happen, the therapist offered the interpretation that, at the very least, this showed that the voice was *not bothered* whether anyone said these prayers or not and therefore that it would not want to harm Richard for not saying them.

The therapist realized she would be able to use the fact that Richard did not wake up every night to say the prayer, and the fact that he felt perfectly well the following day after he had slept through, as evidence to suggest that nothing would happen to him if he deliberately ignored the voice. However, she was careful not to use this too soon for fear that drawing his attention to those nights when he could not say the prayer because he did not wake up might lead him to worry that perhaps he *ought* to wake himself up in the middle of the night to listen for the voice in case it wanted him to pray. To help protect against this happening, she first observed that the voice must be happy when he slept through because surely it would be able to wake him up if it wanted him to pray on those nights. Richard agreed. Therefore, it was agreed that if the voice was powerful, then this must mean it did not *want* Richard to say the prayers every night. This was extended to argue that if it did not want him to say them every night, then it would not want to harm him when he failed to do so.

Later, it was suggested that the voice did not wake him up on these nights because it *could* not wake him up, which meant it was pretty powerless (see goal 4B, below).

Goal 4B: *'The voice is not able to harm me; it has no power.'*

Although Richard was very concerned that the voice might harm him in some way, he was not sure what that harm might be. After discussing this issue it was agreed that it must be something physical that would happen, since even death can only result from a physical change to the body. This was done in order to help protect against the belief being modified to 'The voice can cause me spiritual harm', when it was shown it could not cause physical harm. If this latter dysfunctional modification had occurred, then Richard's new religious beliefs, backed up by the authority of the hospital chaplain, would have been used to refute it.

The therapist gave her opinion that she did not see how a voice could cause any physical harm, and went through her reasons for thinking this. She followed this up with a reality test in which the voice was challenged to make her have an accident that would put her in hospital for six months before the next therapy session a few days later. When nothing happened, Richard agreed that the voice could not harm the therapist – but then concluded that perhaps the voice could harm only him. The therapist countered this interpretation on the grounds that if it could harm only one person out of millions and millions, then this would mean it was a pretty powerless sort of voice. Furthermore, she could see no mechanism whereby the voice could interfere with one set of physical atoms and not with another, almost identical set. She concluded that in her opinion it was much more likely that the voice *could not* harm anyone at all, including Richard.

Following the successful outcome of the reality test of its ability to harm the therapist, the voice had been sufficiently disempowered to enable her to question Richard about previous times when he had disobeyed the voice. This had not been broached earlier for fear it would merely have increased Richard's apprehension of impending punishment. He recalled one recent occasion when he had been so tired that he had just fallen back to sleep within minutes of waking, and another when he had been so cold that he had only prayed for one hour instead of two. The therapist suggested that on the first of these occasions, the fact that the voice had not woken him up again after he fell asleep suggested it did not have the power to wake him when he was deeply asleep, and that this was compatible with his sleeping right through the night on other occasions. She argued that this must mean the voice was very ineffectual and noted that, in contrast, Richard would have no difficulty waking someone up if they were asleep, even if they had taken sleeping tablets. She also argued that the fact that nothing had happened to him after these two occasions when he disobeyed the voice would be consistent with the voice not being able to harm him, even if it wanted to.

At this stage, Richard felt it was safe for him to try the Walkman and earplug to stop the voice if he heard it at night. When these were successful this was further evidence that the voice was not only weak but also considerably weaker than Richard himself.

It was not possible to adopt the 'direct questioning' strategy to disempower the voice until Richard had reached the point of believing that it was almost certainly a product of his own brain. At this point he became confident enough to ignore the voice when it spoke to him in the night and then to directly challenge it by asking *why* he should get up when it was he, not the voice, who would risk getting a nasty cold by so doing. This direct approach usually silenced the voice, which was interpreted as its 'mute submission' to Richard's superior reasoning abilities. And when nothing happened to him, this provided further evidence to support his new beliefs about the nature and powerlessness of the voice.

14 MODIFYING THE RESPONSES TO THE VOICES' COMMANDS

Voices that give instructions can be particularly damaging for the person themself, and/or for other people, if they are unable to resist carrying them out. Instructional voices often seem to come imbued with a sense of significance, power and compulsion, so they may be difficult or impossible to resist even though the person does not want to behave or react in the way that they do.

ASSESSMENT AND GOAL SETTING

The goal for command hallucinations is for the person *to be able to choose whether or not to follow the voice's instructions*. Although in practice this will often mean never doing what it tells them to do, in some cases the voice can give perfectly reasonable suggestions, which is not surprising, given that the voice is the person's own thoughts. For example, a man thought he should always disobey his voice, and on occasions this meant he could not have a cup of tea when he wanted one because the voice had pre-empted him by telling him to make one.

In a minority of cases, the voice's instructions are followed because the person believes that it knows what is best for them. If this is the case, then usually the goal is to modify this belief to 'I know what is best for me' or 'The voice sometimes, but not always, knows what is best for me, so I should consider what it says but then I should make the final decision'.

If the person is trying to resist the voice's instructions, then this suggests they have at least some good reasons for refusing to obey. Equally, if they do sometimes comply, then this suggests there are some advantages or benefits in obeying, even if these advantages are not immediately apparent. In this respect, responding to the instructions given by a voice is no different from any other piece of behaviour, i.e. the person will only act if the advantages of acting outweigh the disadvantages, albeit the balance may be tipped in favour of the advantages for only a very brief time.

In order to change the balance of advantages:disadvantages for obeying or disobeying the voice you need to know what these are, from the person's point of view, so this is very important information to get. Therefore, your assessment should include not only what the voice is instructing the person to do but also whether they try to resist it and if so, how difficult this is, how often they succeed in resisting it, and whether they have developed any strategies of their own to help them do this. Two other very important questions are (a) what happens when they obey the instructions, and (b) what they believe or fear will or could happen if they resist and do not obey. When collecting this information, do not forget to include the very important effects that obeying and resisting the instructions may have on the person's feelings and emotions, as well as the more obvious, objective results of their behaviour.

Alternative, replacement behaviours

It is important to consider what the person could do instead of responding to their voice's instructions. Doing nothing, just listening to the voice and trying to resist it, is likely to be less effective than identifying an active piece of behaviour that, at the very least, will act as a distraction. Ideally, the alternative, replacement behaviour would be incompatible with responding to the voice. For example, someone could not both stay at home and watch a favourite video *and* follow their voice's instructions to throw themself under a car, and someone could not both visit a friendly neighbour *and* take an overdose of the tablets in their bedroom.

Having identified and agreed a suitable replacement behaviour, you should seek to make it as easy as possible for the person to put it into effect. For example, if the replacement behaviour is to listen to relaxing music, then this might involve making sure the person has the discs or tapes and the means to play them available, perhaps with a list of which music to use. Or if the replacement behaviour is to visit someone, then this might involve having a list of options available, perhaps alerting the people on the list to the importance of responding positively if the person phones or calls in.

REMOVING/REDUCING THE ADVANTAGES OF OBEYING THE VOICE

The person may find it difficult to detect or report the advantages of obeying the voice, especially if they normally try hard to fight it and if the resulting behaviour is disapproved of by themself and others. For example, one woman was very hesitant to report the sense of relief and peace she got after obeying the voice's instructions to hit a member of staff. It is important to be non-judgemental and sympathetic about the advantages of obeying, and to acknowledge the adverse effects for the person concerned of not obeying, even if the outcome of the behaviour is undesirable for social or other reasons.

If there is a delusional fear that the voice can cause harm if it is not obeyed, then your first step is to remove this very persuasive reason for obeying it (see Chapter 13, pp. 249–252). An additional line of logical reasoning applicable in this context is '*The voice would not need to tell* **you** *to do that if it was able to do that for itself*'. For example, 'The voice would not need to instruct you to stab that policeman if it had the power to lift a knife and do the act itself. It needs *you* to do it because it is weak and cannot do anything itself other than frighten you with its words. So actually *you* are more powerful than the voice. It cannot harm anyone else, and so it cannot harm you, either'.

Some voices may have to be obeyed because of *who or what they come from*. For example, if the voice is believed to come from some powerful spiritual or alien force, then the person may consider it right and proper to obey its commands even if they conflict with their conscience or normal behaviour. In these cases it is usually necessary to modify the belief about the origin of the voice in order to remove its authority (see Chapters 12 and 13).

For many people, one of the major advantages of obeying their voice is that *it stops bothering them*, at least for the time being. This being so, if the voice can be stopped in some other way, for example by using an earplug or Walkman, then this can effectively remove one of the reasons for obeying it.

Obeying the voice is often accompanied by *a reduction in stress or agitation*. Where the stress or agitation is caused by the feared consequences of not obeying the voice, then CBT to modify these beliefs or fears is a key aspect of the treatment. However, clinical experience suggests that in many cases the high arousal levels are not secondary to what the voice says, though this will serve to exacerbate it, but have a more direct biological origin, i.e. the psychotic brain activity causes both the voice and the increased arousal. Anything that helps the person to relax is likely to be beneficial, not only because reducing arousal level by this alternative method may mean the person no longer has to obey the voice for this reason but also because reducing arousal level may have the secondary benefit of reducing the actual occurrence of the voice.

In some cases, it may be possible to remove the advantages of obeying the voice by *other means*, which are specific to the individual's circumstances. For example, a woman who followed her voice's instructions to hit her fellow patients when they pestered her for cigarettes identified two advantages of this behaviour: (a) the patients concerned stopped putting her under pressure, and (b) she gave fewer cigarettes away. Assertiveness training produced the same end results and so effectively removed these particular reasons for obeying the voice.

One of the disadvantages of always obeying the voice because of the feared consequences of not obeying is that the opportunity *to discover that nothing bad actually happens* does not occur. Put another way, always obeying the voice acts as an avoidance behaviour that maintains the fear. Once the voice has been disempowered sufficiently to allow the person to risk not obeying, and thereby to experience the true consequences of not obeying, then this may lead to a rapid decline in fear and belief in the voice's power.

INCREASING THE DISADVANTAGES OF OBEYING THE VOICE

As a general theoretical principle, increasing the negative consequences for obeying the voice's instructions, i.e. punishing the behaviour, should reduce the probability of this behaviour occurring. The major proviso to this general principle is that if the behaviour is being reinforced by anxiety reduction, then there is a risk that increasing the apprehension about the negative consequences of obeying may increase anxiety levels to such an extent that it actually increases the unwanted behaviour instead of suppressing it. Increasing anxiety levels will also tend to increase the intensity and persistence of the voice, which is undesirable.

Whatever the theoretical considerations, for ethical reasons it is not considered appropriate to administer 'punishment' as part of a treatment programme. However, there are nearly always some naturally occurring punishments that result from obeying the voice, for example having to face questions about the behaviour from staff, having medication increased, having a hostel place cancelled, having feelings of regret for disappointing family members, etc. Unfortunately, these 'natural' disadvantages of obeying the voice may be ineffective in controlling the behaviour, and this may be due in part (a) to the person being unaware or not thinking about the consequences, and (b) to the fact that the disadvantages occur in the longer term and therefore their immediate effect is not as great as the immediate gains of obeying the voice. Therefore, (a) it is appropriate to make the possible consequences known, by discussing them with the person, and (b) it may also be appropriate to make the long-term consequences more immediate by encouraging the person to think about or image them when the voice gives its instructions. For example, when a woman heard her voice telling her to throw a cup of hot soup at another resident, she would visualize telling her partner what had happened and her partner's disapproving reaction to this. Another woman, when instructed by her voice to cut her wrists, would remember how boring it was being confined to the ward after she had done this; she also reminded herself that the voice usually came back within the hour and pestered her just as much again, and she remembered how much she had regretted giving in to the voice the last time it had happened.

INCREASING THE ADVANTAGES OF RESISTING THE VOICE (AND OF USING THE REPLACEMENT BEHAVIOUR)

Imagery may also be used as a positive reward for not responding to the voice. For example, in the cases described above the first woman visualized the pleasure of being welcomed home by her partner and the satisfaction she would get from telling her partner she had resisted the voice, and the second woman remembered how enjoyable it was to be able to leave the ward and walk around the hospital grounds and go to the local shops, and how good she had felt last time when she did not obey and the voice finally went away.

In some cases it may be feasible to construct a behavioural programme wherein not following the voice's instructions for set periods is rewarded in some way, perhaps by interest and social praise from staff or by something more tangible like money or an outing. If an alternative, replacement behaviour has been identified, then positively rewarding this alternative behaviour will help the person to resist obeying, because it changes the balance between the advantages and disadvantages of obeying.

WEIGHING UP THE ADVANTAGES AND DISADVANTAGES OF OBEYING THE VOICE[1]

It is helpful to consider the advantages and disadvantages of obeying and disobeying the voice in terms of short- and long-term effects, since it is common

[1]The same principles can be applied to any other unwanted behaviour caused by the delusions or hallucinations.

for there to be short-term benefits for obeying the voice (often around reductions in feelings of tension or compulsion to act, and stopping the voice) and long-term losses or costs.

As with all cost/benefit analysis work, i.e. weighing up the advantages and disadvantages of something, it is important that you are unbiased with respect to the outcome and do not start off with the assumption that it is 'a bad thing' for the person to obey their voice, even if the resulting behaviour appears to other people to be undesirable. For example, one man felt so much better after obeying his voice's instruction to smash a hole through the wooden fence surrounding the hospital that it seemed unreasonable to try to prevent him doing this unless and until we were able to find another way of reducing his feelings of severe tension when they occurred.[2]

It is generally better to concentrate on the advantages and disadvantages as they affect the person concerned rather than as they affect other people. For example, if the undesired behaviour is hitting a fellow resident, then it is better to concentrate on what effect this will have for the person concerned, for example losing the resident's friendship, being hit back, being taken back into hospital, etc., rather than concentrating on how much it might hurt the fellow resident. This approach makes it clear to the person that in doing this exercise you are primarily concerned for *their* well-being. Furthermore, it is a fact of life that we are all inclined to be particularly concerned with how things affect ourselves, and people who hear voices are no different from the rest of us in that respect.

EXAMPLE OF A COST/BENEFIT ANALYSIS

The example given below shows the advantages and disadvantages of obeying a voice that 'advised' a young man in hospital to punch out windows and cut his arms on the glass.

	Advantages	*Disadvantages*
Immediate	Voice goes away Feel good, less stressed (lasts about five minutes) Attention from nursing staff	Pain Staff cross with me
Long term	Feel people are more interested in me as a patient	Arm hurts for several days Can't go out for walks or go to the shops Wife gets upset with me Feel a failure

[2]We were unable to find an adequate replacement behaviour. When he was threatened with discharge if he continued to damage the fences, he stopped doing it – and started cutting his wrists instead.

In order to reduce the 'advantages' he was given access to a Walkman, which was effective in giving him temporary relief from the voice. The agreed alternative strategy for providing relief from stress and for getting attention from staff was that he would seek out staff to talk to them about how he was feeling. To reduce the long-term advantage of feeling that cutting his arms made him a more important patient, the advantages and disadvantages of people showing interest because of his disabilities rather than his abilities were discussed and he agreed that he would rather people be interested in him as a person than as a patient. There was general agreement within the staff team to take care to show special interest in what he was doing when he was well and to put more emphasis on his non-illness-related activities.

In order to increase the 'disadvantages' we concentrated on the long-term effects of the cutting behaviour, not least because although the young man had put the pain of cutting in the 'immediate disadvantages' section, it appeared from discussion that there were also some advantages to the pain, linked to issues of control. It would not have been beneficial overall to emphasize the 'feel a failure' consequence because this would have countered the work we were doing to build up his self-esteem and to build up his understanding about his illness so that he would become sympathetic and non-judgemental about his own behaviour. Indeed, we argued that refusing to obey the voice was not a matter of 'success' or 'failure' but simply a matter of what served his interests best, taking everything into consideration.

Therefore, we concentrated on the other long-term effects, like being confined to the ward, and strengthened these by identifying and discussing them. At the same time, we identified and discussed the advantages of not cutting, so that all these factors would come to mind when he was making his decision about cutting.

EXAMPLE OF DISEMPOWERING A VOICE AND RESISTING ITS COMMANDS

When his psychosis went into relapse, Nigel heard a voice instructing him to self harm and to commit suicide. Usually he was able to resist its instructions but on a few occasions he had made very serious attempts at suicide, and over the years there were many incidents of significant self-harm. He found it particularly difficult to resist the voice when it threatened to harm members of his close family.

Nigel thought that his voice came from the spirit world. He was a spiritualist and gained great comfort from the positive voices he heard when well, so it would not have been functional to attempt to disempower the voice with a total modification of his belief about its origin. However, a partial modification was undertaken so that he ended up believing some of his voices came from his own brain and reflected his own fears and past experiences (traumatic memories from his time as a policeman) whilst others came from the spirit world. He devised a way of working out which were which, namely that if they were threatening and/or negative and destructive, then they could not be coming from the spirit world because all messages from the spirit world would be encouraging, supportive and helpful. In this way it was possible to disempower the negative voices without disempowering the positive ones.

The various lines of work to disempower the voice were summarized on cards.[3] The details given below are an amalgamation of these cards.

WHEN THE VOICES TELL ME TO DO SOMETHING

The voices are not real (not like my family or people that I know).

It is better *not* to do what the voices tell me.

In the past I have *not* done what the voices have told me – and later I was very pleased about this.

In the past I have harmed myself when the voices told me to (for example, when the voices said I had to put my hands under boiling water to get them clean from germs), and I've always been sorry afterwards.

At the time it seems easier to give in, but I will be sorry later if I do.

The voices are not my friends. They are not helpful. They don't tell me anything that is for *my* good. So I would be better off ignoring them.

THE VOICES HAVE NO POWER TO DO ANYTHING

The voice has predicted things that don't happen

For example:

- changes to the weather (this has happened several times)
- that the phone will ring (this has happened many times)
- that my son would be knocked off his bike
- that my daughter would be attacked on her way home from work if I didn't go to London to warn her

Things I thought had been made to happen by the voice could have happened anyway

For example:
- my sister was mugged
- my son's mobile phone was stolen

(When I was better, I realized when my car broke down that if I had been ill I

[3]This was only part of the treatment programme: the other major part was on the trauma memories that influenced the content of the voice and the threats it made.

would probably have thought the voice had done this, but this sort of thing can happen to anybody, and so can happen to me *without* the voice being involved.)

The voice was ignorant or told lies when it said:
- I would never get out of hospital
- the nurse had put poison in my food
- I was entitled to night-time tablets
- I was responsible for the deaths in the mudslides
- the dishes were still dirty, after I'd washed them.

When challenged, the voice failed to:
- make 'H' hear it
- wake 'H' at night
- stop the old TV from working
- lift a piece of paper from the chair.

It feels as if the voice has power, but I know it doesn't really have any power whatever it says. There is no evidence from the past that it can physically affect me or others. It can frighten and threaten but cannot actually carry out the threats. It is just a bag of nasty wind!

The voice itself cannot do what it instructs me to do. *If it could do it itself, it wouldn't need to tell me to do it.* For example, when the voice told me to pick up a knife and cut myself this was because it was unable to move the knife or cut me in any way.

I am much more powerful than the voice. It needs me to do the nasty things it tells me to do: it cannot do these things itself.

Summary

I do not have to do what the voice instructs for fear it will harm me or somebody else, because although it may threaten harm I know that it cannot do anything itself.

When I do follow the voice's instructions, it may quieten it for a short period but then it always starts up again.

It is for *me* to decide whether the short-term gain of following the voice is worth the long-term disadvantages of following it.

Before following the voice's instructions I should work out what the long-term effects will be, so that I can decide whether doing what the voice says will be the best thing for me or not.

15 DEVELOPING AND ENHANCING COPING STRATEGIES

PRIOR TO TREATMENT: LESSENING THE IMPACT AND DISTRESS CAUSED BY THE DELUSIONS AND HALLUCINATIONS

In the early stages of therapy, in the midst of thinking about the more sophisticated CBT modification strategies that you might use, do not forget to consider whether any plain, simple, practical strategies could help to reduce the adverse effects of the delusional belief or hallucination.

As part of your assessment you should find out if the person is already using some form of coping strategy. People may not think about what they do in terms of 'coping strategies', or even be consciously aware they are doing something that helps to control the unwanted experiences, so possible questions include:

- 'Do you do anything when you feel like this?' '... hear the voice?'
- 'Is it worse in some places than others?'
- 'Have you ever noticed anything special that helps at all when that happens?'
- 'In what way does it make you feel better?'
- 'Do you use it every time, or do you forget sometimes?'
- 'Would it be helpful if you were to use it more often?'

A strategy that the person has discovered for themself is 'safe' to use from the earliest therapy sessions, and you should consider if and how it could be used more effectively (see 'Coping strategy enhancement', below).

If you are suggesting a new strategy, or a significant change to an existing one, then you should consider whether what you are proposing will constitute a challenge to the delusional belief before it is safe to do so, or whether there are any wider implications beyond the immediate benefits. For example, using an earplug to block the critical voice of an archangel would avoid the distress caused by the criticisms, but might cause an increase in distress (a) if this confirms that it cannot really be the archangel talking, but is a sign of mental illness, or (b) if the hearer fears that the archangel will be very angry with them if they dare to block him when he is trying to talk to them, or (c) if they conclude that in order to block the archangel's voice there must be a special device in the earplug, implanted by the Devil, or even (d) if they fear that the earplug could get lost in their ear and travel into their brain. Fortunately, for most people the sort of simple practical strategies described here do not carry any wider implications and therefore can be used from the very earliest stages of therapy. However, an important sign to look out for is any indication of reluctance to use the practical strategy you have suggested. If this occurs, then it is safer to back off until you can ascertain why the person is not as positive about the 'helpful' strategy as you were expecting them to be.

Practical strategies fall into five broad categories. Although simple, they can be very beneficial on occasions; indeed in some cases, notably where people are reluctant or unable to engage in a 'talking' therapy, they may be the only or the most effective CBT treatment strategy that you are able to employ.

1. Distraction activities

As a general principle, the more demanding the task, the more distracting it will be.[1] However, the person may have poor concentration and/or motivation and so it may not be possible to use complex tasks.

It is important that, as far as possible, the person enjoy the distraction activity. This is not only because feelings of pleasure are effective counters to negative emotions such as anxiety and depression but also because the person is much more likely to continue to engage in the distraction task if they positively enjoy it. Therefore, when searching for possible distraction activities to suggest, it is important to explore with the person themself what they have enjoyed in the past and what they feel they might both like and be able to try in the present circumstances.

Activities involving other people are likely to be more helpful than solo activities, firstly because the presence of pleasant others may be reassuring, and secondly because it is easier to give up on a task if one is doing it alone.

In some cases, physical activity seems to have some beneficial effect over and beyond that of mere distraction, though it is not clear how this effect may operate. However, many people with psychosis do not engage with physically demanding activities for a number of reasons, including negative symptoms and other illness effects, and the side effects of the medication.

People with psychosis may become depressed or withdraw from social contacts as a part of their illness and/or in response to their illness, so the use of social distraction activities may also have the secondary benefits of improving mood and reintroducing the person to the benefits of a more involved social life.

For auditory hallucinations, verbal distraction activities are likely to be more effective than non-verbal ones because they use the same language areas of the brain that are needed to produce the voices. For the same reason, activities that require the person to engage in talking are potentially better than those that only require listening or reading. (See Chapter 10, p. 212.)

2. Changing the environment

The delusion or hallucination may be more troublesome in some situations than in others, so making changes to the person's situation may be helpful. For example:

- A woman who ruminated on her paranoid ideas at night was helped by cutting out her afternoon nap and altering her medication regime so that she slept through without waking up.

[1] *Caution:* Overactivity and too much excitement can increase arousal levels and thereby increase delusional thinking and voices even though the activities themselves are enjoyable.

- A man who sometimes misinterpreted the murmur of speech from the street outside as critical comments found he was much less agitated if he spent most of his time in the room at the back of the house.
- A man who heard threatening messages through his TV when his psychosis became active found it was helpful to 'ban' TV when this was happening.

Even in non-psychotic people voices are more likely to be heard in noisy surroundings (e.g. under a hairdryer or on a noisy road), or where there is a background of indistinct speech (e.g. people passing by outside a window or heard from afar), or a confusion of different people talking at the same time (e.g. in a party, crowded ward or canteen). Therefore, these factors should be borne in mind when considering if any changes to the environment might help reduce the hallucinatory voices.

3. Changing other people

Not all the changing needs to come from the person themself. Benefits may be achieved by other people changing what they say or the way they behave and interact with the person. Family therapy goes into this aspect in great depth, but unfortunately this is still a scarce resource and so for the majority of people with psychosis the only changes that can be suggested in this area are the more obvious ones that come up in the individual therapy. For example, a young man would become very agitated when his parents kept telling him that his girlfriend was a fantasy of his imagination, so it was suggested that they stop asking him about her. In another example, a woman's brother took her to a drop-in centre so she could benefit from the company and distraction there.

4. Relaxation and stress reduction

Increasing stress and arousal tends to increase the occurrence of voices and the intensity and preoccupation with delusional ideas, so anything that reduces these aggravating factors is potentially beneficial.

Most people with psychosis seem unable to learn and practise muscular relaxation in a formal training programme, but for those who do it can be very helpful. For example, a man who became very agitated when his psychosis became active and triggered paranoid thoughts and threatening voices learnt muscular relaxation when his psychosis was in temporary remission. To aid his regular practice he was given a 15-minute audio tape describing a peaceful beach scene.[2] During his periods of regular practice he burnt a vanilla candle and spent a short while after the tape had finished saying 'calm and relaxed' in time with his breathing: these latter features were added so that in times of stress he could cue the relaxation response by smelling the vanilla or repeating the mantra. Having learnt these skills during remission he was able to continue to use them to good effect when the paranoia and voices returned. He was undoubtedly helped by his partner in

[2]Ideally, if time permits, audio tapes should be tailor-made for the individual person so that the scene described is both safe and relaxing for them.

this relaxation training, as she practised regularly with him and reminded him to practise when his psychosis was bad.

People may be more willing to use less formal ways of relaxing, in which case the therapist's role is to identify what activities or places the person finds peaceful and relaxing and then to help them put these into effect when required. Often this latter involves making a list of the possible activities and making sure, where necessary, that the list includes details of how to carry them out. For example, one woman had a list that included: going to her bed and listening to a favourite piece of music; stopping the housework and sitting down with a cup of decaffeinated coffee and a book for one hour; taking the dog for a walk; having a bath with a special oil; sitting in the garden for at least 30 minutes.

5. Reassurance

For the reasons described in earlier chapters, the recommended approach for CBT with psychosis is to explore the person's belief(s) and experiences with an open mind, suspending disbelief where possible and accepting their way of looking at things, without disagreement, at least in the early stages of engagement. However, CBT is a flexible therapy and very few, if any, 'rules of therapy' are absolute. Therefore, if the person is very distressed by their delusion or hallucination *and* does not want it to be true, *and* is reassured rather than irritated if other people say they do not believe it to be true, then in these particular circumstances it may be appropriate to deviate from the usual approach and tell the person that *you* do not believe as they do, explaining your reasons. Even though they will probably not find your reasons convincing at this stage, they may find it mildly reassuring that you (and everyone else) are convinced by them. Furthermore, presenting the evidence and arguments against the delusion at this stage may cast just a shadow of doubt in the person's mind, which may be enough to encourage them to think it worthwhile exploring the issues further with you. For example, one of our young female patients believed she had had 20 or more babies and had killed them all. Although she was not persuaded by our arguments that she could not have had so many babies in that time, that someone would have noticed she was pregnant, that she would have required medical treatment that would be recorded in her notes, etc., she did accept that if we were all so sure she could not have done these things, then perhaps there could just possibly be some doubt about it.

You should be cautious about taking the line of giving reassurance because once you have come off the fence and stated your views then you cannot go back to the position of undecided, neutral enquiry. If you know the person well, then it is much easier to judge which approach will be the most useful at this particular time, but if you know the person less well or are unsure how they will react, then you should gently test this out. Using the 'other person' approach (see p. 74) may be a helpful starting point. Other people will have already tried telling the person that things are not happening as they think they are, so you can ask how they feel when people do that: Does it help? What is the most helpful thing that has been said? In what ways was that helpful or unhelpful?, etc.

You can give different levels of reassurance, so if you have decided it would be beneficial to take this line, then you will need to decide how definite your reassurance will be. As part of the assessment process, you will have asked the person about their delusional beliefs and hallucinatory experiences in order to set appropriate goals for modification, so you will probably have a good indication from their responses to these questions about their attitude to being disbelieved. If you are not sure whether they would welcome your reassurance or whether they would take this as a sign that you had failed to listen properly, then you can test the ground by starting with a tentative level of doubt (e.g. 'I'm not in your position, of course, but I don't think I can be as certain as you are that . . .') and getting more definite if the response is favourable (e.g. 'That seems unlikely to me' or 'I'm pretty sure that can't be true'). You need to be sensitive not to push your level of certainty too far, but there are occasions when an unequivocal reassurance is the most helpful: this is more likely to be appropriate and effective when the person already knows and trusts you. For example, a woman who knew she had a mental illness and who had just been readmitted to hospital was terrified by the sounds of gunfire coming from the hospital grounds. In the first few days the only thing that helped her was the reassurance of staff that they could not hear any gunfire and that they were convinced this was an hallucination and that she was safe.

CASE STUDY JANE

(See also pp. 76, 95, 99, 136, 143 and 188.)

Belief: *I am an evil witch.*

Immediate goal: *Reduce the distress caused by the delusional belief using simple coping strategies.*

The coping strategies described below were put into effect at the very beginning of treatment, i.e. before the belief modification work described in Chapter 8 was started (p. 188).

1. Jane's feelings of guilt about the Iraq war were made worse when she learnt about the individual incidents and atrocities that had happened, so as an immediate practical strategy it was recommended she stop watching the news on TV and avoid the daily newspapers.

2. She had noticed that she brooded less about what was going on if she was doing something active, so the occupational therapist devised a full OT programme for her.

3. If Jane went to the shops with someone else, she still noticed some people sticking out their tongues at her, but she felt safer. Therefore, it was suggested that whenever possible she go to the shops with a friend rather than on her own.

4. Jane was distressed when she noticed people sticking out their tongues and this suggested that a possible strategy to reduce anxiety in the immediate situation was to

avoid eye contact and avoid looking at people's faces when she went to the shops. However, when she tried this out she found it difficult and stressful to do. This was because when she checked she saw most people as being non-aggressive, and so looking them in the face provided reassurance of this fact; not having this means of checking meant that everyone who passed by was suspected of making aggressive facial gestures. The strategy was abandoned.

5. A key source of distress for Jane was her belief she was responsible for the events in Iraq. The replacement belief for the total modification was entirely acceptable to Jane from the beginning, and gently testing the waters indicated she welcomed other people's reassurance that they thought this was part of her illness. Therefore, the therapist gave her as many reasons as possible why *she* believed Jane could not be influencing events over there. She also explained how she thought Jane could have developed this belief that she was responsible for a war that had nothing to do with her, namely that her illness might have made her feel a sense of dread, a feeling that she must be responsible for doing something bad, and that this feeling then made her think she must be responsible for the war, not vice versa. In order to maintain the collaborative approach, this was presented as the therapist's opinion only, based on what Jane had told her, not as an established fact. The subsequent CBT treatment explored and established this alternative explanation.

CASE STUDY RICHARD

(See also pp. 204, 214, 226, 246 and 262.)

Goal 1B: *Reduce the distress caused as a result of hearing the voice.*

1. The voice was only a problem for Richard if he woke up to hear it. When he did not wake up he did not feel guilty or under any sort of threat the next day for not having chanted the prayer during the night. Therefore, the first practical strategies to control the voice were aimed at helping him to sleep through the night. It was suggested he go to bed later and omit his final cup of coffee, and his medication regime was changed so that he took more of his sedating medication at bedtime.

2. The voice was more frightening and insistent when it was dark, so arrangements were made for Richard to sleep with a small night light on.

3. One of the distressing aspects of this situation for Richard was that he felt compelled to kneel by his bed to pray, which was uncomfortable and cold. Therefore, arrangements were made for him to have a thick rug to kneel on and for extra heating to be available. This was not expected to have any effect on the voice as such, but was solely for the purpose of making its consequences less distressing.

COGNITIVE COPING STRATEGIES

As the CBT treatment progresses, arguments and challenges to counter the delusional ideas and voices will emerge, as will coping statements. The most effective and useful of these can be developed for use as coping strategies in everyday life; for example, using the reasons why the voice cannot really come from a Mafia boss, or the evidence that shows that the person's partner does *not* want her dead, or the reality test that will check out whether people really are reading the person's mind. Making these available as coping strategies commonly involves writing the key points on cards, so that the person can remind themself of them as and when needed (see pp. 294–295 for examples).[3]

COPING STRATEGY ENHANCEMENT (CSE)

CSE involves identifying a potentially helpful strategy, determining what the effective components of that strategy are and then experimenting to see whether the effective components can be used in a more reliable and targeted way. This applies to strategies the person has discovered for themself and to strategies suggested by the therapist.

What might be the effective component(s) of the strategy?

People may repeat an activity because they found in the past that it helped with a delusional idea or voice, but not all parts of that activity may be necessary. In order to refine and improve the effectiveness of a coping strategy you should try to determine which aspect(s) is the important one.

EXAMPLE OF DEVELOPING AND REFINING A COPING STRATEGY

A woman notices that her voices disappear when she is singing hymns in church, but unfortunately her church has only one service a week so the usefulness of this as a coping strategy is very limited. Consideration of what the key factors of this coping strategy might be immediately suggests some related activities that could be as or more effective and that would be more readily available. The woman could try out one or more of these activities to see how useful they are.[4]

[3]This area of work is covered in more detail in the next chapter, 'Maintaining the therapeutic gains'.

[4]New or changed strategies are usually introduced one at a time to make it easier to assess their use and effectiveness. In the table, the items separated by a slash incorporate different combinations of the factors that might be important and so need to be tested separately.

Possible reasons for effectiveness	*Other possible activities*
The sound of other people singing blocks the voices.	Listen to music/songs/hymns on a radio or CD.
The act of her singing blocks the voices.	Sing along with a CD of songs/hymns. Sing with a choir.
The words of the hymn are comforting.	Read books of a religious nature. Contact the vicar for support.
Being with the other people in the congregation is comforting and distracting.	Join other people at a day centre/church group.
The atmosphere and associations of being in church are comforting.	Visit churches to sit in them during the daytime.

Can the activities be expressed more clearly, or improved?

Vague plans are harder to carry out when needed than precise ones, so it is often helpful to agree (and write down) a specific plan of the 'what, when, where and how' for the coping strategy. For example, if a woman has found that she feels less paranoid if someone rings her up to talk to her, and the coping strategy derived from this is for her to ring someone up when she begins to feel uneasy or under threat, then it will be easier for her to do this if she has a list of phone contacts readily to hand with a plan of who to ring. Alternatively, if she finds she is unable to initiate the contact once she begins to feel paranoid, then arrangements could be made for other people to ring her on a regular basis.

In some cases it may be possible to improve on the coping strategy being used. For example, if a man feels less worried about his arms dropping off when he thinks about the discussions he has had with you in therapy but he cannot recall these in detail, especially when the ideas are at their strongest and causing him to panic, then you could write down the key points or tape record your session so that he could go through the full set of arguments whenever he needed.

Could the strategies be used more frequently and more reliably?

People may notice that something seems to help but then not go on to deliberately exploit it as a coping strategy, so one aspect of coping strategy enhancement is to see if the strategy could be used more frequently. For example, a woman felt better after doing her weekly shopping but had not considered breaking her usual routine and going more often, for smaller amounts, so she agreed to try smaller, daily trips to the shops. In a similar example, a man reported feeling less paranoid when he left his house but only had one regular appointment that he had to attend each week, so other places he could visit were identified and he was given a record sheet to act as a reminder and a motivator to prompt him to go out more regularly.

A coping strategy is not effective unless it is used, but it is not uncommon for people to forget to use their coping strategy(s) when they need it most. Although this can be a frustrating feature of this part of the therapy, this forgetfulness is not as surprising as it might seem, since the person will most need to use their coping strategy when the symptoms are at their worst, which is when the psychosis is at its most active; but the psychosis may also interfere with the person's thinking and memory so that the possibility of using a coping strategy does not come to mind. Ways of working to overcome this problem are discussed in Chapter 16, pp. 296–297.

Another problem that may arise is that when the psychosis becomes more active, and the delusional beliefs or voices become more overwhelming, then the person may feel that the coping strategy stands no chance of success and therefore is not even worth trying. In these circumstances you would try to collect 'evidence' of specific occasions when the coping strategy has been helpful, so that these can be summarized on a card to remind the person and to argue that it is at least 'worth giving it a go'.

Refining the coping strategy and its use: recording the effects

Each possible modification and improvement to the coping strategy is discussed with the person, who chooses which they would like to try in practice. They then try out the agreed plan. If the person is able to keep a formal record of when they use the coping strategy and what happens, then this is very helpful for assessing the usage and effectiveness of that strategy. However, very often people are not able to keep formal records in this way, especially as they are likely to be at their most agitated and/or psychotic when they most need to use their coping strategy, so in practice you often have to make do with an informal report of whether they used it and whether it was 'helpful'.

If you are asking someone to keep a formal record, then you should make it clear that it is entirely up to the person themself to decide whether or not they want to use the coping strategy in everyday situations, as and when these situations arise; otherwise, you run the risk that the person may say they have used it because they feel under pressure from you to do so.

When a strategy has been used, the results are discussed and then further adjustments are made, and so on, until the optimum coping strategy regime is achieved.

MEDICATION ADHERENCE

The large majority of people with psychosis get at least some benefit from taking medication. For many the medication effectively controls their symptoms, whilst for many more the medication provides a partial control. Therefore, taking medication can be a very important coping strategy for very many people; indeed, for many it is *the* most important one. Unfortunately, if people have little or no insight into their illness, then it is quite reasonable from their point of view to consider medication inappropriate, and if they are aware of unpleasant side effects or, as sometimes happens, actually blame the medication for their psychotic symptoms and experiences, then it is understandable if they are unwilling to take it.

Ethical considerations

People may be non-adherent for one of two general reasons: either (a) they want to take the medication but forget, or fail to take it for some other reason, or (b) they do not want to take it. When someone wants to be compliant there are no ethical issues with medication adherence work because, as the therapist, you are following the basic principle of using CBT to help the person achieve their own goals. However, when someone does *not* want to take the medication prescribed, and will very likely have expressed this explicitly as well as implying it by their behaviour, you are faced with an immediate ethical problem: should you embark on a course of therapy where your goal is diametrically opposed to that of your patient/client, especially as you will probably have to keep your goal concealed at the start of therapy? Whilst the resolution of this ethical dilemma will rest on consideration of each individual case, we have found it helpful to consider that our primary aim with people referred for poor medication adherence is not to improve medication taking per se but rather to improve the person's sense of well-being, which may or may not be achieved through taking medication. With this approach you can have an agreed goal (implicit or explicit) with the other person, namely that of trying to find something that would improve things for them in some way. This is genuine and honest on your part but avoids the likely conflict and loss of rapport if you were to immediately broach the medication issue. Of course, this approach does mean you should genuinely keep an open mind about whether or not medication has an overall beneficial result for the person and not just assume it is a 'good thing' because they are 'ill' and your colleague has prescribed it. It has been my experience in just a few cases that medication is not helpful, or causes significantly more negative than positive effects, but if this is the result of your investigation into the effects of the medication, then you should inform your colleagues, giving them all the information that you have, and support the person in their anti-medication position.

Attendance at therapy sessions

An obvious but necessary prerequisite for medication adherence therapy to be successful is that the person attends the therapy sessions, but, by the very nature of this particular patient group, engagement in treatment programmes is problematic. At best, they are likely to be indifferent to the prospect of meeting regularly with you, and at worst they may be actively hostile to the idea of seeing someone associated with the mental health team and/or to talking about the unpleasant 'treatment' for an illness that they do not have. Therefore, more than with any other aspect of CBT with psychosis, in this area of work you will need to be both flexible and very tolerant with respect to appointments and failed attendance.

Developing a rationale for taking the medication that makes sense to the person

Typically, people refuse medication because they do not think they have an illness, so a goal that is often used is to promote the person's understanding of their symptoms in terms of some biochemical abnormality that can be corrected by medication. However, it is not necessary to go for this particular insight to achieve adherence. Medication can be as relevant for helping symptoms attributed to LSD, X-rays, ghosts, etc. as it can for symptoms attributed to illness or psychosis. The rationales given below illustrate the range of insight and reasons that people have given to me for taking their prescribed medication.

Pragmatic
For example:

- I feel better overall for taking it.
- I don't get brought into hospital if I take it.
- My family/doctor/nurse doesn't nag me if I take it.
- The doctor/nurse knows best.

Partial insight; use of an intermediary concept
For example:

- It helps me sleep better.
- It keeps the dust away (it's the dust that makes me ill).
- It keeps me calm.
- It corrects the brain damage caused by the X-rays.

Biological, but not incorporating the notion of illness
For example:

- It stops my voices.
- It makes the biochemistry of my brain normal.
- It stops my brain being oversensitive and jumping to conclusions.

Biological, incorporating the notion of illness/psychosis
For example:

- I get paranoid if I don't take it.
- It treats the illness.
- It makes my psychosis better.

These rationales are not mutually exclusive and it would be normal practice to develop as many as possible in order to strengthen the reasons for adherence. Positive reasons are more likely to produce reliable adherence than negative ones, so where adherence is based on a negative rationale (e.g. 'I avoid arguments with my wife if I take it') you should try to develop a positive rationale(s) to add to it.

Rationales that incorporate some notion of changing or correcting brain chemistry are stronger than those that do not in that they provide a reason for taking medication rather than doing something else that might help. For example, if my rationale for taking medication is that it helps me sleep better, or keeps me calm, then I may decide that having a warm milky drink and listening to relaxing music will be just as effective as the medication. Therefore, wherever appropriate, you should seek to establish that it is the medication that (best) produces the beneficial effects.

Enhancing the existing rationale

When trying to find a rationale that will make sense to the person, a good starting point is to explore why they take the medication when they do, or why they have taken it in the past, as this may suggest a reason that already makes some sense to them and that could be developed and strengthened. For example, if the reason given is 'I sleep better for taking it and that makes me less worried about the police', then it might be helpful to develop this by linking both the poor sleep and the suspicions about the police to 'overactivity of part of your brain', which the medication corrects and returns to normal.

Finding a new rationale

Of course, it is not always possible to develop the existing rationale, for example if the only reason is 'because I am compelled to do so when I am under a section of the Mental Health Act'. In these circumstances you would need to develop a new rationale that would apply and make sense to the person concerned, which (you hope) would emerge from the work on changing the advantages:disadvantages of taking medication (see below).

As a last resort, you can try using the 'consequences' rationale, which looks at what, in practice, the consequences of not taking medication will be for the person, whether or not these consequences are 'fair' or 'justified'. In one case, this meant looking at what would happen if the man concerned got into another fight in the pub after he was discharged. Based on past experience, we noted that if he was *not* taking medication when this happened, then there was a much greater likelihood that the mental health team would attribute this behaviour to re-emergence of his illness (which, rightly or wrongly, they firmly believed he had) and therefore that they would re-section him to hospital, which he heartily disliked. On the other hand, we noted that if he was taking medication when the fight happened, then there was a better chance this would be put down to the effects of alcohol only, so that at least he was given a second chance. The man was indignant and angry about this, despite the therapist's best efforts to explain that the team acted in this way because they genuinely believed he was ill and that he could become dangerous if this illness was untreated. Nevertheless, he did accept the consequences as an accurate prediction.

Changing the balance of the advantages and disadvantages of taking medication

Whether or not the person understands they have a mental illness, at the end of the day someone will only take medication if, for them, the perceived advantages outweigh the perceived disadvantages. This balance becomes particularly important when control of medication is entirely in the person's own hands and there is no social or other pressure to encourage adherence, for example role expectation as a patient in hospital, desire to be seen to cooperate with treatment in order to get early discharge, mother overseeing the medication and getting upset when pills are not taken, etc. Therefore, the essence of this approach is to increase the perceived advantages and decrease the perceived disadvantages of taking medication until the advantages outweigh the disadvantages.

The first step is to *determine the negatives and positives* of taking the prescribed medication as experienced by the person concerned. If you are doing medication adherence work because the person does not want to take the medication (as opposed to just forgetting to take it), then it is more empathic and more productive to *start by asking about the negative aspects* and only later, tentatively, going on to ask about any possible positives. Someone who is being forced to take medication against their will may be very angry about its effects and hotly deny that it has any advantages. If you listen empathically to the disadvantages, and do not try to tell them about the 'good things' that medication can do or is doing for them, then they are likely to feel under less pressure to convince you that the medication is awful and therefore are more likely to admit to its having a possible or slight advantage (if, from their viewpoint, it has one).[5] If a 'possible' or 'minor' advantage does come up in these circumstances, you should resist the temptation to seize upon it and try to use it as a reason for taking the medication, because this would contradict your neutral stance of weighing up the evidence for and against.

You should identify as many of the disadvantages of taking medication as possible, because you will not be able to reduce any disadvantages you are not aware of. *Any perceived disadvantages that are based on delusional or dysfunctional beliefs should be modified using CBT principles* so that the person no longer has these reasons for refusing the medication, for example 'The drugs turn my skin yellow' or 'People look down on me for taking drugs' or 'The medication makes me feel paranoid'. *Where disadvantages are valid, it may be possible to reduce them* by some means; for example, a man who disliked having a 40-minute walk through the rain to get his depot injection was given these injections at home.

Be careful not to minimize the unpleasantness and impact of the side effects of some of these medications as they can be a very real deterrent to adherence. Weight gain and impaired sexual performance can be particularly pernicious,

[5]Obviously you will not be able to adopt this approach if you are the prescribing doctor, or if you have the role in the team of explaining why the medication has been given and persuading them to take it.

having serious adverse effects on the person's self-esteem and personal life.[6] Objections to these side effects should be taken very seriously and every effort made to find an alternative medication, especially when the drugs are being administered to someone who is under a section of the Mental Health Act or who, for some other reason, has no option but to comply. Apart from the side effects that people can describe, for example restlessness and slowed thinking, some antipsychotic medication seems to have some very unpleasant effects that people find very difficult to put into words but that make them reluctant to take it despite appreciating some of the advantages of doing so.

At the same time as reducing the disadvantages of the medication, you should be starting to *develop the perceived advantages*, by helping the person to be more aware of and to understand the beneficial effects of the medication as it affects them. A helpful starting point for getting some of the possible 'beneficial' effects is to ask the person *why* their doctor has prescribed the medication that they have – even if the medication is 'inappropriate' or 'awful' or 'poison', what was the doctor *hoping* it would do for them? Often people seem to have no idea why their medication was prescribed, in which case they are encouraged to ask their doctor about this and then you can discuss with them what the doctor said.[7]

Asking why the doctor prescribed the medication will also enable you to detect if there are any *negative or paranoid beliefs about the doctor or mental health team*. Where these negative beliefs exist it is usually appropriate to try to gently modify them, from 'They are giving me the medication to control or harm me, to experiment on me, to keep the hospital full so that they keep their jobs, etc.' to 'They are doing their best to help me, from the way they see things (even though they have got it all wrong)'. Apart from the obvious benefits of having a trusting rather than distrusting relationship with their doctor, if people see their *doctor as someone who is trying to help* them, then they are likely to be more willing to try the treatment the doctor suggests.

Understanding how their medication works may help people to understand why they need to take it, but by giving this information you will be implying very directly that their experiences or beliefs are manifestations of a mental illness caused by a biochemical abnormality, and it is difficult not to imply that you consider medication to be a 'good thing'. If it is important for you to maintain your stance of neutral, collaborative enquiry regarding the effects and benefits of medication, then another member of the team should take the lead on this part of the work. Alternatively, there are now some excellent leaflets available, for

[6]I do not recommend dieting for weight gain. In my experience it is virtually impossible for people who have put on large amounts of weight as a result of taking antipsychotic medication to lose this weight through dieting. Most of us are sensitive to critical remarks about our size and if you suggest a diet, this will imply that they are unattractive and unacceptable at their heavier weight, and their self-esteem is likely to suffer further when they 'fail' to stick to the diet or lose weight. In my opinion, with so little chance of success, it is better to use your CBT skills to try to weaken the dysfunctional belief that being overweight matters.

[7]If the person repeatedly 'forgets' to ask their doctor why they are on medication, then this suggests they know what the answer will be and are unwilling to confirm or discuss it.

example from The National Schizophrenia Fellowship and The Royal College of Psychiatrists, that describe how the different medications work. A secondary advantage of you not being the one to explain about the medication effects is that it enables you to ask the person about what they have been told, or read, and this enables you to assess how accurately they have understood the information and their attitude towards it.

Another important line of work is to explore with the person how they have been when they have been *'on' and 'off' medication in the past*, so as to establish a *connection between feeling better and being on medication*. This information is obtained not only from the person's own memory but also from the memories of others and from their medical notes. When the information from other sources contradicts the person's own memory, it should be double-checked for accuracy and, when the time is appropriate, introduced very gently.

A major factor that can hinder someone making the connection between being off medication and worsening symptoms is the length of time between the last dose being taken and the illness relapse, a period that can extend to weeks where medication was in the form of depot injection. On first stopping medication, people may actually notice an improvement in their general feeling of well-being because some of the side effects of the medication, for example drowsiness, may clear up quite quickly and so this tends to reinforce the belief that it was the medication making them feel unwell in the first place. It is perhaps not surprising that people do not causally connect events that are separated by days or weeks since in everyday life substances taken by mouth or by injection tend to have much more rapid onset and short-lived effects, as for example with aspirin or alcohol. Information about how the medication works and, in particular, how long it stays in the body will be necessary before the person can understand why something they did several weeks ago can make them feel poorly now, especially if they have felt better in between.

Showing that a connection could exist between missed medication and illness recurrence is particularly difficult where the person has stayed well for weeks or even months after discontinuing medication. In this case, you would have to explain the notion of a fluctuating illness, and the role that medication plays in countering the adverse effects of the illness as and when they re-emerge, and in preventing the illness developing. A relevant finding here is that people who remain on medication and thereby avoid relapses tend to do better in the long run than people who stop their medication and then wait until a relapse occurs before using medication to bring it under control again.

At some stage it may be helpful to *formally record the advantages and disadvantages* of taking the medication to help the person weigh them up. There are likely to be disadvantages associated both with being on and off medication, so at the end of the day the person will probably have to choose between the lesser of two evils. It is in our nature to try to find a positive option so you may need to work specifically on this point, to help the person see that, sadly, unlike other people, what is not possible is for them to be both well and free from the adverse effects of medication.

Note: If at any time this exploratory work suggests to you either that the person is getting no benefit from their medication or that the benefits are outweighed by the side effects, then you should report this finding back to the team and to the prescribing doctor in particular. It may be that a change of medication is indicated or even that the person would be better on no medication at all. *Remember, your role is only to help the person be aware of all the factors so they can make an informed decision for themself about whether or not to take the medication, and only to improve adherence if, on balance, taking the medication makes the person feel better than not taking it.*

Developing good habits for taking medication

Not all the people who fail to take their medication do so because they believe it to be bad for them or even that they would be better off without it. In some cases people fail to take their medication, at least in the first instance, for practical reasons, for example because they forget or because it is not convenient to go for their depot injection, etc. This being so, once the person has decided that, on balance, they are better on medication than off it, you should work with them to find the best possible regime to ensure they do actually take the medication as prescribed. This may involve discussing practical arrangements (e.g. location of depot clinic, days of appointment, etc.) and making appropriate changes around those where possible. If the person is forgetful or disorganized, it may be more fruitful to ask others to make the changes rather than relying on them to do so, for example asking staff at the depot clinic to phone them on the morning of their injection rather than trying to train them in the use of a diary.

As anyone who has been on a course of antibiotics knows, it is surprisingly easy to forget to take medication, so it is important for the person to develop a routine for taking their medication. Helping them develop an appropriate routine may be an important step in establishing adherence. The simpler and more repetitive the routine, the better chance it has of being established as a habit. The other important factor is to establish a trigger or prompt which will remind the person to take their medication when it is due. For example, if they take pills at night and in the morning, it might be effective for them to leave the medication bottle next to the bedside cabinet, or if they brush their teeth regularly twice a day, next to the toothbrush holder. Similarly, if the pills have to be taken at mealtimes and the person takes sugar in their tea, then it might be effective for them to leave a reminder in the sugar bowl to take the medication.

Dosset boxes (which, if necessary, can be filled by someone else) help to simplify more complicated drug regimes and provide an immediate reminder if a dose has been missed. Various electronic aids have been developed that can be useful, for example the pill box that bleeps at regular intervals or the appointments reminder that can be set to ring at specific times during the day.

Whatever the reminder chosen and routine developed, it must be one that fits in with the person's general habits and lifestyle. If the person lives at home or in a hostel, they may wish to include their relative or carer in their medication compliance routine, for example, by asking them to give the person a reminder when medication is due. (See also 'Putting the effective strategies into practice', pp. 296–297.)

16 MAINTAINING THE THERAPEUTIC GAINS

LONG-TERM STRATEGIES

Recognizing the symptoms when they recur

The essence of long-term therapy is for people to be able to identify their symptoms when they recur, so that they can put into effect measures to counter them. After a degree of insight has been achieved during therapy, many people start spontaneously to label their delusions and hallucinations (e.g. 'It's one of my odd ideas', 'It's just a voice'). This is a very positive step forward because it helps the person discriminate more clearly between what is due to 'illness' or 'overactive imagination' (or however they conceptualize their psychotic experiences) and what is not. This (a) helps to reduce the impact of the thoughts or voices (e.g. 'If it's only one of my paranoid ideas, then that means that "X" isn't really trying to poison me'), and (b) provides the person with a clear focus and trigger to apply learnt cognitive and other coping strategies (e.g. 'If it's one of my paranoid ideas, then I will feel better if I leave my room and go to talk to someone'). Whilst some labels may stem from the therapist and be mutually agreed during rephrasing and recapping, wherever possible it is better to use the person's own words for labelling as these are likely to be more accurate in describing their own experiences.

During the course of therapy you are likely to have identified some characteristic features of the delusional ideas and hallucinations that the person can use to help detect when a delusional idea or hallucination has occurred. Note that 'detection' in this context does not necessarily mean the person is immediately able to recognize the idea as definitely delusional or to recognize that what they hear is definitely an hallucination; often the goal is for the person to recognize that this *could* be a delusional idea or hallucination, and therefore that they should apply the various tests and techniques learnt during therapy in order to examine it further before coming to a decision.

When *the content of the delusional beliefs* are quite specific, then it is easier for the person to detect their reoccurrence, for example 'I know that one of my paranoid ideas is that my brother is trying to poison me, so if I get this idea then it is a sign my illness is having a dip again; my brother doesn't want to poison me and I know this because ...' Similarly, someone may learn to be sensitive to and question any thoughts that *follow a particular theme*, for example 'I know that I can develop paranoid ideas about people, so if I get a feeling that someone wants to harm me, this could be one of those paranoid ideas. I must look for objective evidence that would be acceptable in a court of law to back up the feeling, and I might be able to check it out by ... If I can't find any evidence to prove the feeling, then I will know it is one of my paranoid ideas and not really true'.

Or it may be *some other feature associated with the delusional belief or with worsening illness* that is recognized. For example, a man who experienced a sense of 'life speeding up' when he became unwell was able to incorporate this into his coping strategies. Whenever he got this feeling he would rigorously check all ideas he had about people being against him by looking for evidence and asking friends what they thought. In another example, a woman learnt to associate an increase in voices with an increased likelihood of paranoid thinking, 'If I can hear those voices again I must be careful because at these times I am very likely to get the idea that someone is trying to harm me in some way. These feelings are very convincing but when I have checked them out in the past they have proved not to be true in fact, so although the feeling may be very persuasive now I must look for proof to back it up. If I can't find any proof this means it is my brain misleading me and the person doesn't really wish me any harm'. Another woman learnt to be particularly vigilant for the first couple of hours after getting out of bed in the morning: 'I very often get horrible thoughts about the staff interfering with me in the morning, but it goes by lunchtime and in the afternoon I realize that they like me and wouldn't want to harm me.'

Hallucinations are generally easier for someone to detect than delusional ideas. If the person is able to detect something different about *the physical characteristics of the voices*, as compared to the sound of the voices when they come from a real person, then this can help them decide whether or not what they have just heard are 'voices'. Examples of this are: 'If I can't tell which direction it's coming from, then it must be one of my voices' and 'If it sounds as if it's coming from just two or three inches away, then that means it is being produced by my own brain'. In some cases, people may learn to recognize that there is something different about the voices, or some different sort of feeling associated with hearing them, even though they are not able to describe this 'difference' in words. They should be encouraged to recognize this difference when it occurs. For example, one woman found that when she heard her hallucinatory voice, she was only 95% certain it came from a real person, whereas with a real person she was 100% certain. Having identified this feature, she was able to use the check 'If I'm only 95% certain it's real then it's not, it's one of my voices'.

Some voices can be recognized as such because of *the particular words used*. For example, one man's voices always said 'You're a hypocrite' or 'You're talking through your hat' so he learnt that whenever he heard these accusations they were voices and not coming from real people. In another example, a woman noted that her voice was particularly likely to use the words 'well, actually', whilst another woman discovered that being addressed as 'bitch' was typical of the voice but atypical of everyday social contacts. In other cases, the words used may be *atypical of the people they seem to be coming from*, for example when obscene words seem to be coming from strangers, or lewd remarks are heard during a social conversation, and this feature can be used as a sign that they come from a voice.

Voices typically follow certain *specific themes* for individual people, for example, sexual history, sins committed in the past, envy, etc., so once these themes have been identified they can be used by the person as an alert to the possibility or even probability that what they heard came from a voice. For example, having heard something relating to these themes the person may be able to reason 'Be careful, this is the sort of thing my voice says, I need to check where it's coming from before I act on it' or recognizing it as the sort of thing their voice says could trigger them to bring other checking mechanisms into play, like asking a friend if he had heard the voice too, or asking themself if it is likely that the person concerned would have said what they apparently heard him say.

DEVELOP CBT STRATEGIES TO COUNTER AND COPE WITH SPECIFIC DELUSIONAL BELIEFS AND HALLUCINATIONS

The downside of the fact that the new beliefs established during CBT overlie rather than completely eradicate the delusional beliefs they replace is that the person will always be potentially vulnerable to a reactivation of these delusional beliefs, should the conditions be right (see 'Belief modification', Chapter 1). However, the upside is that in times of relapse it is the same delusional beliefs that tend to recur, even if they are disavowed in between, and so it is possible to plan ways of countering them before the relapse occurs. The logical arguments, evidence and reality-testing results, etc. that were found to be useful during therapy are collected together so that they can be used immediately to combat the re-emerging delusions and help prevent them becoming firmly re-established. Similarly, you can take the person through the most effective challenges to their voices. These can be repeated as many times as necessary to ensure that they come to mind naturally and spontaneously whenever the voices reoccur.

Develop coping statements

Coping statements are peculiar to each individual person, being built up from the rational arguments and evidence obtained about the delusions; for example, 'The voice has lied in the past, so I shouldn't believe it now' and 'I know from the experiments we did that no one else can hear the voice, so I don't have to get off the train to ensure that other people won't hear it'. Coping statements are often used to trigger coping behaviours; for example, 'If I am beginning to feel isolated in my room, I am particularly likely to get the feeling that people don't like me any more, but I have found in the past that going down to the day centre helps stop that feeling. So although it feels like a tremendous effort, I must make that effort and go to the day centre; it will be well worth it in the long run. I will treat myself to a cake when I get home'.

Coping during 'bad patches'

Fluctuations in psychosis are common in the medication-resistant population and often, when in relapse, people feel as if they have always felt this bad and that it will never get any better. This is due in part, at least, to the effect of mood-dependent memory, which means that when they feel bad they are literally unable to recall the good times. In these circumstances, it may be comforting as well as helpful for the person if they have developed a coping statement around the duration of these fluctuations or 'bad patches'. By carefully monitoring these periods as they occur during therapy and/or by going through the past case notes, the person, when well, will be able to write a statement along the lines: 'Although I feel as if this will go on for ever, in the past it has usually lasted for about . . . days, so if I can just keep going it will get better.'

Insight into the nature and likely extent of a bad patch may also help to prevent dysfunctional behaviour, the more extreme forms of which can include violence to self or others. For example, one woman who put her arm through windows when she felt bad developed the statement, 'If I can just keep going for another couple of days without putting my arm through a window I will feel better then and be able to enjoy myself again, but if I have put my arm through a window, I may be transferred to the locked ward and then I won't be able to ride my bicycle. If I feel really tense I can go into the garden and shout at the roses'.

Make cards detailing the effective CBT strategies

An obvious but essential requirement for the success of long-term therapy is that the person actually uses the effective strategies when they need to do so, so facilitating this is an important aspect of long-term therapy work. The most common way of doing this is to summarize the key points on cards (often called 'cue cards' or 'flash cards') so that they are readily available to the person. These cards will typically contain summaries of the most effective lines of logical reasoning, evidence evaluation and results of reality tests, together with a conclusion of what these showed, and/or a reminder of coping statements and strategies that can be used.

As far as possible the cards should be written by the person themself and include the things that *they* have found to be most persuasive and helpful and want to include, and they should be expressed in *their* words. Whether the cards are written in terms of 'I' or 'You' is a matter of personal preference and differs from person to person. We have found from experience that the cards should be small enough to be kept in handbags or pockets and strong enough to withstand being crushed against other things; A5 card or file cards are convenient. It is advisable to keep photocopies in your notes, not only for the sake of having an accurate record but also in case the person loses theirs and another copy is urgently required.

EXAMPLE OF A CARD TO HELP DEAL WITH RECURRING VOICES

The following card was developed for a woman who heard voices of unknown origin, usually accusing her of something that was false or instructing her to do something to harm herself. The card incorporates the particular strategies that she had found helpful. Note that, in her case, directly questioning the voices always shut them up for a while, so it was a safe and effective strategy to use.

CHALLENGING THE VOICES

To get rid of the voices:

1 Tell the voices that you know they tell lies and talk nonsense.
2 Tell the voices to go away.
3 Use a Walkman to stop the voices.
4 Go and talk to someone.
5 Go on a brisk walk.
6 Avoid TV, because you may get false 'messages' from it.

To challenge the voices:

1 Ask them for *evidence* to support their claims, for example when the voices are accusing you or other people of something.
2 Go through your individual cards if you need to remind yourself of the evidence *against* what the voices are saying.
3 If the voices tell you to do something, ask 'Why should I?'. Tell the voices 'I don't trust you – you've told me to do some terrible things in the past, for example drink poison – you've never told me anything that's for my good'.
4 If the voices say you are responsible for some event, ask 'How could I be responsible for that?'.

EXAMPLE OF A CARD TO HELP DEAL WITH A RECURRING DELUSIONAL IDEA

The example given below is a card used by a woman who had recurrent feelings that people hated her.

When I get the feeling that people hate and despise me, it's due to my brain chemistry. Therefore, other people do not really hate me, even though I feel that they do.

Evidence that the feeling is due to my brain chemistry

1 It wouldn't make sense that people would change so drastically from day to day about how they felt about me when nothing has happened between us. For example, when I kept a record I noted that it felt as if Maureen hated me on days three and five but on the other days I knew that she liked me.
2 There would be no reason for people who knew nothing about me to hate me.

3 The feelings are worse before my period is due.
4 Whenever I've actually asked people if they hate me, they've told me they don't.
5 When I look for evidence that my friends and family hate me, I can never find anything that would stand up in a court of law. Actually, they continue to do nice things even when I feel they hate me.
6 The only reason I have to think people hate me is the strong intuitive feeling that I get, but even very strong feelings can be quite wrong.

When I get the feeling that people hate me

1 When I get the feeling that people hate me it's my brain being oversensitive and giving me the wrong message. My higher thinking is better able to work things out and tell me what is really happening, so I should rely on what my reasoning tells me, not the intuitional feelings.
2 These feelings only last for a day, or at most two, so if I can stop myself being snappy with people I won't upset them and have to apologize later.
3 Sometimes I feel better if I go off to my room and listen to my music.
4 Also, if I talk to staff about what I feel they can remind me that this is only a feeling, that it won't last and that people really like me.

EXAMPLE OF A CARD TO HELP DEAL WITH FEELINGS THAT ORDINARY EVENTS HAVE SPECIAL SIGNIFICANCE

A man had episodes when everyday situations could suddenly take on a sense of great significance. We discussed how the brain could produce these feelings *without* there being anything significant in the situations themselves, so the card below was developed to help him decide, when he got the feeling of significance, whether the situation really was significant or not.

He also heard voices, which he recognized as a symptom of his illness. These voices could also, on occasions, be imbued with a sense of great significance. However, the situation was complicated by the fact that the religious faith to which he belonged believed that God could communicate directly with people through words, so he was also concerned to have a way of checking whether a 'significant voice', when it occurred, came from God or not.

WHEN THINGS SEEM SIGNIFICANT

This could be an internally generated feeling, caused by your brain.

What other explanations could there be?

- Can you think of any other ordinary (i.e. non-significant) reason(s) why this has happened?
- How would someone else, in the same situation, interpret what was happening?

- Having considered the other possible explanations, which is the most likely to be correct? Which one(s) would other people think most likely to be correct?

Is this a 'voice'?

- Could what you heard be one of your voices, generated by your own brain? Remember that hearing a voice out loud saying something does *not* mean that someone has actually said that.

Is this a message from God?

- Would God choose this way of indicating something to you?
- Is this message or instruction important and meaningful enough to come from God?
- Is it the sort of instruction that would come from God? If it came from God, it would be caring and helpful for you and for others.
- If God can alter things in the environment to indicate something significant for you, could He write it down on paper to make it clear what He wants?

Is this a genuine spiritual experience?

- Since your brain can cause you to experience something as spiritually significant even when it is not, it is important that you do not misinterpret things with respect to the . . . faith.
- To check whether your experience is genuine or not, and to seek further guidance, ring . . . [A senior member of the faith].

Putting the effective strategies into practice

However wonderful the long-term strategies or flashcards may be, they will not benefit the person if they are not used when needed. Therefore, putting in ways of cueing the use of the coping strategies is an important aspect of the work. This will require innovative thinking from the therapist because the cues used have to be tailor-made to the individual person and their particular circumstances and so can vary greatly from person to person.

Frequent repetition of the effective lines of CBT during therapy will help to make these come to mind; for this reason it is helpful to keep to the same terminology (ideally that of the person concerned) when you are repeating these in session rather than succumbing to the temptation to vary or develop them for fear of sounding boring. *Frequent reminders* during the course of therapy to use the challenges and coping strategies in everyday life, in between sessions, will also help to establish them as second nature. If people forget to use their flash cards when needed, then you should consider suggesting they *read the card daily* for a while, firstly to help them remember that they have the card, and secondly to establish the content in memory so that they can recall it when needed without having to read the card. Or it may be helpful to consider *where the card is kept*; for example, it is more likely to be remembered if it is kept on the bedside cabinet than if it is hidden away in a drawer, or it may be more helpful if it is carried around in a pocket or handbag so it is immediately available when needed.

Although it is generally more empowering for people to control their illness themselves rather than relying on help from elsewhere, *using other people to do the reminding* can be an effective way of cueing the use of a coping strategy, so if the person agrees, then this option should also be considered. Some people may find it useful for *someone else to have a copy of the flash cards* (e.g. a relative or hostel staff), but this should only be done with the person's full agreement. This not only ensures that a spare copy is available if required but also means that other people will know and be able to use the most appropriate and helpful lines of reasoning etc., if the person's delusional ideas or voices recur. (When other people are given these cards they should be strongly advised not to elaborate or deviate from the content as this could cause confusion or, even worse, undermine the CBT that has been done.)

Some people become very adept at *knowing what their therapist would say or suggest*. When this occurs it can be very useful as a way of transferring the CBT skills from the therapy sessions to everyday life. One way of encouraging the skills to develop is to ask during therapy 'What do you think I would say to you now?' rather than launching straight away into the appropriate CBT strategy. I have known a number of people who successfully managed their symptoms by asking themselves 'What would Hazel say to me now?'. At some stage, when there is no risk that it will weaken the perceived validity of the strategy, you should feed back that all this CBT wisdom is actually coming from the person themself and has absolutely nothing at all to do with you. This is empowering for the person and also helps encourage them to trust their own thinking and judgement on a wider range of issues.

RELAPSE PREVENTION

Early detection of relapse enables appropriate action to be taken before the effects of the psychosis become overwhelming. Therefore, an important set of coping strategies to develop is the ability (a) to detect the 'warning signs', and (b) to respond appropriately to the early signs of relapse. The warning signs and action plan are discussed and agreed, and written down. Where appropriate, i.e. where the person wants to involve someone else, for example a carer or trusted contact in the care team, and there is a suitable someone else to involve, then it is useful for this person to have a similar (it is unlikely to be identical) set of warning signs and 'action plan', also written down. This is constructed in collaboration with the person themself.

The list of warning signs can be built up when the person is relatively well and written down for them to use, either at regular intervals, as a sort of checklist, or when they begin to feel unwell. Once the possibility of relapse is detected, the person refers to their action plan for what to do. These actions may include items such as 'Read my therapy cards' or 'Tell my carer' or more idiosyncratic items such as 'Cut down on the alcohol' or 'Don't stay indoors on my own'. By the very nature of the illness, the person may not be able to detect relapse in themself and may even be antagonistic towards any intervention at this time, which is why involving someone else can be very useful. In addition to the person's own relapse prevention plan there would be an agreed plan of action for the other person to take should certain signs or criteria be met; for example, a woman's husband would contact the doctor or social worker if she started to hear gunfire from outside the house, and a man's wife would check his dosset box if he became agitated and started talking about the witch doctor upstairs. One advantage of having agreed and formally recorded this plan of action before the person becomes unwell is that it helps the friend or relative to counter any accusation of betrayal (e.g. 'I'm not trying to get rid of you, you asked me to contact your doctor if ...') This may not be very effective at the time but it may help to repair the trusting relationship later.

Having the warning signs of worsening illness identified and written down not only alerts the person to the possibility of a relapse when this occurs but also has the less obvious benefit of helping them and their carers not to immediately attribute everything unusual to worsening of the illness, for example an outburst of temper or not sleeping one night.

The agreed relapse plan is tested in practice the next time the person relapses. Any problems are noted and are discussed when the person is well again to see if there is a way they can be overcome. For example, a man may plan to contact his doctor when he begins to be suspicious about his family but discovers that when this actually happens, he thinks it could really be true this time and therefore that contacting his doctor is inappropriate. With this experience, when he is next well he may decide that if this happens again, it would be better if his sister phoned the doctor on his behalf when he started accusing her of trying to steal his money. This new relapse plan is retested when the person next relapses, modified if necessary, and so on, until a workable, effective plan is developed.

EXAMPLE OF A RELAPSE PREVENTION PLAN[1]

The man whose relapse prevention card is detailed below identified three different levels of illness. The first level symptoms could come and go, so the action plan for this level identified strategies that would help him cope with them when they occurred. The second level (not included here, for the sake of brevity) represented worsening symptoms, but the action plans for himself and his mother were still concerned with helping him to cope with the symptoms *in situ*. The third level signs indicated that the psychosis was in relapse, and by this stage he was relying on his mother to take the effective action. His mother had a similar card, which identified the signs as they appeared to her and included the action plan of how he wanted her to respond to these signs.

[1]Another aspect of this case is discussed on pp. 295–296.

The relapse prevention plan was developed when the man was relatively well. He had a very good understanding of his illness when he was well, and both he and his mother were exceptionally adept at using CBT strategies to control and cope with his psychotic experiences.

SIGNS OF BECOMING UNWELL

Note: Out of the five times I have relapsed, on four of the occasions it happened when I came off medication.

- Therefore, if I have taken myself off medication, I should be particularly vigilant for signs of relapse.
- Also, if I have taken myself off medication, then it is very likely any feelings of significance, etc. I get are due to my brain going off balance.

1st level signs
- feelings of significance about what my commonsense tells me are insignificant or meaningless actions (e.g. feel that I have to buy a bike)
- begin to lose some clarity of thought
- easily distracted, for example by external noises
- rushing around, trying to do several things at once and rushing from one thing to another
- feelings of enhanced suspicion.

What I can do:
1 Play my relaxation tape.
2 Call and talk to mum.
3 If I'm rushing around:
   (a) Stop. Count to 10. Deep breathing through nose.
   (b) Make a list, do one thing at a time. If this is difficult, speak to mum if I want.

What I would like my mother to do:
1 Ask me if I am taking medication; if I am not, for my mother to spell it out to me, i.e. to start taking medication again in order to prevent hospital admission.
2 Talk to me softly and gently. Be sympathetic. Try using CBT to help me look for alternative explanations and regain insight.
3 Encourage me to reread my notes and 'challenge' the voices and suspicious thoughts.

. . . .

3rd level signs
- Voices more or less continuous. They are so convincing that I am unlikely to detect that they are voices or believe my mother if she tells me that is what they are.

- My behaviour becomes more erratic.
- For me, it appears that people really are making unpleasant comments and remarks about me.
- I'm fearful of other people, including my mother.
- I'm convinced that my mother is evil, a black witch or inhabited by a male extra-terrestrial.[2]
- There is a risk that I may obey the voices, even if what is said is very dangerous for me (e.g. stop that car).

What I can do:

1. Try to listen to mum and 'G'. [a friend]
2. Ask for 'E's' opinion. [a senior member of the faith]
3. Look at my folder and all my information on schizophrenia. I wouldn't have this stuff if I didn't have schizophrenia.

What I would like my mother to do:

1. Arrange for hospital admission as soon as possible. By this stage there is too great a danger of my harming myself or someone else. Also, it is very distressing for me to feel so frightened and threatened all the time. If I have reached this stage, only hospital admission will help to get things better again.
2. I would like my mother to do this for me, for my own well-being, even though I will resent it and dislike her for it at the time.

[2]He had a separate sheet detailing the reasons and evidence against this belief, which he constructed when he was well.

17 PUTTING THE THERAPY INTO PRACTICE, SAFELY

FORMAL THERAPY[1]

Warning for therapists: it is easier said than done!

Like many worthwhile things in life, CBT with delusions and hallucinations is easier to describe in principle than it is to achieve in practice. CBT with this client group is *not* easy. Delusions, hallucinations and psychotic experiences come in all shapes and sizes and for a variety of reasons. The development and maintenance of delusions and hallucinations are complex processes, involving many different factors, so case formulation is not easy. Furthermore, there are many different aspects to the psychotic experiences and beliefs, and so there are a correspondingly large number of goals and possible CBT strategies that might be applicable. Every case is truly unique and has to be considered as a special case, so a 'cookbook' approach to this area of work is totally inappropriate. Added to this, by the very nature of the psychosis, engagement and commitment to therapy may be absent or limited and the psychotic experiences may continually reinforce the delusional beliefs and hallucinations you are trying to modify.

In view of the difficulty of this work it is important that you *do not become discouraged by slow or erratic progress, or indeed by no progress at all.* It is dysfunctional in this area of therapy to have high expectations of success, such as 'I ought to be able to help all or most of the people referred to me' or 'I ought to be making faster progress'. Be on the alert for negative thoughts along the lines: 'If I were better at therapy, I would be able to get positive results with this person' and 'If "X" were here, I'm sure *they* would do better and be able to do something for this person.' More functional and realistic underlying beliefs in these circumstances might be:

- 'With such a difficult illness to treat, any progress I can make will be a very positive success.'
- 'It's better to go slowly, even if no progress is made, than to try to push ahead too quickly and risk making the person worse.'
- 'I know that not everyone with psychosis will respond to a CBT approach but since I don't know who will respond and who won't, I can give it a try – that is the best I can do for this person.'
- 'Even if I make no progress in modifying the delusions and hallucinations, it is

[1]Formal therapy refers to the use of CBT in a course of one-to-one therapy sessions conducted by a therapist who has been trained in this area of work.

right that someone should take the time and effort to *try* to alleviate this person's suffering.'

- 'Perhaps the person has benefited in other ways from our relationship and the time we have spent together.'

Because of fluctuations in the underlying psychosis, *progress may be erratic* with gains made in one session appearing to be completely lost by the next. If this happens, you should proceed cautiously as this may not be a good time to try to push the therapy forwards; however, it may be helpful to remember that it will be quicker to regain the ground you have already covered than it was to cover it for the first time.

Conviction in a belief may fall gradually as the challenging work continues but not infrequently the therapist feels as if no progress is being made at all, only to find that *the belief change, when it does occur, occurs quite suddenly*, often between sessions. So do not be discouraged or deterred from continuing with therapy if all your best efforts seem to be getting nowhere. The modification you are working towards could appear quite suddenly.

One effect to be aware of in this area of work is that *the beneficial effect of therapy may not always be recognized* by the person themself. After successful modification some people may dismiss their previously held delusional beliefs as if they had been of no significance for them. This can be disconcerting for the therapist, not least if it causes you to wonder if all the time you spent with the person had really been necessary. I well recall with one of my early cases reporting to our ward team how pleased I was that we had been able to modify a woman's very distressing belief that she would be doomed to eternal damnation. On interview, the woman certainly looked cheerful and agreed that she was not damned, a gratifying moment for me, but then went on to add that she did not think she could ever have really believed such a thing possible! Disconcerting as these denials or minimizing of the previously held delusional beliefs may be for the therapist, from the cases we have seen we are now confident that this can be a sign of a profound and secure belief change and as such should be welcomed. It is as if, looking back with the hindsight of the new firmly held positive belief, the person cannot credit that they could ever have believed differently. It may also be a reassuring sign that you have done your work so slowly and thoroughly that the person is able to attribute their new understanding to their own efforts rather than to your interventions.

In your early days as a therapist it is likely that you will not think of all the possible approaches that could be tried (this is often true for more experienced therapists, too) but *it is better to try some potentially beneficial techniques than none at all*, providing you apply these techniques safely. Some new therapists are worried that by discussing the delusional beliefs and voices with the person, or in attempting to intervene, they may inadvertently make things worse. Whilst you certainly should not be gung-ho in your approach to this work, neither should your apprehension about making a possible mistake prevent you from trying these strategies. As a very general rule, if you are sufficiently sensitive and aware of what could happen to be worried about making things worse, then you will not do so. Undoubtedly an unscrupulous therapist could make someone's symptoms worse by misapplying CBT strategies, but they would need to set about this deliberately and, furthermore, have the expertise to know how to do it. Providing you are sensitive to the other person as a fellow human being and follow the promptings of your sense of kindness, then it is highly unlikely you will make things significantly worse for them by using CBT inexpertly; the worst thing to happen will be that your efforts will be ineffective, not that they will do any positive harm.

The complexity of this work can be daunting, and it is easy to lose track of what you are doing and to confuse the various lines of therapy you are trying to take. For this reason it is suggested that you make frequent reference to the overall summary charts given in Appendix 1 in order to provide a structure for your work. Whilst this is certainly not an exhaustive list of strategies, or the only way of organizing this therapeutic approach, it may provide a useful reminder of some of the different lines of work that could be used, the reasons for doing them, and how they relate and interact with one another.

INFORMAL THERAPY

CBT for psychosis is still a scarce resource so many people with dysfunctional delusions and hallucinations do not have the chance to receive this form of treatment, and amongst those who do, some are not willing to engage in formal therapy settings. Even when someone is receiving a course of CBT, they are likely to spend many more hours each week in informal contacts with other people than they will in formal therapy.

The potential therapeutic importance of informal contacts and the opportunities for informal therapy that these provide should not be underestimated, and professionals who are seeing people for other reasons can use these opportunities to employ the CBT approach to good effect. People who have not been formally trained in the use of CBT with psychosis can make significant therapeutic contributions in these situations. However, whilst some CBT strategies can be used safely in these circumstances, others cannot, so it is important to know which are which.

Probably the single most useful CBT strategy, in both formal and informal therapy, is that of *empathic listening and talking to the person from within their own belief system*. This strategy can be used safely in any situation, with anyone, even in the most casual of contacts with someone you have never met before.[2] It can be used whatever the level of insight, and regardless of whether formal goals of therapy have been considered or set. I feel that I cannot emphasize too strongly the potential therapeutic, as well as human, importance of these contacts. Being prepared to spend time with someone, seeking to understand how

[2] 'Safely' refers to how safe it is for the person you are talking to, i.e. free from risk that your intervention may make them worse.

it is for *them*, indicates your concern and respect for them, and accepting how it is for them, as they tell it, validates their experiences. Furthermore, providing a situation in which the person can talk freely about their experiences, without fear of scepticism or contradiction, may be a sufficient condition for them to make some changes for themself to their understanding of, and response to, their experiences.

It is safe to ask someone about the *coping strategies that they already use* and to suggest ways in which they could use them more frequently or more reliably. It is also safe to suggest *distraction tasks*, though you should be careful that your suggestion does not trivialize or minimalize the person's situation.[3] If someone is hearing voices, then it may be helpful to suggest trying *an earplug or Walkman*, but if the contact is a casual one and you do not know the person, then it is safer to float this suggestion, backing off rapidly if it is not well received.

If you are in fairly frequent contact with the person, then is it appropriate to use informal contacts to *find out more* about their symptoms and to ask questions to help you understand their interpretation of what is going on, their level of insight, and their knowledge of and attitude towards mental illness and psychosis. Although there are nearly always some advantages for the person in understanding their experiences in terms of mental illness, for example seeking appropriate treatment and making appropriate plans for the future, there may be some very significant disadvantages as well. Therefore, *do not assume it will be in the person's best interests to tell them their diagnosis or to try to force acceptance when this is not wanted.* However, even if the person does not see their experiences in terms of mental illness, it is almost certain that other people will have told them that this is their diagnosis and so it is appropriate to use your informal contacts do some *gentle normalizing/destigmatizing work*, as and when the opportunities arise, but being very careful that what you say refers to mental illness in general and is not linked specifically to the person or their experiences.

If the person knows they have a mental illness and is distressed by this knowledge, then it is appropriate and safe to use the strategies summarized in Appendix 3: 'Ways of reducing some of the negative aspects of a diagnosis of "mental illness"'. The one proviso is that the strategies described in section 4, 'Guilt/shame because the voices are "my thoughts"', can only be used safely in informal therapy if the person is also aware that their voices come from within themself.

Belief modification strategies, as applied to both delusions and/or hallucinations, are *not* safe to use unless the goal for the belief modification has been clearly set and you are sure that the identified replacement belief is acceptable (or has been 'prepared' and made acceptable). For this reason, too, it is not safe to do *insight promotion* work with someone who is denying illness unless you are sure that the person is prepared for it and what it implies.

In clinical practice the most common situation in which the replacement belief

[3]For example, suggesting to someone that they join in a game of Scrabble is likely to come across as being very unempathic if they have just told you they are terrified because the satellites overhead are going to kill them with laser beams.

is acceptable and in which, therefore, belief modification work can be safely attempted in an informal therapy setting, is when the person knows they have a mental illness and understands what this means for them but does not think that the particular belief or experience in question can be attributed to their illness.

As a general rule, it is much safer to apply CBT informally with someone who understands that they have a mental illness and how this can affect them than with someone who does not.

COMBINING FORMAL AND INFORMAL THERAPY

If the person is receiving formal therapy, then you *must* speak with the therapist before engaging in any informal CBT work other than listening and responding empathically, to make sure that what you are planning to do will not conflict with the work taking place in formal therapy. If the person is receiving formal therapy, then this may be a good opportunity for you to use some more elaborate CBT strategies than you would otherwise feel competent to use, as part of the overall CBT programme and under the guidance of the therapist. Most therapists welcome support of this kind.

THE ESSENTIALS OF SAFE PRACTICE

1. *Always think about what you are doing before you do it* – do not do it unless you have a good reason for doing it. Think about the possible wider consequences of what you are saying or doing as well as the more obvious ones that you intend.

2. *Go slowly*. Be prepared to back off if there is any evidence of resistance or distress, especially if you were not expecting this reaction. Do not be tempted to press ahead too quickly because you are concerned about lack of apparent progress. If something of potential significance comes up during therapy that you are not sure how to use, it is better to go away and think about it in between sessions rather than pushing on straight away.

3. *Be gentle, be kind*. Imagine how the person feels being at the receiving end of your therapy. Do not use a strategy that increases their distress, even if only temporarily, unless you have good therapeutic reasons for doing so.

4. *Set the goals of belief modification and ensure that any replacement beliefs are acceptable and functional* **before** *making any attempt to challenge or modify a delusion or hallucination*. In my experience, absent or inadequate goal setting and goal preparation are the most common causes of problems brought to clinical supervision.

5. *Have access to supervision*. Peer supervision is a minimum requirement if you are engaging in formal CBT, with at least one of the supervision group being a qualified CBT therapist with experience in CBT with psychosis. It is recommended that therapists new to this area of work also have access to consultation or supervision by phone, in case of need.

If you do not have formal training in the use of CBT, it is recommended you seek supervision even if you are only using the basic CBT approach and strategies on an informal basis. If you are under the supervision of an experienced therapist, then you will be able to use more of the strategies that are used in formal therapy, and be able to use them more effectively and safely.

18 EVIDENCE-BASED PRACTICE

INTRODUCTION

The published literature concerning the use of CBT with people with psychosis is a very extensive one, as is the literature concerning the nature and development of psychotic symptoms and experiences. This chapter is intended to be an introduction to some of the issues that are most closely related to and relevant for the use of CBT with delusions and hallucinations in clinical practice. The aim is to provide some of the more recent, key references that would serve as a starting point for someone wanting to obtain more information on a particular topic of interest. References for note cues within the text can be found on p. 317.

THE RESEARCH LITERATURE

THE EFFECTIVENESS OF CBT FOR DELUSIONS AND HALLUCINATIONS

Early studies

The earliest report of the application of CBT principles to the symptoms of psychosis dates back to the early 1950s. In 1952, Aaron T. Beck[1] reported the case of a man with a chronic paranoid delusion that was modified by introducing him to an alternative understanding of the content of his delusion and why this had developed. In a fascinating review of this early case,[2] he looks back and considers the treatment he used from 50 years on. Unfortunately, the very large majority of clinicians did not appreciate the importance of this original study, just as they failed to appreciate the importance of the report by Fraser Watts and colleagues in 1973.[3] This was due in no small part to the fact that delusions were defined as being irrational and not amenable to change through psychological intervention, so most psychologists and other clinicians working with this client group assumed that any attempt to modify a delusional belief using cognitive strategies would be a pointless waste of time. As a consequence, psychologists concentrated on helping people to cope with their symptoms rather than change them, though by the 1970s the use of a cognitive strategy, namely self-instruction, as a way of coping with the effects of the illness had been reported.[4]

Controlled trials of CBT with chronic/persistent psychosis

Apart from isolated cases, it was not until the late 1980s and early 1990s, with the groundbreaking work of Chadwick and Lowe,[5–6] that reports of single case studies of CBT applied directly to delusions and hallucinations began to appear in the research literature. Small group studies followed until, by the late 1990s, larger, controlled trials, often involving several centres and research teams, were being planned and carried out.[7–15] The results from these clinical trials provide a very solid foundation for evidence-based practice.

CBT in routine clinical practice

The conditions under which controlled trials are carried out are necessarily different in certain respects from routine clinical practice. For example, in order to reduce the number of spurious, uncontrolled factors that could influence the outcome, criteria are set for who is eligible to receive the treatment; this has the effect of excluding a number of people who would be seen in routine practice. Furthermore, additional resources of a clinical trial ensure that there is adequate skilled therapist time to complete the courses of treatment being investigated. On the other hand the therapist has to adhere closely to the particular treatment package being assessed and therefore cannot include any other treatment strategies that might be advantageous in the individual case. Recent studies have confirmed that the CBT approach can be used effectively in routine clinical practice, both in formal therapy settings[16] and in more informal, everyday settings,[17–19] as well as under research conditions.

CBT with acute psychosis

Although most of the clinical trials have been conducted with people who are so-called medication resistant (i.e. who have some persistent or recurrent symptoms despite being on optimal levels of medication), in non-hospital settings, there are now enough studies with people in the acute phase of the illness to indicate that CBT can be usefully applied at this stage as well.[20–25] Results from these studies have generally indicated that the addition of CBT can, in some cases, make the recovery faster and more complete, with a better chance of staying relapse-free for longer, though the benefits may dissipate with time.[22]

CBT with first- and early-episode psychosis

In 2000, the Department of Health in the UK designated early detection and intervention in psychosis as a priority[26] because clinicians had successfully argued that early intervention could significantly improve long-term outcome.[27] Although medication has a critical role to play in the early treatment, psychosocial strategies including CBT[23–24, 28] are also considered to be important, though not all studies report good results.[29] A number of recent books report the evidence and describe the approach,[30–33] which has been used with adolescents as young as 15 years of age.[34]

CBT in a group format

The effects of psychosis and the form that delusions and hallucinations can take can vary dramatically from person to person, so in order to be able to select and target the most appropriate CBT strategies for the individual's experiences, beliefs and needs, most people who received CBT for psychosis are treated on an individual basis. However, there are cost implications of individual therapy, both in terms of the monetary cost of providing so many hours of individual therapy and in terms of using up the scarce resource of skilled therapist time. Therefore, it may be cost effective to provide some aspects of CBT, such as coping strategy work and psychoeducation, in a group format.[35–36]

Reviews of CBT with psychosis and the effective components of treatment

The actual strategies that comprise the 'CBT treatment' in the efficacy studies vary considerably from trial to trial, reflecting the broad range of treatments that are included under this label in clinical practice. As well as emphasizing different aspects of the CBT approach, the trials may also use different control groups and different ways of assessing the treatment effects, so it is no easy task to try to combine and make sense of the various results. Fortunately, there have been a number of excellent comparative studies, narrative reviews and meta-analyses which look at the effectiveness of the CBT approach and at what the effective components of the therapy might be.[37–46]

PUTTING THE CBT TREATMENTS INTO PRACTICE

CBT with psychosis is not a uniform treatment; it is probably not too great an exaggeration to say that there are as many varieties as there are therapists who practise it. This is not a criticism of the treatment or the people who apply it, nor is it a weakness. The wide variety of CBT treatments available reflects not only the complexity of psychosis and the very wide range of individual differences in the ways that people can be affected but also the flexibility of the CBT approach to adapt and treat each person's experiences and beliefs as unique.

Practice manuals and casebooks

There are a number of books available that describe how the CBT approach can be applied to the symptoms and effects of psychosis[47–53] but the extensive range of CBT strategies and the different points of intervention that can be used does mean that different authors tend to emphasize different aspects of the treatment. For example, some authors put more emphasis on understanding the symptoms in a more helpful way, often through decatastrophizing and normalizing the experiences and beliefs,[51, 54] and psychoeducation,[55] whilst others put more emphasis on belief modification,[49, 50] and yet others stress the importance of developing coping strategies[56, 57] and relapse prevention.[58] All writers stress the importance of case formulation as the basis for effective therapy.[48] One particular approach or set of treatment strategies is not better or more correct than another; it depends on the individual person's problems and present position, and what you are hoping to achieve.

When attempting to learn 'how to do CBT with people with psychosis' the complexity and variety of approaches described can seem both daunting and confusing. This is not helped by the fact that writers may use some of the terms rather differently; for example, whilst some writers make a distinction between belief modification strategies and coping strategies others include belief modification strategies under a broader definition of 'coping strategy'. But despite the apparent differences of the various approaches, they *are* compatible, and in clinical practice it is entirely appropriate to use and integrate these different approaches. However, therapists new to this area of work may find it easier to concentrate on one approach until they feel confident with that before integrating other models of working into their practice.

Additional resources

This manual focuses on the engagement and belief modification aspects of working with people with delusions and hallucinations. As described in Chapter 15, *medication adherence* can be a very important coping strategy and so readers are referred to the practice manual produced by Kemp and colleagues for a more detailed exposition of this aspect of the treatment.[59] As described in Chapter 4, using formal *homework* tasks with people with psychosis can strengthen the therapy but is often problematic; this issue is dealt with in more detail in a recent book about the role of homework in CBT.[60]

RELATED THERAPEUTIC ISSUES

Integrating CBT strategies from other models into the CBT for psychosis

Psychotic symptoms can have an overwhelming impact on someone's life.[61, 62] *Depression* and *suicide* are significant risks,[63] which, if present, may be amenable to a CBT approach.[64] Recent reports have described the integration of CBT strategies for *anxiety*[65] and *anger*[66] into the treatment for psychosis.

The wide-reaching, negative consequences that psychosis can have on people's social and personal lives can have substantial effects on their *self-esteem*. In these circumstances, using strategies to improve self-esteem[67] is likely to be an important part of the overall therapy.[68] Closely related to this are issues of *sense of social position* and *shame*.[69]

In keeping with the stress-vulnerability model of schizophrenia,[70] *trauma* may predispose to and/or precipitate the development of psychosis, and the experience of psychosis may, of itself, constitute a trauma. The relationship between trauma and psychosis has now been recognized[71] and CBT treatments for *PTSD* and psychosis have been combined.[72]

Substance misuse is common amongst people with psychosis; prevalence may be as high as 60%.[73–74] Where the substance abuse causes significant problems, either as a direct result of the substance abuse or because of its adverse effects on the psychosis, then strategies to modify the substance abuse should be used together with the strategies to modify the psychotic symptoms.[75–76]

Recent reviews of *therapy with the families* of people with psychosis[43, 40] have confirmed that it can confer long-term benefits in terms of relapse prevention and reduced stress in other family members. Despite the fact that good practice manuals have been available for a number of years[e.g. 77–78] and the argument that family intervention reduces the need to access costly mental health services later, family therapy is still a poorly resourced area of work and it is only the lucky few who receive it at present.

Psychosis and CBT from the recipient's perspective

Given the collaborative nature of CBT it is perhaps surprising that the experiences of the people who actually receive the CBT treatments for psychosis have not received more attention.[79] The dropout rate from CBT treatments is relatively good compared with other types of treatment for psychosis but, nevertheless, some people do fail to *engage* or to *continue with treatment* for a number of different reasons.[80]

There is now recognition of the importance of *empowering* people with psychosis,[81–82] both with respect to the treatment they receive and to the control they have over their own lives.

The books written by Peter Chadwick about his own experiences[83–84] not only provide a rich insight into the *subjective experiences of worsening psychosis* but are also, as the title of the later book indicates, an invaluable source for providing a more *positive perspective* on the illness and symptoms for other people who have been given this diagnosis.

Other therapies

Social skills training used to be a core feature of rehabilitation programmes for people whose social skills had been eroded by years of institutionalization and illness, and some positive results from trials were reported.[85] However, a recent review of the evidence[86] has indicated that any benefits are minimal and the authors have concluded that it cannot be recommended as a treatment.

This same review has also concluded that there is not yet enough evidence to validate the use of *cognitive remediation therapy*,[87] a treatment that is aimed at improving the cognitive deficits in thinking, including memory and concentration, that are common features of psychosis.

The possible positive and negative effects of *psychodynamic approaches* to schizophrenia have been considered[88] but in a Cochrane review[89] the authors were unable to find any clinical trials of psychodynamic psychotherapy with schizophrenia and therefore concluded that at present there was no evidence to validate the use of these approaches in clinical practice.

SOME THEORETICAL ASPECTS OF DELUSIONS AND HALLUCINATIONS THAT HAVE IMPLICATIONS FOR THERAPY

In a seminal paper published in 1999,[90] Philippa Garety and Daniel Freeman reviewed the evidence relating to three factors that have been suggested to be key to the development of delusional beliefs, namely deficits or biases in reasoning, deficits in theory of mind and in recognizing intentions and actions as one's own, and unusual attributional style. This was followed by important theoretical papers describing multifactorial models for the development and maintenance of delusions and hallucinations.[91–93] A recent paper from the same group has highlighted the importance of developing plausible alternative explanations to replace the delusional beliefs.[94]

In line with standard CBT theory,[95] there is increasing evidence that emotions can contribute to the formation of delusional beliefs and hallucinations[96] and that the emotional reactions to the delusions and hallucinations can be an important maintenance factor.[96–99]

The multifactorial models highlight the need to take the full range of potential factors into account when constructing a case formulation prior to planning therapy. In particular, since the principal aim of CBT with psychosis is to reduce the person's distress and improve their quality of life, it is essential that the CBT programme devised for the individual person is targeted specifically at those factors responsible for the distress and other adverse consequences of the delusional beliefs and hallucinations.

MEASURING THE EFFECTS OF THE CBT INTERVENTION ON DELUSIONS AND HALLUCINATIONS

GENERAL PSYCHOPATHOLOGY SCALES

Many of the clinical trials of CBT with psychosis use one or more general psychopathology scales, administered pre- and post-treatment, to measure the effects of the treatment. Commonly used for this purpose are the **Present State Examination (PSE)**,[100] the **Brief Psychiatric Rating Scale (BPRS)**,[101] the **Scale for the Assessment of Positive Symptoms (SAPS)**,[102] and the **Scale for the Assessment of Negative Symptoms (SANS)**.[103] The PSE is a long and detailed interview and it is necessary to receive formal training in its administration before you can use it in clinical practice. The BPRS is a shorter interview that was developed to measure change in 16 aspects of psychotic symptomatology. The SAPS and SANS focus on positive and negative symptoms respectively and use information from other sources (e.g. other people who know the person concerned) as well as an assessment interview.

A major drawback of these general scales as a means of assessing change due to a CBT intervention is that they were developed in order to assess the full range of psychotic symptoms and as such provide only relatively crude measures of the particular symptoms or aspects of symptoms that might be targeted for modification in a CBT programme, and different aspects of the symptoms (e.g. conviction and preoccupation with a delusional belief) may be combined in a general 'severity' measure.

The general nature of these assessments is an advantage for large group studies because it enables the results from different individuals to be combined for statistical analysis, but necessarily it also means that the measures cannot be targeted specifically to measure aspects of the symptoms that might be significant for the individual person. Measures that can be adapted to the individual case (see below) are more sensitive and, therefore, better for assessing the effects of CBT with an individual person in routine clinical practice.

FORMAL MEASURES OF DELUSIONS AND HALLUCINATIONS

Psychotics Symptom Rating Scales (PSYRATS)

PSYRATS[104] comprises two structured interviews that use five-point scales to quantify different aspects of delusional beliefs (amount of preoccupation, duration of preoccupation, conviction, amount of distress, intensity of distress and disruption to everyday life) and hallucinations (frequency, duration, location, loudness, beliefs about origin, amount of negative content, degree of negative content, amount of distress, intensity of distress, control and disruption to everyday life). The scales are particularly useful for clinical practice because they can be used for individual delusions and voices, and although the subscales can be combined to give an overall score for the delusion or hallucination being rated, it is possible to use just the subscales that are relevant for the particular aspect(s) that you are targeting for modification.

Although the form is filled in by the person who is conducting the interview, it is the person themself, in discussion with the rater, who evaluates each aspect of the symptoms being measured. The subscales have the advantage of being quick and easy to administer, though having only three points between the two extremes means they are not sensitive to small changes. As happens with any attempt to quantify subjective experiences, people may find it difficult to use and decide between some of the percentage options.

At a purely practical level, be careful not to expose the form if you are using the scales with someone who does not recognize their delusional beliefs or hallucinations as such, because the titles of the scales and some of the subscale headings use the terms 'delusions' and 'hallucinations' in large print. In these circumstances you would also need to be sensitive about how you phrase some of the questions, for example those regarding conviction.

Characteristics of Delusions Rating Scale

This scale[105] is applied to a single delusion and measures 11 aspects of the delusion chosen (conviction, preoccupation, interference with behaviour, resistance, dismissability, absurdity, worry, unhappiness, reassurance seeking, self-evidentness and pervasiveness). The subscales used are line scales, each of which is completed by the person themself, after discussion with the rater if clarification is necessary, and this is converted into a 10-point scale. The advantage of using this formal form of line scaling is that it is a good reminder of the many different factors that might be relevant and important in the individual case.

The revised Beliefs About Voices Questionnaire (BAVQ–R)

The BAVQ-R[106] comprises 35 statements about the voice, which the person has to respond to with a 'yes' or 'no' option. The statements fall into five subscales (malevolence, benevolence, omnipotence, resistance and engagement) that assess how the person feels about their voice. The questionnaire is completed separately for each different voice.

Power Scale (Voices)

The power that is invested in a voice may be one of the most significant factors in determining its ability to cause distress and command behaviour, so reducing its perceived power is often an important part of the therapy. The Power Scale (Voices)[107] assesses how the person rates the power of their voice relative to themself on seven dimensions (powerfulness, strength, confidence, respect, ability to harm, equality and knowledge). Each dimension comprises a five-point scale, which is scored by the person themself. (*Note*: the 'respect' item is reversed, so its scoring should be reversed if the subscales are to be summed to give a total 'power' score.)

MEASURES CONSTRUCTED FOR THE INDIVIDUAL CASE

The advantage of constructing measures that are specific for the individual case is that they can target precisely the aspect of the belief or hallucination being targeted for modification and as such will be both more relevant and more sensitive to the effects of the CBT treatment than general measures. Idiosyncratic measures are usually not appropriate for research trials, where results from individuals have to be combined for statistical analysis.

Simple, numerical rating scales

The particular aspect(s) of the belief of hallucination being targeted for modification by the CBT can be rated by the person on a simple numerical rating scale. 0–10 or 0–100% are often used in practice, but the range of the scale depends on what the person themself finds easiest to use. The thing being rated is expressed in the person's own terms; for example, a 0–10 scale might be used to measure 'the determination of my neighbour to poison me' or 'how sure I am that my neighbour wants to poison me' or 'how nervous it makes me feel when I go out', etc. Although these scales sound simple and easy to use, some people may find it difficult to put a number to their subjective experiences and beliefs.

Line Scales

For example:

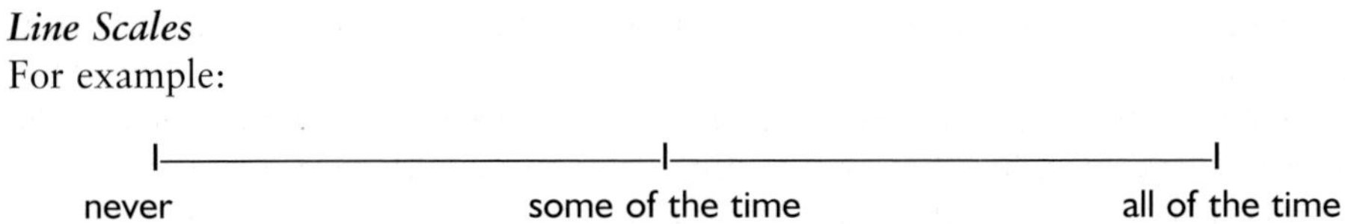

Type 1: The person puts a cross on the line in the position that represents how they are with respect to the factor being measured. The point in time used is often 'how I am *now*' but in some cases it may be more appropriate to use other time periods such as 'how I have been in the last hour/day/week'. The score is obtained by measuring the length of the line from the left-hand end, and change is assessed by the difference between these scores on different occasions. Note that although in theory it would appear that this method could be used to detect very small changes, in practice human beings are not precise enough for small changes to be considered reliable; i.e. if you were to ask someone to repeat the mark they had made a few minutes before, then their second mark would not be in exactly the same place as the first one even though they 'felt' exactly the same on the two occasions.

Descriptions are allocated to the endpoints of the line. Anchor points in between, i.e. verbal descriptions of different points along the line, help to make the judgements more stable and reliable. The descriptions used are expressed in the person's own words. It is common to use one, three or five anchor points between the end points.

Type 2: This type of line scale is very similar to that described above but in this variation the person circles the anchor point that most closely describes how they are with respect to the factor being measured: this produces a scale with the same number of points as there are anchor points. The more points there are on the scale, the more sensitive it is to detect change.

SOME GENERAL CONSIDERATIONS ABOUT THE USE OF RATING SCALES

The general psychopathology scales use the interviewer to assess the presence and severity of psychotic symptoms in the other person. Although this may confer some advantages with respect to reliability, having someone else assess what is essentially a subjective experience will inevitably affect the validity of the measure. Furthermore, because the assessments rely on subjective judgements on the part of the assessor there is always the potential for the scores given to be biased, albeit unintentionally, towards what is expected or hoped for. This latter is particularly likely to occur if it is the therapist who is conducting the pre- and post-treatment assessments. For this reason, in research trials these measures are always done by people who are not involved in the therapy and who do not know whether the person being assessed received CBT or one of the control treatments. It is usually not possible to have the luxury of an independent rater to conduct the measurements for routine clinical work and so in clinical practice you will often find that you have to complete any pre- and post-assessment measures yourself, as well as conduct the therapy. In these circumstances you should try to select measures that are less open to potential distortion.

Involving the person themself in determining the ratings helps to avoid the 'wishful thinking' effect: the more control the person has over the ratings, the less likely it is that the therapist will inadvertently bias the measures obtained.

Nevertheless, the follow-up measures may still be biased if the person feels they *ought* to have improved for some reason, or is seeking to please the therapist, or is just trying to be optimistic. These biases are more likely to occur where the therapist has made it very obvious to the other person that they are expecting or hoping for improvements.

If the person is chaotic or difficult to engage, then this may affect the accuracy of any self-report measures obtained, especially if the assessment is long or complicated, and in these circumstances you should check the answers obtained for consistency with what you know through your informal discussions with the person. In these circumstances, keeping the formal assessment short and uncomplicated will help to minimize the potential inaccuracies and unreliability.

Formal measures help the therapist to measure change in a formal quantitative way and as such are necessary in research projects or to justify the effectiveness of treatment services for service planning purposes. However, measuring the change brought about by the treatment does not of itself improve that treatment or increase its effectiveness for the person receiving it, so if there are significant negative aspects to using formal ratings to assess change, then, for the purposes of routine clinical practice, you should not use them.

EVALUATING POTENTIAL TO BENEFIT FROM CBT

Reaction to hypothetical contradiction (RTHC) and ability to consider an alternative point of view

When people were asked about a hypothetical situation in which something that contradicted their delusion was true (a piece of appropriate, concrete evidence was suggested), those who reported that the contradictory evidence would cause them to reconsider their belief had a better response to subsequent CBT belief modification strategies[108] than those who said it would not affect their conviction in their belief. This finding has been replicated,[109] though not in all studies.[8] In this later study,[8] people who answered 'yes' to a simpler question about the possibility of being mistaken in their delusional belief had a better response to CBT than those who said 'no'.

It is not known how accurately these types of question predict response to CBT in the individual case, so they should not be used as exclusion criteria for routine clinical work.

ASSESSMENT OF DEPRESSION AND ANXIETY

Depression and anxiety often occur in people with psychosis, either as associated features or as a result of the psychosis itself. Therefore, it is useful to have good measures of depression and anxiety available, both for assessment purposes and to measure change with treatment. The **Beck Depression Inventory**[110] and the **Beck Anxiety Inventory**[111] are recommended for this purpose.

REFERENCES

1. Beck, A.T. (1952). Successful outpatient psychotherapy with a schizophrenic with a delusion based on borrowed guilt. *Psychiatry*, 15: 305–12. Reprinted in A.P. Morrison (ed.) *A Casebook of Cognitive Therapy for Psychosis* (pp. 15–18). Hove: Brunner-Routledge.
2. Beck, A.T. (2002). Successful outpatient psychotherapy with a schizophrenic with a delusion based on borrowed guilt: A 50 year retrospective. In A.P. Morrison (ed.) *A Casebook of Cognitive Therapy for Psychosis* (pp. 15–18). Hove: Brunner-Routledge.
3. Watts, F.N., Powell G.E. & Austin S.V. (1973). The modification of abnormal beliefs. *British Journal of Medical Psychology*, 46: 359–63.
4. Meichenbaum, D. & Cameron, R. (1973). Training schizophrenics to talk to themselves: a means of developing attentional control. *Behavior Therapy*, 4: 525–34.
5. Chadwick, P. & Lowe, C. (1990). Measurement and modification of delusional beliefs. *Journal of Consulting and Clinical Psychology*, 58: 225–32.
6. Lowe, C. & Chadwick, P. (1990). Verbal control of delusions. *Behaviour Therapy*, 21: 461–79.
7. Kuipers, E., Garety, P., Fowler, D., Dunn, G., Bebbington, P., Freeman, D. & Hadley, C. (1997). London-East Anglia randomised controlled trial of cognitive-behavioural therapy for psychosis. I: Effects of the treatment phase. *British Journal of Psychiatry*, 171: 319–27.
8. Garety, P., Fowler, D., Kuipers, E., Freeman, D., Dunn, G., Bebbington, P., Hadley, C. & Jones, S. (1997). London-East Anglia randomised controlled trial of cognitive-behavioural therapy for psychosis. II: Predictors of outcome. *British Journal of Psychiatry*, 171: 420–26.
9. Kuipers, E., Fowler, D., Garety, P. A., Chisholm, D., Freeman, D., Dunn, G., Bebbington, P. & Hadley, C. (1998). London-East Anglia randomised controlled trial of cognitive-behavioural therapy for psychosis. III: Follow-up and economic evaluation at 18 months. *British Journal of Psychiatry*, 173: 61–8.
10. Freeman, D., Garety, P., Fowler, D., Kuipers, E., Dunn, G., Bebbington, P. & Hadley, C. (1998). London-East Anglia randomised controlled trial of cognitive-behavioural therapy for psychosis. IV: Self-esteem and persecutory delusions. *British Journal of Clinical Psychology*, 37: 415–30.
11. Tarrier, N., Yusupoff, L., Kinney, C., McCarthy, E., Gledhill, A., Haddock, G. & Morris, J. (1998). Randomised controlled trial of intensive cognitive behaviour therapy for patients with chronic schizophrenia. *British Medical Journal*, 317: 303–7.
12. Tarrier, N., Wittkowski, A., Kinney, C., McCarthy, E., Morris, J. & Humphreys, L. (1999). Durability of the effects of cognitive behavioural therapy in the treatment of chronic schizophrenia: 12-month follow-up. *British Journal of Psychiatry*, 174: 500–4.
13. Tarrier, N., Kinney, C., McCarthy, E., Humphreys, L., Wittkowski, A. & Morris, J. (2000). Two-year follow-up of cognitive-behavioural therapy and supportive counselling in the treatment of persistent symptoms in chronic schizophrenia. *Journal of Consulting and Clinical Psychology*, 5: 917–22.
14. Sensky, T., Turkington, D., Kingdon, D., Scott, J. L., Scott, J., Siddle, R., O'Carroll, M. & Barnes, T.R.E. (2000). A randomised controlled trial of cognitive-behavioral therapy for persistent symptoms in schizophrenia resistant to medication. *Archives of General Psychiatry*, 57: 165–72.
15. Trower, P., Birchwood, M., Meaden, A., Byrne, S., Nelson, A. & Ross, K. (2004). Cognitive therapy for command hallucinations: randomised controlled trial. *British Journal of Psychiatry*, 184: 312–20.
16. Jakes, S., Rhodes, J. & Turner, T. (1999). Effectiveness of cognitive therapy for delusions in routine clinical practice. *British Journal of Psychiatry*, 175: 331–5.

17. Turkington, D., Kingdon, D. & Turner, T. (2002). Effectiveness of a brief cognitive-behavioural therapy intervention in the treatment of schizophrenia. *British Journal of Psychiatry*, 180: 523–7.
18. Durham, R., Guthrie, M., Morton, V., Reid, D., Treliving, L., Fowler, D. & MacDonald, R. (2003). Tayside-Fife clinical trial of cognitive-behavioural therapy for medication-resistant psychotic symptoms: Results to 3-month follow-up. *British Journal of Psychiatry*, 182: 303–11.
19. Morrison, A., Renton, J., Williams, S., Dunn, H., Knight, A., Kreutz, M., Nothard, S., Patel, U. & Dunn, G. (2004). Delivering cognitive therapy to people with psychosis in a community mental health setting: an effectiveness study. *Acta Psychiatrica Scandinavica*, 110: 36–44.
20. Drury, V., Birchwood, M., Cochrane, R. & MacMillan, F. (I996a). Cognitive therapy and recovery from acute psychosis: a controlled trial. I: Impact on psychotic symptoms. *British Journal of Psychiatry*, 169: 593–601.
21. Drury, V., Birchwood, M., Cochrane, R. & MacMillan, F. (1996b). Cognitive therapy and recovery from acute psychosis: a controlled trial. II: Impact on recovery time. *British Journal of Psychiatry*, 169: 602–7.
22. Drury, V., Birchwood, M. & Cochrane, R. (2000). Cognitive therapy and recovery from acute psychosis: a controlled trial. III: Five-year follow-up. *British Journal of Psychiatry*, 177: 8–14.
23. Lewis, S., Tarrier, N., Haddock, G., Bentall, R., Kinderman, P., Kingdon, D., Siddle, R., Drake, R., Everitt, J., Leadley, K., Benn, A., Grazebrook, K., Haley, C., Akhtar, S., Davies, L., Palmer, S., Faragher, B. & Dunn, G. (2002). Randomised controlled trial of cognitive-behavioural therapy in early schizophrenia: acute-phase outcomes. *British Journal of Psychiatry*, 181: (suppl. 43), S91–7.
24. Tarrier, N., Lewis, S., Haddock, G., Bentall, R., Drake, R., Dunn, G., Kinderman, P., Kingdon, D., Siddle, R., Everitt, J., Leadley, K., Benn, A., Grazebrook, K., Haley, C., Akhtar, S., Davies, L. & Palmer, S. (2004). Cognitive behavioural therapy in first episode and early schizophrenia: 18-month follow-up of a randomised controlled trial. *British Journal of Psychiatry*, 184: 231–9.
25. Startup, M., Jackson, M. & Bendix, S. (2004). North Wales randomized controlled trial of cognitive behaviour therapy for acute schizophrenia spectrum disorders: outcomes at 6 and 12 months. *Psychological Medicine*, 34: 413–22.
26. Department of Health (2000). *The National Plan: A Plan for Investment, a Plan for Reform*. London: Department of Health.
27. Birchwood, M. (2000). The critical period for early intervention. In M. Birchwood, D. Fowler & C. Jackson (eds.) *Early Intervention in Psychosis: A Guide to Concepts, Evidence and Interventions*. Chichester: Wiley.
28. Haddock, G., Tarrier, N., Morrison, A. P., Hopkins, R., Drake, R. & Lewis, S. (1999). A pilot study evaluating the effectiveness of individual inpatient cognitive-behavioural therapy in early psychosis. *Social Psychiatry and Psychiatric Epidemiology*, 34: 254–8.
29. Jackson, H., McCorry, P., Henry, L., Edwards, J., Hulbert, C., Harrigan, S., Dudgeon, P., Francey, S., Maude, D., Cocks, J. & Power, P. (2001). Cognitively oriented psychotherapy for early psychosis (COPE): A 1-year follow-up. *British Journal of Clinical Psychology*, 40: 57–70.
30. Gleeson, G. & McGorry, P. (2004). *Psychological Interventions in Early Psychosis: A Treatment Handbook*. Chichester: Wiley.
31. French, P. & Morrison, A. (2004). *Early Detection and Cognitive Therapy for People at High Risk of Developing Psychosis: A Treatment Approach*. Chichester: Wiley.
32. Birchwood, M., Fowler, D. & Jackson, C. (eds.) (2000). *Early Intervention in Psychosis: A Guide to Concepts, Evidence and Interventions*. Chichester: Wiley.

33. McCorry, P. & Jackson, H. (eds.) (1999). *Recognition and Management of Early Psychosis: A Preventative Approach*. Cambridge: Cambridge University Press.
34. Wragg, A. & Whitehead, R. (2004). CBT for adolescents with psychosis: investigating the feasibility and effectiveness of early intervention using a single case design. *Behavioural and Cognitive Psychotherapy*, 32: 313–29.
35. Wykes, T., Parr, A. & Landlau, S. (1999). Group of treatment or auditory hallucinations. Exploratory study of effectiveness. *British Journal of Psychiatry*, 175: 180–5.
36. Bechdolf, A., Knost, B., Kuntermann, C., Schiller, S., Klosterkotter, J., Hambrecht, M. & Pukrop, R. (2004). A randomised comparison of group cognitive-behavioural therapy and group psychoeducation in patients with schizophrenia. *Acta Psychiatrica Scandinavica*, 110: 21–8.
37. Bouchard, S., Vallieres, A., Roy, M. & Maziade, M. (1996). Cognitive restructuring in the treatment of psychotic symptoms in schizophrenia: A critical analysis. *Behaviour Therapy*, 27: 257–78.
38. Dickerson, F. (2000). Cognitive behavioral psychotherapy for schizophrenia: a review of recent empirical studies. *Schizophrenia Research*, 43: 71–90.
39. Garety, P., Fowler, D. & Kuipers, E. (2000). Cognitive-behavioral therapy for medication-resistant symptoms. *Schizophrenia Bulletin*, 26: 73–86.
40. British Psychological Society Division of Clinical Psychology (2000). *Recent Advances in Understanding Mental Illness and Psychotic Experiences*. Leicester: British Psychological Society.
41. Gould, R., Mueser, K., Bolton, E., Mays, E. & Goff, D. (2001). Cognitive therapy for psychosis in schizophrenia: an effect size analysis. *Schizophrenia Research*, 48: 335–42.
42. Rector, N. & Beck, A. (2001). Cognitive behavioral therapy for schizophrenia: an empirical review. *Journal of Nervous and Mental Diseases*, 189: 278–87.
43. Pilling, S., Bebbington, P., Kuipers, E., Garety, P., Geddes, J., Orbach, G. & Morgan, C. (2002). Psychological treatments in schizophrenia. I: Meta-analysis of family intervention and cognitive behaviour therapy. *Psychological Medicine*, 32: 763–82.
44. Rector, N. & Beck, A. (2002). Cognitive therapy for schizophrenia: from conceptualisation to intervention. *Canadian Journal of Psychiatry*, 47: 39–48.
45. Lecomte, T. & Lecomte, C. (2002). Toward uncovering robust principles of change inherent to cognitive-behavioural therapy for psychosis. *American Journal of Orthopsychiatry*, 72: 50–7.
46. Turkington, D. & McKenna, P.J. (2003). Is cognitive-behavioural therapy a worthwhile treatment for psychosis? *British Journal of Psychiatry*, 182: 477–9.
47. Wykes, T., Tarrier, N. & Lewis, S. (eds.) (1998). *Outcome and Innovation in Psychological Treatment of Schizophrenia*. Chichester: Wiley.
48. Morrison, A., Renton, J., Dunn, H., Williams, S. & Bentall, R. (2004). *Cognitive Therapy for Psychosis: A Formulation-based Approach*. Hove: Brunner-Routledge.
49. Chadwick, P., Birchwood, M. & Trower, P. (1996). *Cognitive Therapy for Delusions, Voices and Paranoia*. Chichester: Wiley.
50. Fowler, D., Garety, P. & Kuipers, P. (1995). *Cognitive Behaviour Therapy for Psychosis*. Chichester: Wiley.
51. Kingdon, D. & Turkington, D. (1994). *Cognitive-behavioural Therapy of Schizophrenia*. Hove: Lawrence Erlbaum.
52. Kingdon, D. & Turkington, D. (eds.) (2002). *The Case Study Guide to Cognitive Behaviour Therapy of Psychosis*. Chichester: Wiley.
53. Morrison, A. (ed.) (2002). *A Casebook of Cognitive Therapy for Psychosis*. Hove: Brunner-Routledge.
54. Turkington, D. & Kingdon, D. (1996). Using a normalising rationale in the treatment of

schizophrenic patients. In G. Haddock & P. Slade (eds.) *Cognitive-behavioural Interventions with Psychotic Disorders*. London: Routledge.
55. Pekkla, E. & Merinder, L. (2001). Psychoeducation for schizophrenia. *Cochrane Database of Systematic Reviews (Issue 1)*. Oxford: Update Software.
56. Tarrier, N. (2002). The use of coping strategies and self-regulation in the treatment of psychosis. In A. Morrison (ed.) *A Casebook of Cognitive Therapy for Psychosis*. Hove: Brunner-Routledge.
57. Yusupoff, L. & Tarrier, N. (1996). Coping strategy enhancement for persistent hallucinations and delusions. In G. Haddock & P. Slade (eds.) *Cognitive Behavioural Interventions with Psychotic Disorders*. London: Routledge.
58. Birchwood, M., Smith, J., Macmillan, F. & McGovern, D. (1998). Early intervention in psychotic relapse. In C. Brooker & J. Repper (eds.) *Serious Mental Health Problems in the Community: Policy, Practice and Research*. London: Baillière Tindall.
59. Kemp, R., Hayward, P. & David, A. (1997). *Compliance Therapy Manual*. London: The Maudsley.
60. McLeod, H. & Nelson, H. (2005). Using homework assignments in CBT for delusions and hallucinations. In N. Kazantzis, F. Deane, K. Ronan & L. L'Abate (eds.) *Using Homework Assignments in Cognitive Behavioral Therapy*. Hove: Brunner-Routledge.
61. Bayley, R. (1996). First person account: Schizophrenia. *Schizophrenia Bulletin*, 22: 727–9.
62. Close, H. & Garety, P. (1998). Cognitive assessment of voices: Further developments in understanding the emotional impact of voices. *British Journal of Clinical Psychology*, 37: 173–88.
63. Rossau, C. & Mortensen, P. (1997). Risk factors for suicide in patients with schizophrenia: nested case-control study. *British Journal of Psychiatry*, 171: 355–9.
64. Birchwood, M., Iqbal, Z., Chadwick, P. & Trower, P. (2000). Cognitive approach to depression and suicidal thinking in psychosis. I: Ontogeny of post-psychotic depression. *British Journal of Psychiatry*, 177: 516–21.
65. Williams, S. (2002). Anxiety and associated physiological sensations, and delusional catastrophic misinterpretation: Variations on a theme? In A. Morrison (ed.) *A Casebook of Cognitive Therapy for Psychosis*. Hove: Brunner-Routledge.
66. Haddock, G., Lowens, I., Brosnan, N., Barrowclough, C. & Novaco, R. (2004). Cognitive-behaviour therapy for inpatients with psychosis and anger problems within a low secure environment. *Behavioural and Cognitive Psychotherapy*, 32: 77–98.
67. Mruk, C. (1999). *Self-esteem*. London: Free Association Books.
68. Hall, P. & Tarrier, N. (2004). Short-term durability of a cognitive behavioural intervention in psychosis: Effects from a pilot study. *Behavioural and Cognitive Psychotherapy*, 32: 117–21.
69. Birchwood, M., Meaden, A., Trower, P. & Gilbert, P. (2002). Shame, humiliation, and entrapment in psychosis: A social rank theory approach to cognitive intervention with voices and delusions. In A. Morrison (ed.) *A Casebook of Cognitive Therapy for Psychosis*. Hove: Brunner-Routledge.
70. Zubin, J. & Spring, B. (1977). Vulnerability: A new view on schizophrenia. *Journal of Abnormal Psychology*, 86: 103–26.
71. Morrison, P., Frame, L. & Larkin, W. (2003). Relationships between trauma and psychosis: A review and integration. *British Journal of Clinical Psychology*, 42: 331–53.
72. Callcott, P., Standart, S. & Turkington, D. (2004). Trauma within psychosis: using a CBT model for PTSD in psychosis. *Behavioural and Cognitive Psychotherapy*, 32: 329–44.
73. Lehman, A. & Dixon, L. (1995). *Double Jeopardy: Chronic Mental Illness and Substance Use Disorders*. Chur: Harwood Academic Publishers.
74. Linszen, D. & Lenoir, M. (1999). Early psychosis and substance abuse. In P. McGorry &

H. Jackson (eds.) *The Recognition and Management of Early Psychosis*. Cambridge: Cambridge University Press.

75. Barrowclough, C., Haddock, G., Tarrier, N., Lewis, S., Moring, J., O'Brien, R., Schofield, N. & McGovern, J. (2001). Randomised controlled trial of motivational interviewing, cognitive behaviour therapy and family intervention for patients with co-morbid schizophrenia and substance use disorders. *American Journal of Psychiatry*, 158: 1706–13.
76. Graham, H., Capello, A., Birchwood, M., Orford, J., McGovern, D., Atkinson, E., Maslin, J., Mueser, K., Tobin, D. & Georgiou, G. (2003). *Cognitive-Behavioural Integrated Treatment (C-BIT): A Treatment Manual for Substance Misuse in People with Severe Mental Health Problems*. Chichester: Wiley.
77. Falloon, I. (1985). *Family Management of Schizophrenia*. Baltimore: John Hopkins University Press.
78. Barrowclough, C. & Tarrier, N. (1992). *Families of Schizophrenic Patients: Cognitive Behavioural Interventions*. London: Chapman and Hall.
79. Messari, S. & Hallam, R. (2003). CBT for psychosis: A qualitative analysis of clients' experiences. *British Journal of Clinical Psychology*, 42: 171–88.
80. Tarrier, N., Yusupoff, L., McCarthy, E., Kinney, C. & Wittkowski, A. (1998). Some reasons why patients suffering from chronic schizophrenia fail to continue in psychological treatment. *Behavioural and Cognitive Psychotherapy*, 26: 177–81.
81. Birchwood, M., Meaden, A., Trower, P., Gilbert, P. & Plaistowup, J. (2000). The power and omnipotence of voices: Subordination and entrapment by voices and significant others. *Psychological Medicine*, 30: 337–44.
82. Repper, J. & Perkins, R. (2003). *Social Inclusion and Recovery*. London: Baillière Tindall.
83. Chadwick, P. (1997). *Schizophrenia: The Positive Perspective. In Search of Dignity for Schizophrenic People*. London: Routledge.
84. Chadwick, P. (1992). *Borderline: A Psychological Study of Paranoia and Delusional Thinking*. London: Routledge.
85. Marder, S., Wirshing, W. & Mintz, J. (1996). Two-year outcome of social skills training and group psychotherapy for outpatients with schizophrenia. *American Journal of Psychiatry*, 153: 1585–92.
86. Pilling, S., Bebbington, P., Kuipers, E., Garety, P., Geddes, J., Martindale, B., Orbach, G. & Morgan, C. (2002). Psychological treatments in schizophrenia. II: Meta-analysis of randomized controlled trials of social skills training and cognitive remediation. *Psychological Medicine*, 32 (5): 763–82.
87. Wykes, T. & van der Gaag, M. (2001). Is it time to develop a new cognitive therapy for psychosis – cognitive remediation therapy (CRT)? *Clinical Psychology Review*, 21: 1227–56.
88. Fenton, M. & Glashan, T. (1995). Schizophrenia: individual psychotherapy. In H. Kaplan & B. Sadock (eds.) *Comprehensive Textbook of Psychiatry*. Baltimore: Williams and Wilkins.
89. Malmberg, L. & Fenton, M. (2002). Individual psychodynamic psychotherapy and psychoanalysis for schizophrenia and severe mental illness (Cochrane Review). In *The Cochrane Library (Issue 3)*. Oxford: Update Software.
90. Garety, P. & Freeman, D. (1999). Cognitive approaches to delusion: A critical review of theories and evidence. *British Journal of Clinical Psychology*, 38: 113–54.
91. Garety, P., Kuipers, E., Fowler, D., Freeman, D. & Bebbington, P. (2001). A cognitive model of the positive symptoms of psychosis. *Psychological Medicine*, 31: 189–95.
92. Freeman, D. & Garety, P. (2004). *Paranoia: The Psychology of Persecutory Delusions*. Taylor and Francis.

93. Freeman, D., Garety, P., Kuipers, E., Fowler, D. & Bebbington, P. (2002). A cognitive model of persecutory delusions. *British Journal of Clinical Psychology*, 41: 331–47.
94. Freeman, D., Garety, P., Fowler, D., Kuipers, E., Bebbington, P. & Dunn, G. (2004). Why do people with delusions fail to choose more realistic explanations for their experiences? An empirical investigation. *Journal of Consulting Clinical Psychology*, 72: 671–80.
95. Beck, A., Rush, A., Shaw, B. & Emery, G. (1979). *Cognitive Therapy of Depression*. New York: Guilford Press.
96. Freeman, D. & Garety, P. (2003). Connecting neurosis and psychosis: The direct influence of emotion on delusions and hallucinations. *Behaviour Research and Therapy*, 41: 923–47.
97. Freeman, D., Garety, P. & Kuipers, E. (2001). Persecutory delusions: Developing the understanding of belief maintenance and emotional distress. *Psychological Medicine*, 31: 1293–1306.
98. Freeman, D. & Garety, P. (1999). Worry, worry processes and dimensions of delusions: An exploratory investigation of a role for anxiety processes in the maintenance of delusional distress. *Behavioural and Cognitive Psychotherapy*, 27: 47–62.
99. Birchwood, M. & Chadwick, P. (1997). The omnipotence of voices: Testing the validity of a cognitive model. *Psychological Medicine*, 27: 1345–53.
100. Wing, J., Cooper, J. & Sartorious, N. (1974). *The Measurement and Classification of Psychiatric Symptoms*. Cambridge: Cambridge University Press.
101. Overall, J. & Gorham, D. (1962). The brief psychiatric rating scale. *Psychological Reports*, 10: 799–812.
102. Andreasen, N. (1984). *The Scale for the Assessment of Positive Symptoms (SAPS)*. Iowa City: The University of Iowa Press.
103. Andreason, N. (1981). *The Scale for the Assessment of Negative Symptoms (SANS)*. Iowa City: The University of Iowa Press.
104. Haddock, G., McCarron, J., Tarrier, N. & Faragher, E. (1999). Scales to measure dimensions of hallucinations and delusions: The psychotic symptom rating scales (PSYRATS). *Psychological Medicine*, 29: 879–89.
105. Garety, P. & Hemsley, D. (1987). Characteristics of delusional experience. *European Archives of Psychiatry and Neurological Science*, 266: 294–8.
106. Chadwick, P., Lees, S. & Birchwood, M. (2000). The revised Beliefs About Voices Questionnaire (BAVQ-R). *British Journal of Psychiatry*, 177: 229–32.
107. Birchwood, M., Meaden, A., Trower, P. & Gilbert, P. (2002). Shame, humiliation, and entrapment in psychosis: A social rank theory approach to cognitive intervention with voices and delusions. In A. Morrison (ed.) *A Casebook of Cognitive Therapy for Psychosis*. Hove: Brunner-Routledge.
108. Brett-Jones, J., Garety, P. & Hemsley, D. (1987). Measuring delusional experiences: A method and its application. *British Journal of Clinical Psychology*, 26: 257-65.
109. Chadwick, P., Lowe, C., Horne, P. & Higson, P. (1994). Modifying delusions: The role of empirical testing. *Behaviour Therapy*, 25: 35–49.
110. Beck, A., Steer, R. & Brown, G. (1996). *Beck Depression Inventory-II (BDI-II)*. Harcourt.
111. Beck, A. (1993). *Beck Anxiety Inventory (BAI)*. Harcourt.

APPENDIX 1
SUMMARY OF TREATMENT STRATEGIES

COGNITIVE-BEHAVIOURAL STRATEGIES WITH DELUSIONS

1 ENGAGEMENT

2 ASSESSMENT and CASE FORMULATION

3 REDUCE THE IMPACT OR DISTRESS USING PRACTICAL STRATEGIES

4 SET THE GOAL FOR THE MODIFICATION
- (a) Specify the belief to be modified.
- (b) Consider the possible goals.
- (c) Check whether the most functional goal(s) is acceptable.
- (d) Set the optimal goal.

5 PREPARE FOR THE BELIEF MODIFICATION

For a total goal:

(a) Prepare for the negation of the delusion:

Establish 'Believing something to be true does not mean that it is true.'

- *misinterpretations of everyday events*
- *beliefs that are no longer held to be true*
- *misperceptions at a physiological level*
- *use of dream analogy*

Replace any positive aspects of the delusional belief (if possible).

(b) Prepare the replacement belief:

Replacements in terms of mental illness: 'Insight' promotion within a destigmatizing, normalizing framework

- *sharing experiences of 'odd ideas'*
- *factors that increase vulnerability to odd ideas*
- *discussing the meaning of 'psychosis', 'schizophrenia', 'delusions', etc.*
- *giving information and correcting any misunderstandings*
- *taking a positive perspective*
- *famous people who have had psychosis*

Replacements in terms of oversensitivity/overactivity of the brain

- *'Part of my brain is dreaming whilst I am awake'*
- *2-route model*
- *Something happened to make my brain this way' (e.g. illicit drugs)*

Replacements in terms of psychological factors

- *Explain and normalize automatic thoughts*
- *Remove guilt/shame for automatic thoughts*
- *Explain and normalize the factors involved in belief formation and maintenance.*

For a partial goal:
Consider whether the partial modification could bring about an unwanted total modification.

6 (IF IT APPLIES) MODIFY THE BELIEF(S) THAT UNDERLIE THE 'DEEP' MEANING OF THE DELUSION
  (a) Speculate about possible underlying beliefs.
  (b) Check out which, in any, of these beliefs is relevant.
  (c) Set a functional goal(s) within the socio-cultural-religious group (if possible).
  (d) Modify the belief(s).
    - *evidence evaluation*
    - *logical reasoning*
    - *reality testing.*

7 MODIFY THE DELUSIONAL BELIEF
  (a) Work directly on the delusional belief
  Evidence evaluation
    - *Reinterpret evidence supporting the delusion.*
    - *Build up evidence against the delusion.*

  Logical reasoning
  Reality testing
  (b) Modify the underlying belief(s) that are* necessary *in order for the delusion to be possible.
  Deduce what the necessary belief(s) are.
  For each necessary belief:
    - *Specify what the ideal goal would be.*
    - *Consider whether this is achievable in practice.*
    - *Attempt the modification, if feasible.*

COGNITIVE-BEHAVIOURAL STRATEGIES WITH HALLUCINATIONS

1 ENGAGEMENT

2 ASSESSMENT and CASE FORMULATION

3 REDUCE THE IMPACT AND/OR DISTRESS USING PRACTICAL STRATEGIES
  Walkman®
  Earplug

4 MODIFY THE BELIEFS THAT UNDERLIE AND INFLUENCE THE CONTENT OF THE VOICE
  Deep meaning
  (a) Consider why the voice says what it does.
  (b) Set the goal(s) for the belief(s)/fears that underlie what the voice says (as described in 'Delusions' 4, above).

(c) Modify the belief(s)/fears that underlie what the voice says (as described in 'Delusions' 6, above).
(d) Use CBT with any issues/memories that underlie what the voice says.

Surface meaning

Establish that what the voice says is wrong (if it applies).

- *the voice is ignorant/tells lies*

Correct any misinformation or inaccurate knowledge that underpins what the voice says.

The voice expresses a delusional belief

CBT with the delusional belief.

5 DISEMPOWER THE VOICE AND TAKE AWAY ITS AUTHORITY

Move the belief about the invoice's intent from malign to benign (if possible).
Re-evaluate any evidence supporting the voice's power/authority.
Establish that the voice cannot cause harm.
Build up evidence that the voice makes mistakes and is ignorant.
Logical reasoning

- *'Claiming to have power is not the same as having power.'*
- *Voices cannot affect solid substances.*
- *If an earplug/Walkman/medication works, then the voice cannot be powerful.*

Reality testing – challenge the voice to:

- *do to you what it appears to do to the hearer*
- *do to you what has been threatened or is feared*
- *do something it ought to be able to do if it had real power*
- *answer questions it ought to be able to answer*

Show that the person has more power/knowledge than the voice.
Modify the belief about the origin of the voice (as described in 6, below).

6 MODIFY THE BELIEF ABOUT THE NATURE/ORIGIN OF THE VOICE

*(a) Set the goa*l (as described in 'Delusions' 4, above).

(b) Prepare for the negation of the belief about the voice's origin.

Perceiving something to be so does not mean that it is so'
(as described in 'Delusions' 5, above).
Replace any positive aspects of the belief about the voice'*s origin.*

(c) Prepare the replacement belief.

Replacements in terms of '*my own thoughts heard out loud*'

- *the inner-speech loop model*
- *vivid imagery*
- *remove guilt/shame because 'the voices are my thoughts'*

Replacements in terms of memory
Replacements in terms of mental illness

- *sharing experiences of voices*
- *factors that increase vulnerability to voices*

- *discussing the meaning of 'psychosis', 'schizophrenia', 'hallucinations', etc.*
- *giving information and correcting any misunderstandings*
- *taking a positive perspective*
- *famous people who have heard voices*

(d) Modify the belief about the voice's origin.
evidence evaluation
logical reasoning
reality testing

7 STRENGTHEN THE ABILITY TO RESIST THE VOICE'S COMMANDS
The goal: to be able to choose whether or not to follow the voice's commands.
(a) Identify an alternative, replacement behaviour(s).
(b) Reduce the advantages of obeying the voice.

- *Establish that the voice cannot cause harm if disobeyed.*
- *Block/reduce the voice using coping strategies.*
- *Find alternative means of stress reduction (e.g. relaxation, pleasant distraction).*

(c) Increase the advantages of the replacement behaviour.

- *Make aware of and rehearse the consequences of obeying the voice.*
- *Make aware of and rehearse the consequences of using the replacement behaviour.*

LONG-TERM STRATEGIES FOR DELUSIONS AND HALLUCINATIONS

Encourage recognition and labelling of delusional ideas and voices.
Develop sets of 'challenges' to counteract specific delusional beliefs and/or what the voice says. Flash cards may contain:

- logical reasoning
- results of evidence evaluation and reality testing
- reality tests to check out the validity of the ideas and/or voices should they recur
- coping statements
- coping strategies

Develop/enhance coping strategies.
Improve medication adherence (if appropriate).
Develop a relapse prevention plan.

APPENDIX 2
THE FEELING BRAIN⟷LOGICAL BRAIN MODEL

This appendix comprises the diagram and accompanying sheet that we normally use in clinical practice, but they can be freely adapted to meet the needs of the individual case. Examples from everyday life should be given to illustrate the model in action.

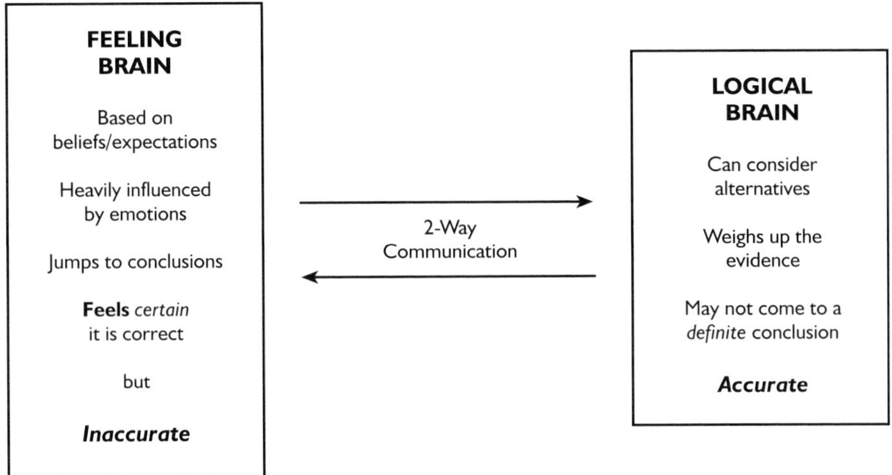

Figure A.1 *Feeling Brain⟷Logical Brain model*

FEELING BRAIN AND LOGICAL BRAIN

Our human brains do not operate like computers. Although part of our brain (let us call it 'Logical Brain') thinks and reasons calmly and rationally, there is another part (let us call it 'Feeling Brain') that thinks and reasons emotionally about things. So, unlike computers, our brains can misinterpret things and our reasoning can bring us to wrong conclusions.

Feeling Brain

Feeling Brain looks at the world through a filter that interprets everything it sees in terms of its *beliefs and expectations* about itself and the world. It is also heavily influenced by its *emotional state* such that its thoughts and interpretations tend to be in keeping with that emotional state.

Feeling Brain can *jump to conclusions* on the basis of little or no evidence. Indeed it can come to a conclusion based on its beliefs and expectations without any fact at all to back it up.

- The stronger the belief about a particular subject, the more likely it is that Feeling Brain will jump to a conclusion without any evidence.
- Similarly, the stronger the emotion felt, the more likely it is that Feeling Brain will jump to a conclusion that is consistent with that emotion.

When *Feeling Brain* comes to a conclusion, it *feels* convinced that this conclusion is absolutely correct and that this is how things really are; but this 'gut feeling' of certainty can be quite *wrong in fact*.

Thus Feeling Brain can be *very inaccurate* or even completely wrong in fact, even though it gives the convincing *feeling* of being sure it is correct.

Logical Brain

Logical Brain can look at the facts *objectively* and can *reason* about them. It can speculate about possible *alternative interpretations* and weigh up the evidence for and against. It can think in terms of *possibilities* and *probabilities* so it does not always come to a definite conclusion, but may decide only that something is 'most likely' to be true.

Logical Brain is not directly linked to the emotions, so when it comes to a conclusion, it does not give the gut feeling of certainty in the way that Feeling Brain does.

Thus Logical Brain comes to the *most accurate* conclusions, though it *may not feel* the most correct.

Interaction between Feeling Brain and Logical Brain

Ideally there should be fluid two-way communication between Feeling Brain and Logical Brain as this leads to the best thinking and most accurate conclusions. This is sometimes called 'Wise Mind'. With good two-way communication between the two parts of the thinking brain, Logical Brain is used to monitor, correct and refine the more powerful emotional thinking of Feeling Brain.

However, Feeling Brain may respond so quickly and strongly that it swamps Logical Brain. When this happens, Feeling Brain feels so sure it is correct that Logical Brain never gets brought into it. Unfortunately, as we have seen, Feeling Brain on its own can be very biased and inaccurate and, on occasions, completely wrong, so without Logical Brain to question and reason about Feeling Brain's conclusions we may be completely convinced our ideas are correct even when they are grossly inaccurate.

The stronger the beliefs involved, the more likely it is that Feeling Brain will overwhelm Logical Brain, without Logical Brain even being aware of it, so that we come to the wrong conclusions but *feel certain* they are correct.

Similarly, the stronger the emotional state at the time, the more likely it is that Feeling Brain will swamp Logical Brain and bring us to the wrong conclusions.

People appear to differ in the relative strength of the Feeling and Logical parts of their brains, and life events and circumstances can alter the balance between the two. Furthermore, the two-way communication may work less well in some conditions, for example when stressed, tired or under the influence of street drugs.

How do we know if Feeling Brain has brought us to an incorrect conclusion?

We can help Logical Brain to work more efficiently by asking the question '*Is there any hard evidence to support this conclusion?*'[1]

If Logical Brain cannot come up with any hard evidence, then this means that Logical Brain was not involved in coming to the conclusion. This means that the conclusion was the result of Feeling Brain's reasoning alone – and this means that the conclusion could be completely wrong.

Warning: If Feeling Brain responds very strongly, then it may overwhelm Logical Brain and force it to agree. When this happens, instead of acting to restrain and correct Feeling Brain, Logical Brain is now forced to provide 'evidence' and 'reasons' to support Feeling Brain's conclusions.

Someone else may be able to see the way that we are distorting the facts. It is very much easier for someone else to do this because they can use their Logical Brain without being swamped by the strong beliefs and emotions that are powering our Feeling Brain. However, when someone tells us that we are distorting the facts, we are likely to react irritably or angrily because our Feeling Brain assures us we are correct and our Logical Brain can even come up with some hard evidence to support it. We cannot see that this evidence is distorted so it is not surprising if we find it hard to accept that we could be wrong – even though we are wrong!

[1] i.e. the sort of unbiased evidence that would be accepted in a court of law.

Appendix 3[1]
Ways of reducing some of the negative aspects of a diagnosis of 'mental illness'

1. *The diagnosis of illness/psychosis/schizophrenia is accepted but is disturbing*:
   (a) Because of the stigma.
   - **Normalize** the symptoms, i.e. treat the symptoms as extreme forms of essentially 'normal' experiences. The symptoms are different in severity from those experienced by 'normal' people but the person is not weird or peculiar or essentially different from the rest of mankind because of these experiences. Useful strategies to support this position include:
     - The therapist sharing their own and colleagues' experiences of 'odd ideas' and voices.
     - Looking at factors that increase everyone's vulnerability to delusions and voices, for example high temperature, sleep deprivation, food/water deprivation, high anxiety.
     - Sharing information about the frequency of voices in the normal population.
     - Using the 'dream' analogy, i.e. that in dreams everyone has weird, bizarre experiences that are not recognized as such at the time.
     - Understanding how thoughts, feelings and beliefs interact so that the 'delusional' conclusions are seen to be reasonable, given the experiences and circumstances.
   - Decatastrophize 'mental illness'/'psychosis'/'schizophrenia'.
     - Describe psychosis/schizophrenia as a collection of different and only loosely-related disorders, which are of different severity and which affect people in different ways.
     - It can affect anyone.
     - It does not imply some moral or personality weakness or defect.
     - It does not imply suddenly going berserk or becoming violent.
     - The rich experiences of psychosis are often associated with artistic creativity.
     - Some people pay a lot of money for illegal drugs to get these types of experiences.
     - Some famous people have had psychosis.

[1]This appendix refers specifically to how strategies used to prepare people for the understanding that they have a mental illness can be used with people who already know that this diagnosis applies to them. When used in this way, the work does not require the same cautious approach as is necessary for 'insight promotion' with people who deny having an illness.

- Find an alternative explanation for 'part of my brain is overactive/not functioning properly' that avoids 'being ill'.

(b) Because the course and prognosis of the illness is feared.

- Discuss the meaning of 'mental illness or 'psychosis' and give information to correct any misunderstandings. It may be helpful to make the following points:
  - For the person concerned it implies no more than the experiences they have; there is nothing worse.
  - Psychosis does not infect every cell of the body – most of the person and their brain works entirely normally.
  - The person is unlikely to develop other symptoms which they do not have already.
  - Likely to fluctuate, *not* a downward deterioration.

2. *Implies 'I've been wrong'.*
   May imply 'I've been stupid/foolish to believe what I have', or 'Other people must think I am stupid/foolish to have believed that'.
   - If it is understood why the delusion has developed in the way that it has, explain to the person why they were perfectly reasonable to come to the conclusion they did, given their experiences, both internal and external, and their circumstances.
   - Discuss the normality and desirability of people changing their views about things when they learn more about them.
   - Share your own experiences of having been wrong about things in the past and changing your ideas later, or those of your friends and colleagues.
3. *Implies wasted opportunities/relationships over the years when the delusion was held and acted on. (This is likely to be a particularly relevant factor for delusional beliefs held for a long period that have significantly affected the person's lifestyle.)*
   - Understanding how the delusional beliefs came about may help the person to understand that, in the circumstances, this was entirely reasonable and therefore inevitable. The consequent adverse effects on their life were also inevitable and unavoidable.
   - If the delusion is still held to be true, another option is to go for the partial modification: '[The delusion] may have been true in the past but it is not true now.'
4. *Guilt/shame because the voices are 'my thoughts'.*
   - Give information about automatic thoughts.
     - We all have unpleasant, shocking and even bizarre thoughts on occasions. Normalize this phenomenon and explain why it happens.
     - Our brains tell us what might be *possible*, based on our knowledge, experience and memories, not necessarily what is probable or what we want.
     - Thinking does not equal doing (e.g. the common automatic thought

of pushing someone under a train). We are morally responsible for our acts not our thoughts.

- If someone has seen, read, heard or knows about something, or can imagine something, then it is possible for them to get an automatic thought about it. This automatic thought can be 'heard' as an auditory hallucination or can influence the formation of a delusional belief.
- We cannot control our automatic thoughts and, therefore, should not feel guilty/ashamed for what they are about.
    - the 'think of nothing for 20 seconds' test
    - the 'think of anything *except* the pressure of your chair, for 20 seconds' test
- If we have a strong emotional response to a thought, or try to suppress it, then this is likely to cause the thought to come back more strongly.

INDEX

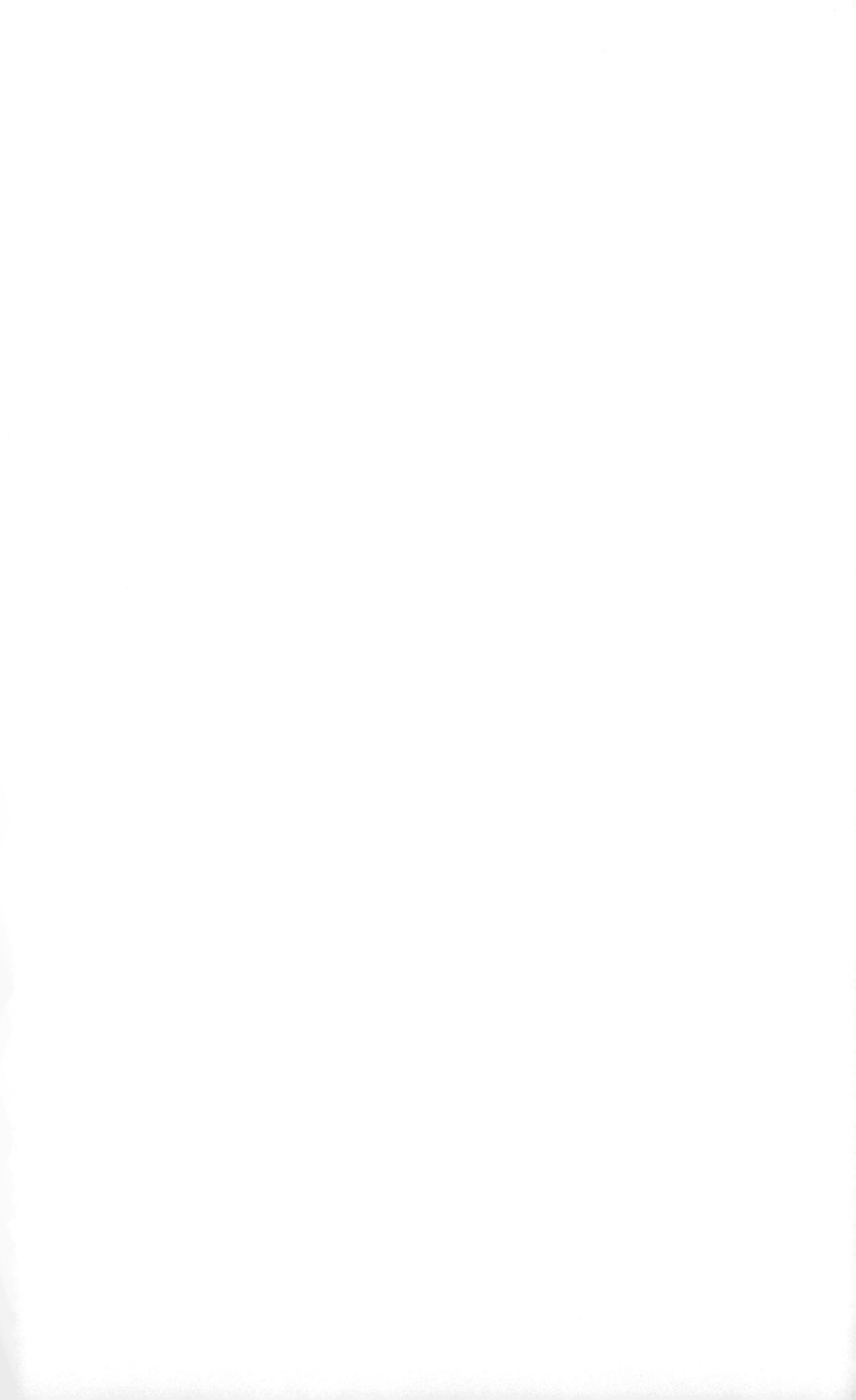